THE
PATIENT
GROUP
HANDBOOK

First Print Edition: January 2016

Published by Findacure Publications

Contents

THE PATIENT GROUP HANDBOOK

A PRACTICAL GUIDE FOR RESEARCH AND DRUG DEVELOPMENT

EDITED BY

Anthony HALL

AND

Nicolas SIREAU

FINDACURE PUBLICATIONS

Introduction

Anthony Hall
Findacure

It has taken almost two years from the first inception of this book to reach the final printed version that you are now reading. It was a complex project, involving some 52 authors contributing 25 chapters between them and we're hugely grateful to all the authors who have contributed. The idea for this Handbook came about as a result of the work I was doing with Nick Sireau and the AKU Society to develop a treatment for the ultra-rare inherited disease alkaptonuria (AKU), which affects both of Nick's sons. Like many parents faced with the prospect that their children may not be able to have the normal lives they had hoped for, he wanted to do something about it. Much of this inspiring story unfolds in the first rare diseases book, edited by Nick, which was published in 2013.[1] Nick had managed to bring together a phenomenal consortium, from top clinicians and researchers, to patient advocates and industry people, in order to expand research into AKU, develop animal models and work towards a treatment. One of the results was the DevelopAKUre consortium, which raised 6 million Euros from the European Union's 7th Framework Programme (FP7) in order to fund the repurposing of nitisinone for the treatment of AKU. I am honoured to have been a part of that consortium and pleased to say that the first clinical trial has now been completed and the second is underway and on track. If this is successful, it will lead to an application for regulatory authorization.

The DevelopAKUre consortium was ultimately able to raise a significant amount of money and get a drug into clinical development, but we realized the problems that Nick had faced along the way were not unique to AKU. They were repeated a thousand times over by those struggling to find a treatment for any of the 5,000 or so rare diseases for which no drugs are available. Despite recent improvements, thanks to the explosion in social media making it easier for patients to connect, rare diseases patients and their families still often experience severe isolation and exclusion. The large, well-funded patient organisations are the exception rather than the rule and many patient support groups are no more than a 'kitchen table' organisation set up by someone living with a rare disease or by a family member of an affected individual.

We therefore decided to put together this Handbook to give other patient groups an insight into how these issues might be tackled. Realizing that there is no single recipe for success, this book is not intended as a step-by-step guide, but instead shares the experiences of others and how they have tackled their own unique problems, as well as detailing some of the more formal elements such as those relating to clinical trials and regulatory approval. Depending on the size and stage of development of their organisation, different people will want to use different parts of this Handbook.

The book is intended to complement the series of workshops run by Findacure, the charity that we founded to help empower patient groups to themselves become effective campaigners for change and spearhead the development of treatments for rare diseases. With a small but highly talented group of staff members based out of a small office in Cambridge, Findacure has so far held patient group workshops on (to name but a few) crowdfunding for rare diseases, raising largescale funding, how to work with pharma, drug repositioning for rare diseases, identifying rare diseases patients, managing a small patient group, communications and PR and running clinical trials, as well as organizing a host of other activities. These topics, plus many others, are covered in this Handbook.

As noted earlier, many small patient groups are run by a parent or patient out of their home and it can be difficult to make any progress. In order to address this need, Findacure also runs a peer mentoring scheme, whereby struggling and/or small patient groups are matched with experts in the field, who have the knowledge and experience to mentor the small patient groups and help them achieve their goals. We hope that the information in this Handbook, particularly the chapters on setting up a patient group, small fundraising and engaging with industry will further assist such groups.

For the larger, more established patient organisations, the chapters on building a research consortium, raising larger funding and those on the drug development aspects might be especially useful.

One of the most difficult gaps for patient groups who have been able to raise finance to support research is in understanding the pathways that need to be followed to take a candidate treatment through development and ultimately to patients. This has traditionally been the sole jurisdiction of the pharmaceutical industry and is where the expertise and knowledge still resides in large part. But this has started to change in recent years, with the expansion of (rare diseases) patient groups and umbrella organisations such as EURORDIS, which runs an annual summer school for patient groups to learn about these aspects. Furthermore, patient organisations are seemingly no longer afraid to take on the daunting task of identifying promising research, raising funding to support it and finding the appropriate partners to take a promising candidate drug into development.

Nevertheless, there may be many research projects ongoing in academia that could be funded by a patient group and it can still be difficult for the organisation to separate the good projects from the bad or to see which are most likely to make it through development and ultimately reach the patients. This is a crucial factor that needs to be tackled to ensure that hard-won funds don't go to waste. To this end, many patient groups, even quite small ones, have been able to attract top specialists to their Advisory Boards. By carefully selecting appropriate members, the patient organisation can ensure that the Advisory Board is able to provide advice on which research projects to support financially and to advise on next steps once a project is completed. We hope that this book will further supplement that knowledge and expertise.

My foray into the world of rare diseases began in 2009. It has been a fascinating, challenging and rewarding journey, during which I have met some of the most interesting and driven people of my life, many of whom I can now count among my friends. I am happy that we have been able to bring together the collective knowledge of a few of these remarkable people into this Handbook for patient groups. We hope you find it useful.

Anthony Hall
Leiden, October 2015

Reference

1 Sireau N. (Ed). 2013. Rare Diseases: Challenges and Opportunities for Social Entrepreneurs. Greenleaf Publishing Ltd.

Foreword: What Issues Do Patient Groups Face?

Yann Le Cam
EURORDIS, the European Organisation for Rare Diseases

Patient Empowerment

Hoping for a cure? We all are. Patients and their families hope for a cure, a treatment, some relief. Everyone can have hopes, wishes and dreams. One can trust science and progress, believe in society and solidarity, have faith in the mercy of their god and walk with confidence in life; all sensible things to do. But that is not what patient empowerment is about. Empowering patients to drive research and medicine development is not about promoting hypothetical hopes or believing in better futures that are beyond our control. Patient advocates are much more pragmatic and ambitious than that. In Letters to Lucilius, Senèque wrote, *"When you will have unlearned to hope, I'll teach you to want."* We want to act now in the present moment and have an impact where we can. Empowered patient advocates have the willingness, desire, audacity and courage to act now. Patient advocate empowerment is about knowledge, experience, process, actions and results. Empowering patients to drive research and medicine development is only about what we can and want to achieve.

Patient empowerment transforms the tragedy of our lives into an individual and collective adventure to create positive change, and to improve the survival and quality of life of people living with severe, debilitating, life-threatening diseases, whether rare or not.

Empowerment is the process of enhancing the awareness, self-confidence, autonomy, strength and capacity of individuals or groups to act, to make choices and to transform those choices into desired actions that generate individual and collective benefits. Patient empowerment creates public goods that address their own issues but in turn also benefit society at large. To quote Margaret Mead, American cultural anthropologist: *"Never doubt that a small group of thoughtful, committed citizens can change the world. Indeed, it is the only thing that ever has."*

A critical mode of action is the promotion of ideas, new concepts and innovative approaches. *"If the domain of ideas is revolutionized, reality cannot remain as it is"*, said G W F Hegel in the Age of Enlightenment. In research and drug development, some ideas spring to mind.

Every human's life is of equal worth to any other human's life. There is no acceptable reason to leave any part of humanity without the opportunity of health research progress. It is desirable and possible to take all necessary actions to develop medicines for those patients affected by diseases that have no treatment yet. When one human suffers, another human cares for him to relieve him of his pain. Care and hospitality are core principles of action.

Patient Involvement in Medicines Research and Development

Patient-centric research is a useful compass to improve patients' health and public health. By putting the patient (the end user) at the centre, the utility (the societal value) comes first before the scientific aspects of product, characteristics, innovation, and before the economic aspects of cost, price, market, revenue and budget impact. A drug addressing an unmet medical need is more challenging to develop but has a much higher utility than another similar drug or a drug with a tiny incremental benefit. Focusing drug development on patient outcome measures which are clinically meaningful to patients, triggers progress towards medicines with higher therapeutic added value. Patients are best placed to discuss the levels of risks they are ready to accept for a potential benefit. Article 2 of the 1997 *Oviedo Convention of the Council of Europe* states, *"The interests and welfare of the human being shall prevail over the sole interest of society or science."*

Patients are experts when it comes to experience of their disease. They have the capacity to bring a useful perspective on what it means to live with their illness in relation to various aspects: consequences of the disease, daily care requirements, appropriate expectations, the right medical centres/ experts and which constraints are acceptable or not for patients, etc.

Through their involvement in the research and drug development process, patient advocates are the catalyst of the multi-stakeholder approach and create a shared value between all stakeholders. By putting the patient (the person we care for and listen to with compassion and empathy) at the centre, relationships between all stakeholders are reshuffled and the processes of research collaborations, scientific assessments and access are progressively redefined.

Empowered patient advocates create favorable conditions and a better environment for the research and development of medicines. Patients continue to advocate on legislation and policies regulating development, approval and access to medicines. This includes legislation on clinical trials, data protection, transparency, pre-approval access, adaptive licensing, orphan medicinal products, paediatric use of medicines, advanced therapies, safety, pharmacovigilance, heath technology assessment, off-label use and shortages of medicines. This advocacy includes the promotion of: research, public funding to stimulate scientific progress, economic incentives to stimulate private investment, public-private partnership and patient advocates' fundraising.

Empowered patient advocates can be actively engaged in the development and assessment of, and access to, medicines. Patient advocates: enhance the self-consciousness of those affected by diseases in their status as patients and as the families of patients; create patient communities through patient groups, web-based social media, their networking and further outreach; raise awareness of scientific and medical experts as well as of policy makers and pharma and biotech companies; help establish centres of expertise, wide-scale harmonised data collection and registries; promote natural history studies, evaluation scales and other measurement methods; organise patient information, patient therapeutic education and capacity building of patient advocates in research and drug development; and support basic research, clinical research and fellowships. Increasingly, patient advocates are full members of hospital boards, advisory boards of research institutions, ethical committees for clinical trials, scientific committees of the European Medicine Agency or health-technology assessment bodies. More often than ever they are being consulted as experts to provide scientific advice or take part in scientific assessment. Pharmaceutical and biotech companies are consulting more patients as part of their methodology of development and sometimes establish a dialogue with patient advocates.

Perspective on Patient Advocacy Groups

This active role of empowered patients in research and drug development stems from other initiatives that began over thirty years ago. The HIV epidemic prompted the emergence of patient advocacy characterised by the appropriation of scientific and medical knowledge and the drive to take an active part – both critically and constructively – in addressing this new health challenge. In turn, the AIDS advocacy movement has generated a new generation of patient advocates in cancers, starting with breast cancer, parents with children affected by cancers and cancer survivors, then expanding to several rare cancers and later frequent cancers. These new areas of empowerment are rooted in, and run in conjunction with, other citizen movements including civil rights and antidiscrimination, new humanitarian actions, feminism, abortion rights, the right to die with dignity and more. In parallel, some patient groups directly allocated the funds they raised to conscious strategic choices; the French AFM-Téléthon funded major game-changers such as the first genome map and the first gene therapies; the US Cystic Fibrosis Foundation created a completely new model of partnership with academia, industry and the NIH 25 years ago, which is still leading to breakthrough therapies by biotech companies today; the international Parent Project Muscular Dystrophy movement is carrying out a comprehensive intervention at all levels of drug development and approval; top executives with a child affected by a disease are creating research-based biotech companies, such as John F. Crowley for Amicus in the USA and Karen Aiach for Lysogene in France; and the AKU Society in the UK is creating a research consortium of public and private partners for a disease where no research has been done before. Behind each of these initiatives there is a parent or patient affected by a disease that has become a patient advocate, a leader and developed a clear vision for change. More of these people are coming forward year on year as the patient advocacy movement only grows stronger.

Resistance and Risks Encountered by Patient Groups

A major issue is to gain a more robust recognition of the value that empowered patients can bring to research and drug development. These thirty years of progress are fragile. The claim of Michel Foucault, "*Where there is power, there is resistance*" fully applies to this new patient empowerment. Many idealist and dogmatic counter powers stiffly oppose our pragmatic realism. We should beware of idealism – reality is truth, the ideal is a mirage and not attainable. We need to make more visible how we aim to forge compromise to reach the best choice for all through our conditions of interaction and the processes of regulation/ negotiation in which we engage as powers and counter-powers.

Some experts feel their status is challenged by patient advocates, provoking a conservatism according to which those experts would prefer the scientific advice and assessments process to be 'pure', to be based only on scientific truth. Patients, even more if empowered, are perceived as intruders, scientifically incompetent and emotionally driven. Such experts seem to forget that there is no truth in science, that nothing is definitive and that knowledge is composed of facts, figures and judgements; patients are part of this knowledge and are entitled to form part of these opinions. Some experts would like to avoid engagement of patients in risk-benefit assessment, particularly for early or conditional approvals, and consider patient advocates as agents of the pharmaceutical industry, incapable of an independent opinion and prone to taking irresponsible risks. Others, brought together in a coalition of consumer movements with members of parliaments and the media, are preaching for a zero-risk society. But a trend to zero risk in medicine does more harm than good to patients; obviously, no one wants to take risk when there is the 6th or 7th medicine for a disease that already has satisfactory treatments. But patients with severe life-threatening diseases are ready to trade off higher potential risks for benefits in the context of a well-informed discussion that includes strategies to reduce uncertainties while monitoring safety.

An obvious challenge facing patient groups in the coming years is how to maintain or enhance their financial capacity and independence. This requires diversified sources of funding, primarily from their own fundraising through donations, events and grants, or services. Some patient groups refuse to be funded by any health company. Others are funded through grants from pharmaceutical or biotech companies, usually unrestricted, or dedicated to a project. The more patient groups engage in research and drug development, the higher the number of medicines that will be available or in the pipeline, and hence the easier it will be to create opportunities to partner with companies and to get funding. This trend is good. It shows that health companies are taking their corporate social responsibility more seriously. Patient groups and industry have interests in common, and it is to the benefit of patients to discuss them. Experience shows that the quality of interaction between a company and patient groups, even when confrontational, is better when the company also provides support to patient groups, an interesting paradox. The best ways to minimise risk are: firstly, and most importantly, to have a good governance structure in place within the patient group; second, to have clear rules and respect them; and third, to be transparent and always declare all potential conflict of interest.

Another issue faced by patient groups and advocates in coming years will be how to maintain unity and solidarity in an increasingly complex environment. As patient engagement will require patients to have more knowledge, training and time, there is a risk that patient advocates will disconnect from real patient life, even though this is the primary reason that they become advocates. This risk can be addressed with good governance processes within patient groups and by enlarging the number of empowered patients able to play an active role. Also, as therapies, either chronic treatments or cures, will come to the market for only some diseases (or some subsets of patient populations based on genetic profiling), there is a risk of new egoisms from individual patient groups wanting to secure their share of the healthcare budget. After years of exhausting battles, when the first major solutions appear there is a risk of demotivation and demobilisation of volunteers in patient groups, which can in turn impact the wider community. This risk can be addressed by always unveiling the veil of ignorance, by regularly revitalising our values and reminding advocates of the reasons to maintain solidarity. History has proved that solidarity is socially, economically, politically more efficient.

The Future of Patient Involvement in Medicines R&D

To gain recognition and a more active role for patient advocates in the long term, we need to establish robust concepts, principles, methods and tools for the engagement of patients all along the medicine life cycle and with all stakeholders. We need to evaluate the real impact of this patient engagement on the stakeholders, the drug development process, clinical trials, scientific opinions and investment. We need to scale up this engagement of patients at different points of time along the research and development pathway, with more stakeholders (more companies, much more academia, more public agencies, payers etc.) and on a more frequent basis, so that they gain experience.

Key success factors to ensuring a more active role for patient advocates include building their capacities through training, information, networking and support. This in turn means that all stakeholders, and industry in particular, need to accept that patient advocacy groups play this empowering role, without trying to disrupt the relationship by reaching out directly to patient experts.

Another important factor will be to find appropriate ways to mitigate potential conflicts of interest. In the long run, patient empowerment and patient engagement will be trusted only if we act in ways which are safe and transparent for all. We will need to accept to work in other ways than giving our time as a charitable contribution – we need to develop a business model that makes patient engagement sustainable on a large scale and over a long period, and which in turn will enhance the expectations and quality of this engagement.

Increased patient engagement in research and drug development enables a more patient-centric research and therapy strategy, as discussed above, but also aims to de-risk research and to accelerate the translation of research into actual therapies.

We want private investment to be attracted to research and drug development and we want these resources to be allocated to assets with optimal chances of success. Patient advocates should therefore dare to play a role in very early dialogue with biotech and pharmaceutical companies, so as to inform their choices based on patients' needs. We want early, multi-stakeholder, open and confidential dialogue that enables discussion of the best conditions for research on a medicine. An early uptake will improve the targeted population, registries, natural history studies, clinical endpoints, surrogate endpoints, measurement methods. We want all public funding and tax incentives for drug development to be granted under the condition that the company must seek scientific advice from regulatory and HTA agencies. This will again help to de-risk the investment and optimise the research outcome.

The Future of the R&D Model for Rare Diseases and Beyond

Rare diseases and orphan medicines are leading the way on precision medicines, also called stratified therapies (and abusively personalised medicines). But a successful strategy, which enabled the approval of over 150 rare disease therapies at an accelerated pace of 15 to 30 new therapies per year, is insufficient to address today's challenges. Scientific knowledge is growing rapidly but not translating into therapies quickly enough. Patients are facing major hurdles to access approved new therapies. The sustainability to provide an increasing number of rare disease therapies is an issue for national healthcare budgets that are already under high pressure. Issues are similar for all therapies intended for small populations: paediatric medicines, upcoming gene and cell therapies and genetically-targeted precision medicines. Society, patients, experts, healthcare systems and the pharma industry need to think outside the box to address new challenges facing the rare disease community.

Scientific innovation cannot be disconnected from access to medicines. If a scientific innovation only translates into an innovative medicine being approved, and not into a societal advancement reaching all patients who need it, it fails on its primary objective. New R&D and business models are needed to connect innovation with patient access to medicines. Our common objective should now be more, better and cheaper innovative treatments accessible to patients, and faster.

The new R&D model relies on several key elements:

- adaptive clinical trial design and innovative statistical methods;
- animal modelling on new species and alternatives to animal models, such as *in silico* modelisation;
- new surrogate endpoints to capture evidence which is meaningful to patients, such as patient-reported outcome measures; and
- a recognition that data generation is a continuum.

The production of robust data on new medicines should no longer be for the purpose of the marketing authorisation, rather to capture data all along the medicine's product life cycle (from R&D to patients' real-life use of the medicine), hence generating real-world evidence. This larger and more clinically relevant data set also captures the variations deriving from the highly heterogeneous clinical expression of complex rare diseases. This reduces the level of uncertainty around the medicine and means it is easier to refine the optimal target population, treatment regimen and right use of the medicine in the therapeutic strategy. Patients' expert opinions and active engagement in these new models are needed.

For severe or life-threatening diseases, and in the absence of a satisfactory existing treatment but in the presence of a promising product, conditional approvals of medicines should be implemented to save patients' lives. Earlier approvals enable earlier capture of real-life evidence. The appreciation of these higher levels of uncertainties on safety and efficacy require the participation of patient representatives in the assessment of the benefits and risks of a new medicine; only patients as experts on their diseases can legitimately determine how much risk or harm they are willing to accept for a given benefit of a medicine.

This adaptive R&D model makes it possible to recruit many less patients for clinical trials, shortens the time of development from 7-15 years to 5-7 years and de-risks and reduces investment. Through early and increased involvement in medicines R&D process, patient advocates can accelerate the emergence of this new model.

Early approval saves investment in late-stage product development; the cost and price of innovative medicines at the time of initial approval would be much cheaper and the cost of real-life evidence generation would be transferred to healthcare systems. This transfer is an opportunity as it calls for a more fruitful dialogue and closer collaboration between all stakeholders that have a role in ensuring access to a medicine and in all stages of the medicine development pathway: marketing holder, regulators, health-technology-assessment bodies, payers, experts and patients.

The medicines development decision-making process should be based first and foremost on (i) the therapeutic value and (ii) the value for money of a new treatment. This is only possible through European collaboration mechanisms that are inclusive of all stakeholders involved along the life cycle of medicines.

Patients are calling for a smarter Europe. We urgently need a seamless approach to European cooperation on medicines development so that we can bridge the gap between EU regulatory decisions and fragmented national/local pricing and reimbursement decisions. And we need patients to be engaged in all these processes.

Some key mechanisms supported by the EU Commission and Member States should be strengthened so that it is possible to overcome specific issues surrounding rare disease therapies, such as limited disease knowledge and scarce medical expertise. European common value assessment reports by the European

HTA Network should be the norm, at least for orphan medicines. New mechanisms should include the creation of a European table for price negotiation and market access, to be established by National Competent Authorities in Pricing & Reimbursement. This 'table' should be voluntary for both EU Member States and companies, while decisions on the level of reimbursement of a medicine should remain with the national authorities.

Focusing only on budget reduction measures or legal constraints will not solve the issue of patient access to medicines. We as patients need the sector of medicine development to be attractive for investment. The reality is that the future of our therapies is driven by the market (for investment) and the economy (for healthcare budgets), as much as it is by science. Public policy can regulate the market to attract more investments with incentives and can work on its policy framework and processes to create optimal conditions of development and access. But ultimately, the main driver to improve access is embedded in the R&D and business models.

European Reference Networks of national/ regional centres of expertise will be created from 2016, a transformative opportunity that also presents new challenges for the years ahead. These networks will bring together selected centres of expertise, healthcare providers and diagnostic laboratories of high-level medical expertise across Europe. Patient advocates will play a key role in the governance and activities of these networks. These networks will be at the core of future clinical research and trials and long-term data collection.

Towards an Ecosystem Geared at Patient Health Outcomes and Innovation

The main goal of patient groups for future therapies in Europe should be improved patient health outcomes. This is possible with a comprehensive approach combining these European Reference Networks with adaptive R&D and business models, integrating quality infrastructures for clinical trials and data collection at the hospital point of care. Research, drug development and healthcare provision do not exist in silos. A better structured approach to drug development and market access will create a more attractive and simplified environment for investors and sponsors.

Science budgets are under constraints, far below the ambition of a European Union of innovation, competitiveness, jobs and growth. Different fields of research are in competition for public money. To address this issue, patient groups need to advocate for an increased health research budget. They need to articulate good arguments on why society should invest more in research and drug development so as to address patients' and public health needs, as well as the challenges of a healthcare system and budget under demographic and economic pressures. This can be best achieved through public-private partnership involving all stakeholders.

We, patient advocates, are smart, caring, dedicated and resilient to all challenges. *"Be the change you wish to see in this world."* Mahatma Gandhi.

Yann Le Cam is CEO at EURORDIS, the European Organisation for Rare Diseases
Written with the support of Eva Bearryman – Junior Communications Manager, EURORDIS

Chapter 1

How to Set up and Manage a Patient Group (a US Perspective)

Nicole Boice & Andrea Epstein
Global Genes™

John F. Kennedy said it best – "The rising tide lifts all boats". This quote resonated with those of us who started the Global Genes effort at its inception just five short years ago. At the time, a handful of rare disease patient advocates, all representing different rare diseases, came together to develop an organization and campaign that would unify a very segmented community. Why? Because, together, working towards the common goal of 'eliminating the challenges of rare disease' globally, those in the room agreed that 'we' could accomplish so much more then going it alone – and that the result would also allow for more success for individual disease efforts as well. How? Through a model that keeps the rare stakeholder at the core of its mission, and fosters collaboration, shared expertise and resources between and among rare disease stakeholders, each of whom may have very specific rare disease goals but at the same time share a broader mission to advance the collective voice of the rare community.

Unity – The Pink Ribbon Effect

Breast Cancer and the Pink Ribbon are synonymous with finding a cure for a disease that has been brilliantly marketed to promote its broad impact on all women; friends, family, loved ones, sisters, mothers, nieces, daughters. Considering the fact that rare disease impacts more people on the planet then all cancers and AIDS patients combined, this community of 350 million people deserves the same level of awareness and support. The Blue Genes Denim™ Ribbon has become the unifying global symbol of support for those affected by one of the 7,000 rare conditions. The Blue Genes Ribbon™ (Jeans for Genes) has been used by many advocates around the globe to help promote their condition as part of this massive community. It provides patients and advocates the opportunity to share with the world that they are not alone, that their disease is not rare in the context of the larger rare disease community, and that it deserves more attention and support to help them in their fight for the disease that they care most about.

Awareness

Awareness is key to the future success of rare disease patients globally. A coordinated effort is needed to gain substantial interest by major media, consumer brands, and the general public. The aggregate, sheer mass of patients affected by rare disease is shocking to those that are not aware of the plight of this community. Awareness and education are key factors in helping raise the level of understanding about the needs of the rare disease community and how people can get engaged to help. It takes a village -and no one patient advocacy organization can go it alone. It is the collective impact that this community can have that becomes large enough to raise eyebrows and get people thinking, 'Wow. This could happen to me or my loved ones'. 'Rare is not so rare'.

Collaboration within Advocacy Community

At the grass roots level, we know that collaboration is critical for the many rare disease-specific non-profit organizations that have been established by parents, friends, and caregivers to push the envelope for funding research, support programs, treatments and ultimately cures for their loved ones. With only 15% of the 7,000 rare diseases represented by a disease-specific foundation or support organization, we know that that the vast majority of conditions have no designated support at all. Global Genes with its mission of 'Eliminating the Challenges of Rare Diseases', is making an impact by equipping patients to be successful advocates, and through education and empowerment, to become 'activists' for their disease. Global Genes does this through a growing portfolio of educational tools and resources, events, building out critical connections and funding innovations in science and technology that will impact patients within their lifetime.

Starting A Non-Profit – Options, Choices

When one learns that a loved one (or him/herself) has been diagnosed with a devastating disease, one way to respond is to channel frustration or sadness into action. Goals for starting a rare disease group can range from building a support network to a singular focus on advancing rare disease research and treatment, or building a hybrid, broad based organization that focuses on addressing all avenues to advance the progress for disease awareness, support and science.

In the United States, setting up a non-profit organization, or 501(c)3, will require an investment of time, funds and the services of an attorney. Before one decides whether or not to take this leap, there are a number of key questions to be answered. These include:

- Are there other non-profits that exist with a similar mission, addressing the same rare disease with similar goals?
- If yes to the above, are they dedicated to my rare disease and my focus area? (ie. research for a cure, support services, etc.)
- Where are they located and would it be feasible for me to join their existing efforts?

- Is establishing a non-profit a sustainable venture? Can I build both the organizational and financial support to make this work?

Key to the success of a new non-profit will be engaging someone who can help you build out a business plan or road map to chart the first several years of your organization. Whether you choose to rely exclusively or heavily on volunteers in the early stage, it will still be critical to identify sources of funds, as well as initial programs that your organization will support, develop or fund.

Based on your research of the existing work being done for the specific rare disease you want to address, you may choose to go another route. Options include:

- Working for an existing non-profit. Potentially adding a local support group or bringing a new perspective to the organization, such as added programs, resources or fundraising opportunities;
- Organizing a support group or network through social media;
- Creating a local chapter of an existing non-profit. This option provides a sense of name recognition for the public, allows you to be part of a bigger network, and may give you access to broader resources. Similar to a franchise model, you may have limited autonomy in terms of program creation, but you are able to access existing best practices, resources and tools that allow you to focus on the cause versus running a business.

"Being part of a national organization means that you benefit from the credibility of the organization. In the case of Huntington's Disease Society of America, that means more than 40 years of brand recognition and a track record of success, verified by independent auditors, which are important to donors."

Louise Vetter, CEO Huntington's Disease of America

Interim Approach: Fiscal Sponsorship

In America, some non-profits choose to become established through a "fiscal sponsorship." In essence, this entails working through another non-profit without going through the process of establishing a separate 501(c)3. The benefits of this approach clearly are the savings in time and money to get up and running. Without a 501c3, even a separate Board is not necessary. The downside here is that donors cannot direct funds directly to your organization, but rather donations are made to the sponsoring organization, which channels the funds to your entity. Often, a new organization will set up a fiscal sponsorship as an intermediary step to setting up a 501(c)3.

More detailed resources about the process of deciding whether to start a non-profit – and the basic steps to get started – can be found in two Global Genes™ toolkits:

- So You Think You Want to Start A Non-Profit,[1] and
- Starting A Non-Profit: The First Steps.[2]

RARE Resources So You Don't 'Reinvent the Wheel'

For those rare diseases that do have a foundation or NPO already established, collaboration is imperative, so that each group is not re-inventing the wheel to push progress forward. Global Genes™ has moved the needle in patient advocacy collaboration in multiple ways, and it is evidence of the need and desire for these partnerships.[3] Today, nearly 200 patient foundations represent our RARE Foundation Alliance and membership is continually growing. Our annual RARE Patient Advocacy Summit also continues to increase in both participation and demand for content – expanding this year to a 1½ day event with more than 400 projected attendees. Strategies for fundraising, advocacy, resource development and research are shared needs that clearly benefit from collaborative strategies and programs.

Rare Disease Alliance Case Study – Sanfilippo – Collaborations In Advocacy

Sanfilippo Syndrome is a rare, deadly genetic disease that results in the body being unable to properly break down certain sugars. Symptoms often appear early in the first year of life and the disease causes progressive muscular and cognitive decline in children after the age of two. While there are currently no approved treatments for Sanfilippo disease, the goal of discovering a cure has been at the core of nonprofit investment and collaboration worldwide. Many of the leading Sanfilippo research organizations have joined forces to support this research and ensure that it moves into clinical trials, requiring a global coalition to address multiple sub-types of the disease. Through this joint effort, the patient groups together will ultimately contribute over a million dollars towards clinical trials set to begin in the coming year.

Central to this collaboration was Nationwide Children's Hospital (Columbus, Ohio), whose 20 year history of research set the stage for identifying a treatment with strong potential to help patients suffering from Sanfilippo Syndrome. Rallying around this potential breakthrough therapy were a range of foundations including Ben's Dream: The Sanfilippo Research Foundation (US); the Sanfilippo Children's Research Foundation (Canada); Stop Sanfilippo (Spain); Fondation Sanfilippo (Switzerland); and Team Sanfilippo (USA). These foundations are supporting the Children's Hospital with a natural history study for patients with Sanfilippo, and driving the funding for the clinical trials that will take place at the hospital as well.

This collaboration also involved Abeona Therapeutics, formed in early 2013 to focus on a cure and provide a unifying voice for patient advocate groups, researchers, clinicians and investors. Today Abeona is positioned to become a leader in developing treatments for Sanfilippo Syndrome.

Bringing together industry, science, a clinical center and the academic community, with the support and funding from a coalition of patient foundations, demonstrates the true power of collaboration. In 2013, Global Genes™ honored this entire Sanfilippo community of stakeholders with the RARE Champion of Hope – Collaborations in Advocacy award, in recognition of the power that such a multifaceted and global collaboration – with patient advocacy groups at the core – can have on the future of a rare disease.

The Future

Get Connected – Be Counted

Another major initiative underway at Global Genes™ for the worldwide rare community, is to continue to identify new patients. Many affected by rare disease do not consider themselves a rare disease patient or part of the global rare disease community. Our hope is that more patients will self-identify and be counted and become connected so that they can be supported. Global Genes™ is working to partner with major consumer brands and looking at various opportunities to identify more patients, with the aim of plugging them in to the network and community, so that their needs can be supported. Having worked with over 800 patient advocacy organizations, partnering with over 200 patient groups as part of the Global Genes RARE™ Foundation Alliance, and connecting with thousands of individuals, we have still identified less than 5% of those impacted by rare disease. We have a lot of work to do as a community and the goal is to exponentially grow that number of connections over the next five years. It is through this process that we can truly empower an army of rare disease activists for their disease – and build the collective voice to impact the rare community on a global scale.

Doing Well by Doing Good

Slowly, but surely, we have seen traction and momentum related to new support for rare disease patients and their families.

The goal is to continue to build and grow a support community that is not only made up of those impacted by rare disease, but the general public. Progressive companies, consumer brands, celebrity, healthcare philanthropists are all starting to recognize the opportunity to make an impact today on a community desperate for support. Smart companies and individuals are also recognizing that innovation is happening in rare disease and that successes in this community will have an upstream effect on more common conditions. In other words, investing in rare disease is not only a good investment but also the right thing to do for the millions suffering and challenged by these conditions.

Patient Advocates at the Core

Awareness, Education, Empowerment, Engagement, Unity, Strength, Support, Results. It has begun: Patients are driving this success, they are the 'change agents', they are unifying and learning from each other, and they are helping build disruptive new business models. What does this mean in the long run? Those rare disease organizations that embrace this change – whether their origins are in advocacy, industry, science, academics or government – will do well, and will do good by doing what is right by those rare disease champions who are catalyzing this revolution in healthcare.

Nicole Boice
President/Founder
Global Genes™
nicoleb@globalgenes.org

Andrea Epstein
Strategic Advisor – Science
andreae@globalgenes.org
www.globalgenes.org
www.globalgenes.org/toolkits

References

1 So You Think You Want to Start a Nonprofit Toolkit. Global Genes™ Project 2015. (Accessed September 2015). https://globalgenes.org/toolkits/so-you-think-you-want-to-start-a-nonprofit/so-you-think-you-want-to-start-a-nonprofit-2/

2 Starting a Nonprofit: The First Steps Toolkit. Global Genes™ Project 2015. (Accessed September 2015). https://globalgenes.org/toolkits/starting-a-nonprofit-the-first-steps/where-to-begin-what-paperwork/

3 RAREDaily. Global Genes™ (Accessed September 2015). https://globalgenes.org/raredaily/

Chapter 2

How to Set up and Manage a Patient Group (a UK Perspective)

Emily Crossley
Founder and Director, The Duchenne Children's Trust

Introduction

Our son's diagnosis of Duchenne Muscular Dystrophy (DMD) opened my husband and I up to a world of grief and despair we hadn't known was possible. At first it was unbearable to even say the words: Duchenne Muscular Dystrophy. They symbolised such utter heartbreak and devastation, they felt like dagger wounds to the heart.

We were sick with grief, and the doctors were very bleak about the prognosis. I cannot begin to describe the utter devastation we felt, imagining what lay ahead.

Through this fog of grief, we fought to find a way forward. It took us a year to get ourselves together and gather the strength to begin the long and challenging journey of setting up our patient group, the Duchenne Children's Trust.

Why did we do it? Why did we take on the challenge of launching a patient group? Because we felt we had to.

We did it because we believed that we could really make a difference – that we could raise the large amounts of money needed to help fund early phase clinical trials that would mean the difference between life and death not just for our son but for all boys and children with Duchenne Muscular Dystrophy. That was our goal and that is what keeps us going.

Factbox: What Is Duchenne Muscular Dystrophy

Duchenne Muscular Dystrophy (DMD) is the most common fatal genetic disorder to affect children. They cannot produce dystrophin, a protein necessary for muscle survival. As a result, every skeletal muscle in the body deteriorates.

The disease is caused by a mistake in the genetic code in a gene called dystrophin, which is found on the X chromosome. Although girls may carry the mistake, they have 2 X chromosomes, so the healthy one cancels out the faulty one. But boys have only one X chromosome so they are more likely to be affected.

- Duchenne Muscular Dystrophy is 100% fatal – there is no cure
- Most children die in their early 20s from heart or respiratory failure
- Every child ends up in a wheelchair by the age of 10 -12
- One third of all Duchenne Muscular Dystrophy cases are the result of random *in utero* mutation, with no warning until the child is born
- Approximately one in 3,500 boys are born with Duchenne Muscular Dystrophy.

There are around 300,000 sufferers worldwide

First Steps:

Decide on your Message and Decide on your Mission:

From early on I was given some very good advice: look upon setting up your foundation in the same way as you would a company or business. Be absolutely clear on your mission and on your message. You need to appeal to your donors' hearts. But also their minds, with commitment, professionalism and a very clear message.

Our message is simple: we have to save our son, and this generation of children. And we have to do it quickly. The science is almost there. We just need money to bring it to patients.

Our mission was also straightforward: We had to fund these early stage trials NOW – we had only limited time to make this happen.

I remembered the story of HIV. How, in 1986, World Aids Day, HIV was a disease you died from. But within ten years, thanks to science and the power of patient advocacy groups, therapies were being approved that fought the disease and held it at bay. Today if you are lucky enough to live in a country that can afford medicines, HIV is no longer fatal. It is a chronic but manageable disease.

We wanted to do the same for Duchenne. Yes, DMD is a rare disease. Yes we are a tiny, tiny charity compared to others. But why can't we set ourselves the target to 'End Duchenne in Ten'? Of course, it is not us alone. There are some incredible DMD patient groups in the UK and globally, who have been in this fight for decades. The breakthroughs we are seeing today, are happening BECAUSE of them, because they funded that early research, so many years ago, which is finally bearing fruit.

It was a rallying cry to me. But it's ended up being the thing donors keep coming back to – that their money will make a real difference and they will see it happen in their lifetimes. Our message of hope has resonated. The idea that people will give us money and that one day, hopefully in their lifetimes, that money will have helped end the biggest genetic killer of children has proven to be very powerful.

Use Your Network

Had we not felt so positive about the research, and if we didn't think we could make a big enough difference, I think it's fair to say that we probably wouldn't have set up our foundation. We were also motivated to do something because we had an amazing group of friends and family, and felt that with their support we could really achieve something.

We set ourselves an ambitious target of raising £1million a year for 10 years. We chose this amount partly because we felt it was achievable – but also because we had discovered that this was the amount of money needed to enable us to start co-funding early stage clinical trials.

Our charity launched in October 2012, with a dinner for 370 people. We raised £180,000 in one night. But almost more important than that, we created a family of people, a group of core supporters, most of whom have stayed with us on our journey so far. At the time of going to press, our foundation has raised just over £3 million in two and a half years.

How did we manage to make that night such a success? Three months beforehand we held a "Friends Night" at a friends' house, to which we invited 70 of our closest friends and family. We didn't ask them for money. We asked them for help. We asked them to open up their networks to us, we asked them to come to the launch event and bring guests with big hearts and deep pockets who might be inspired to help us.

Help came in other ways too that night. One of our friends organised and paid for the development of the website, which is absolutely crucial to get right from the start.

Another made a series of introductions for me to meet people high up in charities, politics and fundraising, to make sure we got everything right from the beginning. And I cannot emphasise enough the importance of getting good advice and getting your foundation and message right, RIGHT FROM THE BEGINNING. It's no use launching yourselves to your supporters without a clear vision and a truly professional approach. After all they are giving you their money, and they need reassurance that you are going to spend it in the best way possible.

Get the Right Support

Our launch was also a success because we surrounded ourselves with dynamic, connected, motivated and big-hearted friends and family. We chose three trustees alongside my husband and me. One is a lawyer who ensures that all our projects are properly vetted and has set up the charity's governance structure. Our second trustee is an events and branding consultant, who planned our events to perfection, and our third trustee was at that time the Financial Director of a charity, and her advice on governance issues, finance and fundraising has been invaluable.

We also set up a group of patrons, friends who would be ambassadors for the charity and who have proven invaluable in hosting events, offering advice and opening up their networks to us.

My own work network also turned out to be key. I gave up my job as a TV reporter and presenter, believing that the skills I had would be non-transferable. I was wrong. It turned out that the ability to communicate is absolutely crucial to any foundation. And my former friends and colleagues in broadcasting have been remarkable in what they have done to help the charity raise money.

You need to embrace all forms of fundraising:

- Events can raise the profile and earn contributions but are tiring and can be a high risk strategy;
- Pursuing funding from trusts and grant makers should be considered but can be complex and frustrating if you are turned down. See EU funding for clinical trials.

Do NOT embark on this journey unless you have the proper support from friends and family. Running a patient foundation can be a very lonely place, and you need your friends and family around you.

The Benefits of Being a Registered Charity

It was on the advice of one of our trustees that we initially set up our patients group as a charity and a company limited by guarantee. The reason for this is to protect the assets of the charity and protect the trustees.

If a company is limited by guarantee, it means that all the assets are locked into the company. As a consequence, no trustee is entitled to those assets. It also means that if the charity is sued for whatever reason, the liability is limited to the charity and so trustees can't be sued for their personal assets.

You can apply to be a registered charity in the UK once you have raised £5,000. In the UK, registration is through the Charities Commission. This involves filling out a lengthy and quite complex form. Seek advice before you complete the form, especially when it comes to the Articles of Association that lay down the remit and purpose of the charity. This is effectively legally binding, so try not to make the wording too specific, otherwise you might create barriers further down the line if you want to fund things that lie outside any strict criteria that have been previously outlined.

There are huge financial advantages to registering as a charity, but there are stringent protocols that need to be followed so get good advice.

Collaboration / Working Together

Finding Friends

Being the parent of a child with a devastating and life-limiting illness is a lonely, dark and frightening place. Add to that the demands and responsibility of running a patient group, and you can sometimes feel overwhelmed.

I genuinely do not believe I would have had the strength to stay in the fight without meeting three other mothers, all of whom are remarkable and inspirational women. Two run foundations in the UK; Alex Johnson from Joining Jack and Kerry Rosenfeld from the Duchenne Research Fund. In the US, Annie Ganot, who works with Solid Bioscience, a company set up by her husband, Ilan Ganot, to find treatments for DMD. The four of us have an amazing bond – we talk all the time and help each other get through the challenging times. Find friends. You will need them.

One very good piece of advice came from a former Cabinet Minister, who told a friend and me that people in power do not want lots of different groups in the same arena knocking on the door and asking for vastly different things. It's important to speak as one voice. Make friends with organisations that may have similar goals to you.

Conclusion

What I have learnt:

- It seems to take as much time and effort to raise £5,000 as £50,000, so be clear about the events you are developing
- Understand that you are only human and don't wear yourself out
- Get a good team around you and learn to delegate – you can't do everything yourself
- Keep on top of the paperwork and financial management
- Make sure you keep in touch with your donors.

Setting up a patients group can be very demanding – think it through carefully before you commit yourself.

Top Ten things to do:

1. Get as much expert advice as you can before you set up – and keep getting it;
2. Define your mission and set your goals;
3. Find strong and supportive Trustees, Patrons and Friends;
4. Create a brand, a website and embrace social media;
5. Register as a charity;
6. Set up efficient financial and business procedures from the outset;
7. Ensure that someone in the group understands about all aspects of communication and keep in touch with

your donors;

8. Keep up to date with the science that is happening in your group's specific arena and form links with groups working within the same field;

9. Develop a fundraising strategy that includes events, grant applications and a network of Friends who will set up their own fundraising activities to support you;

10.   Stay strong and never stop believing that you can make a difference.

The Duchenne Children's Trust: www.dc-trust.org

Chapter 3

How to Build an International Research Consortium

Stephen Lynn†, Annemieke Aartsma-Rus†*, Hanns
Lochmüller†, Volker Straub† and Kate Bushby†
† Institute of Genetic Medicine, Newcastle University. *
Leiden University Medical Centre.

Introduction

Why do we need an international research consortium for collaborative drug development in rare diseases? To add value to the process leading from research to medical and nursing practice (translational research), a consortium should address the likely bottlenecks. In the drug development process for rare diseases, such bottlenecks might include:

- Lack of cellular or animal model data. This may include a limited understanding about how cell or animal studies might translate to humans;
- Lack of knowledge about patient availability and characteristics;
- Lack of a number of appropriately trained sites with similar levels of standards of care and qualified staff to run trials;
- The time taken for proper protocol design, especially with a lack of generally accepted ways to measure the outcomes;
- Lack of natural history data;

- Lack of major drug company involvement;
- Some of the organisations funding preclinical studies do not understand what makes a trial able to demonstrate or refute efficacy – the appeal of the "pilot trial" as a possible quick fix;
- Lack of regulatory precedent and health economic data.

We have had extensive experience of building TREAT-NMD to address these and other bottlenecks for neuromuscular diseases (NMD). The major achievements of the TREAT-NMD network are in providing the tools for trial readiness and therapy delivery in NMD, especially Duchenne muscular dystrophy and spinal muscular atrophy. The tools include:

- Good communication and networking (website and newsletter);
- Ethics and regulatory engagement;
- Patient registries;
- A registry of expert care and trial sites;
- Harmonized outcome measures in animal models and patients;
- Support to biobank resources and therapy development.

In this way, the TREAT-NMD network has targeted the areas where clinical trials for NMD could be accelerated by collaborative working right from the start.

TREAT-NMD as an EU funded network

Neuromuscular diseases form a large group of diseases, each of which is individually rare (prevalence less than 5 in 10,000). However, collectively they affect approximately 1 in 2,500 of the population (around 200,000 NMD patients in the EU and 3 million worldwide).[1] They are present in all populations and affect both sexes, children and adults. Many cause significant long-term disability and reduced life expectancy, with death often resulting from cardiac and respiratory involvement.[2]

There are currently no curative treatments for any genetic NMD, but knowledge of disease causing genes has begun to clarify the molecular pathological mechanisms underlying NMDs. This has lead to plans for specific gene based therapies or targeted pharmaceutical approaches.[3] Some of these treatment options are now in human studies. Examples that are closest to clinical application include:

- Antisense oligonucleotide and stop codon read-through treatments for Duchenne Muscular Dystrophy (DMD) and spinal muscular atrophy (SMA);
- Myostatin inhibition in a range of muscular dystrophies;
- Gene therapy approaches to DMD;
- Pharmacological approaches to survival motor neuron gene (SMN) upregulation in SMA.[4,5]

While scientific developments were universally welcomed amongst scientists, clinicians and patient organisations, they exposed the lack of harmonisation of possible routes to beneficial therapeutics in NMD. These hinder a smooth move into clinical trials. TREAT-NMD was established to address this lack of harmonisation. It created a model, in which the development of the network's tools would enable delivery of new treatments through a long-term vision. It would also support optimal care for patients. Based initially on DMD and SMA, this model has also been successfully rolled out to other neuromuscular diseases, as new therapies come closer to clinical application.

TREAT-NMD was initially established in January 2007 as an EU-funded 'network of excellence'. Its remit was 'reshaping the research environment' in the translational approach to the neuromuscular field. It was funded through the 6th Framework Programme (FP6), where a specific call addressed this particular problem. The TREAT-NMD (Translational Research in Europe – Assessment and Treatment of Neuro Muscular Diseases) network has subsequently developed from its European roots to become a global organisation. It brings together leading specialists, patient groups and industry representatives. It ensures preparedness for the clinical trials and therapies of the future while promoting best practice today.

The activities of TREAT-NMD address the bottlenecks delaying the development of treatments. These range from assessing animal models, patient registries and outcome measures for clinical trials, to standards of patient care.[6] The overall philosophy is to create the infrastructure to ensure that the most promising new therapies reach patients as quickly as possible. The initial EU-funded network linked over 350 researchers and clinicians in 22 European organisations, with a large number of collaborators. This was not only in Europe, but also around the world. The initial 22 partner organisations included universities, patient organisations, and industrial partners from 11 countries (United Kingdom, Germany, France, Italy, Spain, The Netherlands, Sweden, Finland, Belgium, Hungary and Switzerland). These partners were:

- University of Newcastle upon Tyne, UK (Project Coordinator)
- Institut National de la Santé et de la Recherche Médicale, France
- Leiden University Medical Centre, The Netherlands
- European Neuromuscular Centre, The Netherlands
- Association Française contre les Myopathies and Institut de Myologie, France
- Biozentrum, University of Basel, Switzerland
- European Organisation for Rare Diseases, France
- Karolinska Institute, Sweden
- King's College London, UK
- Santhera Pharmaceuticals (Switzerland) LTD Liab.Co.
- Helsingin yliopisto, Finland
- Medical Research Council, UK
- Fondazione Telethon, Italy
- Université Catholique de Louvain, Belgium
- Universitat Autònoma de Barcelona, Spain

- GenoSafe SAS, France
- NOVAMEN, France
- National Institute of Environmental Health, Hungary
- Genethon, France
- University College London, UK
- University Klinikum of Freiburg, Germany
- Ludwig-Maximilians-University, Munich, Germany.

Each partner was responsible for a specific activity or work package, depending on their areas of interest and expertise. This work was the foundation of the TREAT-NMD infrastructure summarised in Figure 1. In addition, TREAT-NMD attracted a large number of members, made up of individuals and organisations representing key stakeholders, collaborators and supporters.

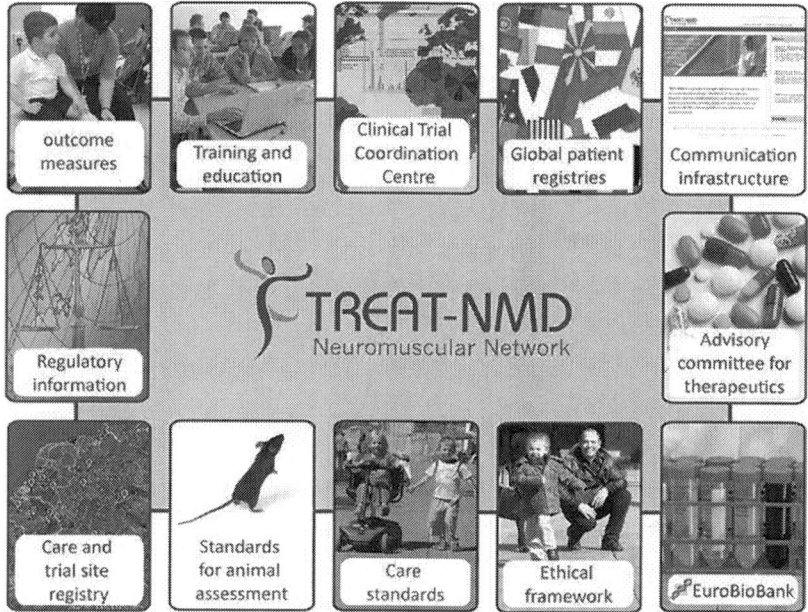

Figure 1. The TREAT-NMD activities, tools and resources developed through the FP6 'network of excellence' funding mechanism

Networking such a diverse group of participants across a wide range of activities needs clear governance. To provide governance and oversight of the network, one of the early tasks for TREAT-NMD was to establish the TREAT-NMD Coordination Centre (TNCC). It was based with the network co-ordinators, Volker Straub and Kate Bushby at Newcastle University, UK. The strategic management of the network was initially provided through the Governing Board. Each partner was an active member of the Governing Board. They were committed to creating the TNCC step by step, by the integration of their research efforts in the neuromuscular diseases field. Any additional institutions or industrial companies linked to the network, but not committing resources directly to the TNCC, were partners of the Club of Interest. The Governing Board, chaired by Newcastle University, was responsible for defining and implementing the TREAT-NMD policy and strategy.

An advisory body was established in order to facilitate the work of the strategic management. This body, the Scientific and Technological Advisory Council (STAC), was made up of several independent worldwide recognised scientists and industrialists. The STAC monitored the neuromuscular diseases research of the partners and benchmarked it against the worldwide state-of-the-art. It also suggested methods to improve the efficiency of research and the transfer of new knowledge to industry. The STAC was a mix of expertise, including patient advocacy and scientists from outside Europe, and senior European scientists working in adjacent areas. The STAC also advised the Governing Board on issues such as network sustainability and expansion, to include new members and disease groups. Representation of such diverse groups undoubtedly created a vibrant culture for the network to develop.

Sustainability beyond EU funding

The sustainability of the network was a major point of focus from the outset of the EU funding period, as no renewal of a 'network of excellence' grant was possible under EU funding rules. Various models of sustainability were explored. In September 2010, TREAT-NMD carried out a wide-ranging public consultation attracting 430 responses from over 60 countries. The aim of the consultation was to determine the key areas of activity to be included in its long-term strategy. The most popular priority for respondents was 'facilitating international collaborations between research groups'. Ninety one percent of responders agreed this as an ongoing priority for TREAT-NMD. It has been at the core of many TREAT-NMD activities, and continues to be the philosophy of the network.

The TREAT-NMD Task Force was set up in response to the consultation to help define a clear, focused strategy with defined goals and objectives. Its aim was to oversee the transition from the network's EU funding status to the TREAT-NMD Alliance. The Task Force, consisting of key clinical and scientific experts from around the world, guided the transition from EU funded network to global Alliance. It continues to play an important role in current and future activities of the TREAT-NMD Alliance.

The establishment of the TREAT-NMD Alliance and the end of the EU funding period meant that a new charter and governance structure were required. This would enable the network to continue to grow and develop scientifically and geographically. In January 2012, the TREAT-NMD Executive Committee, made up of both academic and patient representatives, took over governance of the network. The first chair of the TREAT-NMD Alliance was Professor Hanns Lochmüller. As of January 2015, the members of the TREAT-NMD Executive Committee are:

- Annemieke Aartsma-Rus (Chair) (Leiden University Medical Centre, The Netherlands)
- Eric Hoffman (Vice Chair) (Children's National Medical Centre, USA)
- Filippo Buccella (Parent Project Onlus, Italy)
- Kevin Flanigan (Ohio State University, USA)
- Janbernd Kirschner (University Medical Centre Freiburg, Germany)

- Anna Kole (Eurordis, France)
- Eugenio Mercuri (Università Cattolica del Sacro Cuore, Italy)
- Ichizo Nishino (National Center of Neurology and Psychiatry, Japan)
- Kathy North (Murdoch Childrens Research Institute, Australia)
- Alejandra Pereda Alonso (Duchenne Parent Project, Spain)
- Jes Rahbek (The Rehabilitation Centre for Neuromuscular Diseases, Denmark)
- Thomas Sejersen (Karolinska Institute, Sweden)
- Mathew Wood (University of Oxford, UK).

The members of the Executive Committee are elected from the TREAT-NMD Task Force and from member patient organisations. They are made up of 9 academics and 4 patient organisation representatives. The members of the committee then elect their Chair and Vice-Chair. The governance model is described in the TREAT-NMD Alliance Charter. The Executive Committee is responsible for providing overall policy and strategic direction to the TREAT-NMD Alliance. It also oversees activities and progress, and delegates responsibility for day-to-day operations to the representatives of the various activity groups. The Executive Committee is supported by a Secretariat at Newcastle University that provides the administrative and project coordination necessary for the TREAT-NMD Alliance. The Executive Committee has monthly conference calls and meets with the Task Force in person once every two years. The Secretariat is responsible for implementing the decisions of the Executive Committee.

Membership is open to individuals, academic institutions and patient organisations. As of January 2015, TREAT-NMD has 124 organisational members from 51 countries and 336 individual members in 54 countries. Over 3,500 people receive the monthly TREAT-NMD newsletter and over 30 countries are members of the TREAT-NMD Global Registry initiative.

Membership criteria are defined in the TREAT-NMD Alliance Charter.

To continue to develop the work streams within the TREAT-NMD EU funded period, a three-year rolling work plan of activities was developed by the TREAT-NMD Task Force. The specific targets, milestones and timelines were, for example, as outlined in the current work plan (2014-2016) (www.treat-nmd.eu/about/network/action-plan-2014-2016/).   Working groups continue to advance their activity area. They do this with broad collaboration in newly funded projects under the International Rare Diseases Research Consortium (IRDiRC) initiative. Many of the individual activities have secured, or are in the process of securing, funding as separate projects from other sources. These include national, EU and private funding bodies. The international coordination, communication and registry coordination is carried out by the Secretariat. This work plan is reviewed and updated every two years.

Across both the EU and post EU periods of TREAT-NMD, there have been several specific priority areas, as described below (with further details on the website). These have contributed to the aim of increasing clinical trial readiness for NMD and have acted to facilitate collaborative drug development pathways.

Communication infrastructure

The network communication infrastructure is core to all activities of the network. It unites clinicians and researchers in the neuromuscular field worldwide. This communication infrastructure is also core to our interaction with the patient community. It helps us inform and disseminate the work of the network.

The TREAT-NMD website (www.treat-nmd.eu) has been a major focus of the networking activities. The website and e-newsletter are now recognised as leading sources of up-to-date information on neuromuscular translational research and patient care. The newsletter appears monthly and is read by more than 3,500 recipients. The website is extensive, with over 1,000 pages of static and database driven content, and receives more than 6,500 unique visitors per month resulting in excess of 25,000 page views. The site hosts approximately 400 pdf documents and these were downloaded about 10,000 times during 2014. The site is visited from 182 different countries and territories around the world (as of January 2015).

The TREAT-NMD website acts as a go-to resource for industry. It provides valuable and efficient information, promotes the TREAT-NMD services and tools and facilitates therapy development. The website fosters collaboration between neuromuscular stakeholders and engages the community in meetings and events through its calendar and events pages. There is no doubt that an effective tool for outreach and communication is key to networking activities such as these.

Networking for optimal care

Experimental methods needed to be harmonised to enable drug development for NMD. At the same time, efforts had to be made to ensure that care standards were uniform enough across different sites to enable the delivery of clinical trials. Such efforts also support the adoption and spread of optimal care for all patients, even those not in the initial target groups for therapy development. The TREAT-NMD strategy for the development and spread of care guidelines was very much to work together with disease specific and other initiatives going on in the area. The key aim was to promote the idea of developing single internationally agreed guidelines.

In 2009 there was a worldwide effort to generate care guidelines for DMD. This involved patient organisations, the Centre for Disease Control in the USA and TREAT-NMD. In advance of the full consensus document, TREAT-NMD generated a set of brief standards of care for DMD.[7] The full publication of the international consensus standards of care for Duchenne muscular dystrophy (DMD) was published in January 2010 in The Lancet Neurology. It marked the culmination of a three-year process led by the US Centres for Disease Control and Prevention (CDC).[8,9] Kate Bushby, was the TREAT-NMD Network Coordinator at the time. Under her managing editorship, 84 international experts in all areas of DMD care rigorously reviewed more than 70,000 clinical scenarios to create the consensus guidelines.

Subsequently, a 'Family Guide' was created through close collaboration between TREAT-NMD, advocacy groups and healthcare professionals. The Family Guide sets out the care recommendations in lay terms. As of 2014, this has been available in over 30 languages, with additional translations in progress.

Both the Lancet recommendations and the Family Guide have been used around the world for lobbying and negotiations with healthcare authorities for better care provision. They are included as part of the CARE-NMD project in Europe. The recommendations are also supported by pharmaceutical companies. They recognise that standardised baseline care and full genetic diagnosis of all patients is critical to successful multi-centre clinical trials.

In 2014, the CDC began a review process to ensure that the care recommendations reflected the latest clinical knowledge of DMD, and included additional areas of care such as emergency and adult care. TREAT-NMD is closely involved in this process, in close collaboration with healthcare professionals and patient advocacy organisations.

The work to develop the Family Guide for DMD involved collaborations with the Muscular Dystrophy Association (USA), Parent Project Muscular Dystrophy and United Parent Project Muscular Dystrophy (worldwide). It has been mirrored by efforts for SMA, involving the International Coordinating Committee for SMA (USA), Muscular Dystrophy UK and SMA Support UK. For CMD, it involved Cure CMD (USA), Association Française contre les Myopathies (France) and Telethon Italy.

The generation of guidelines is never sufficient to impact care. For this reason, TREAT-NMD has had a focus on a major dissemination programme. Family guides are generated from the various recommendations and translated into multiple languages (31 for DMD, 17 for SMA). In 2014, the DMD Family Guide was downloaded 2,011 times, while the SMA Family Guide was downloaded 525 times.

These efforts were supported by training programmes, particularly in Eastern Europe and more widely (including Brazil and China). They included the EU funded project CARE-NMD, with the aim of improving access to best-practice care for DMD across 7 EU countries. It includes analysis of current treatment practices and identifies inequalities between and within participating European countries. Information and training workshops for medical professionals and families are also hosted. The aim was to ensure the dissemination and implementation of international consensus treatment recommendations for DMD at national and European levels (www.care-nmd.eu).

Across rare diseases, information on care standards is frequently lacking. This presents a risk for the set-up of the international studies which are often necessary for these conditions. For this reason, as well as raising awareness of care for patients even in advance of clinical trials, emphasis on care standards is very important. This effort is supported broadly now by the FP7 project Rare Best Practice (www.rarebestpractices.eu).

Project Ethics Council

TREAT-NMD also recognised that drug trials in children engage with many ethical issues. These range from drug-related safety concerns to communication with patients and parents, to recruitment and informed consent procedures. Trial design must not only address issues of equal access. Researchers must also think through the implications of using a personalised medicine approach which requires a precise molecular diagnosis. This is in addition to considering other implications of developing orphan drugs. The Project Ethics Council (PEC) was established within TREAT-NMD as a high level advisory group drawing on the expertise of its interdisciplinary members. This includes clinicians, lawyers, scientists, patients and parents, representatives of patient organisations, social scientists and ethicists. The PEC has responded to important ethical issues raised within the TREAT-NMD consortium. PEC has provided a wider resource for any concerned parent, patient, or clinician asking questions of ethical concern. These reports from the PEC are available on the web site (www.treat-nmd.eu/resources/ethics/). Matters raised range from science related ethical issues and issues related to hereditary neuromuscular diseases and the new therapies, to questions concerning patients' rights in the context of patient registries and biobanks.[10]

Clinical trial platform

The Care and Trial Site Registry (CTSR) was established to be a worldwide registry of clinical sites as part of its 'trial-readiness' strategy. These sites have expertise in neuromuscular disease or see neuromuscular patients. As of January 2015, detailed information on more than 320 clinical trial sites is captured in CTSR. In total, the clinical sites can identify over 45,000 neuromuscular patients that have been mapped to a set of diagnostic categories. Examples include, DMD, SMA, CMD (Congenital Muscular Dystrophy) and LGMD (Limb-Girdle muscular dystrophy). Mapping the location, expertise and patient cohorts of these clinical centres is proving key to finding sites capable of running planned clinical trials. Both the CTSR and Global Patient Registries have already been instrumental in supporting both feasibility studies and trial recruitment. However, this network of sites with neuromuscular expertise is important in other ways too. It is also valuable as a platform for spreading best practice in patient care and looking at care standards as shown in the EU Health project CARE-NMD.[11]

CTSR and patient registries are used by industry as well as academics. They are used to support feasibility enquiries for drug development plans and to identify sites for clinical research. The combined use of patient registry and CTSR data provides useful information for planning clinical trials in rare NMDs. As these infrastructures have expanded and developed, their utility has been recognised, especially by industry. Both large pharma and smaller SMEs now make the most enquiries to these resources. In 2014 alone, there were four enquiries with another three in the early planning stage.

As pharma has become interested in the neuromuscular field, the CTSR has served as a useful route for companies to identify key opinion leaders and viable sites. The role of the registry is extending to other neurological diseases as a part of the EU FP7 funded project Neuromics. A resource of this kind is a signal that the field is organised and addressing the issues of accountability and good clinical practice required for setting up trials. In addition such a network provides the backbone for spreading other knowledge and activities. Alongside patient registries, it is a core part of translational research infrastructure.

Patient registry development

A global patient registry for DMD and SMA is one of the key TREAT-NMD infrastructures that has been set up. It is made up of more than 50 national patient registries worldwide.

Before 2007, there was a small number of independent national registries (UK, Czech Republic, France, and USA). Each collected varying data elements. Discussions with these registries, patients, patient advocacy groups and clinicians highlighted the need for a more harmonized approach to patient registries and how they can support clinical trials. These discussions led to a framework for existing and emerging registries[12,13,14] and the development of a 'charter' for registries led by TREAT-NMD. The aim for disease registries through TREAT-NMD was:

- To define data content for each disease/gene;
- To define the regulatory and ethical framework;

- To identify and analyse existing national registries;
- To train curators for quality control of new and existing registries.

The primary aim of this TREAT-NMD activity was to allow feasibility assessment, planning and recruitment for clinical trials. Other secondary objectives included:

- Collecting epidemiological data;
- Establishing genotype-phenotype correlations;
- Defining natural history;
- Assessing burden of illness;
- Treatment outcomes;
- Standards of care.[15,16]

Through TREAT-NMD, this led to the development of the required and highly encouraged data items that all registries are required to collect. The registries in TREAT-NMD also agreed to adhere to legal/ethical best practices. They allowed for patient feedback, possibility of data withdrawal from a registry and encryption of data sets.

The charter for the TREAT-NMD registries was approved by the newly formed TREAT-NMD Global Database Oversight Committee (TGDOC). This is made up of representatives from all national registries in the TREAT-NMD registry initiative. The committee meets annually to discuss registry issues. Through this work these registries now contribute data to the centralised TREAT-NMD Global Registries.

The DMD and SMA registries now hold more than 13,500 and 5,000 individual patient entries respectively. They have standardised items and consent that facilitate and accelerate clinical research and clinical trials, while giving patients improved access to relevant information on standards of diagnosis and care.[17,18]

Most innovative therapies for patients suffering from rare NMDs are expected to act on gene-specific molecular pathways. In some areas, the specific mutation will determine how applicable a particular therapy is. Therefore, patient registries for

NMDs must be gene-based and it is very important to annotate each patient's mutation correctly. Clinical information must be captured in a standardised way and updated regularly. Disease experts are required to curate genetic and clinical information.

TREAT-NMD is supporting similar developments for other rare NMDs. For example, the Congenital Muscular Dystrophies and Congenital Myopathies, Limb Girdle Muscular Dystrophies, Facioscapulohumeral Muscular Dystrophy (FSHD) and Myotonic Dystrophies. Each represents several genetic entities. These registries have either been established on a national or international level, depending on the size of the patient population. For those very rare neuromuscular diseases it is more efficient to establish a single international registry in which all patients can be registered. However, like all TREAT-NMD registries, they require that defined core datasets are collected and that there is appropriate oversight. TREAT-NMD has also provided extensive documentation and resources to help support these and other new registries through the Registries Toolkit. This is freely available on the TREAT-NMD web site (www. treat-nmd.eu/resources/patient-registries/tookit/).

Preclinical research

The research activities in TREAT-NMD contribute to the overall objectives of the network. They have been designed to tackle areas suffering from fragmentation and their own unique (shared) and standardised approaches. The development of novel therapies has been hampered by the fact that there is no standardisation of the parameters for pre-clinical efficacy data and protocols used to measure the results in animal models. It is therefore not possible to compare different treatment options and to prioritise them prior to clinical trials. TREAT-NMD created guidelines for the conduct of preclinical efficacy experiments. They also created a collection of standard operating procedures (SOPs) that can be made available to the scientific community. These offer the possibility for preclinical research to be done under more standardised conditions.[19,20,21] Working groups of European and non-European experts have also been established to evaluate and modify recommended SOPs. Furthermore, a web-based system has been created to allow regular addition, updating and distribution of the recommended SOPs.

It is vital to develop potential therapies and efficacy testing in animal models that are relevant to a particular disease. They need specific endpoints and accurate data evaluation. The limited number of patients with rare diseases and the high costs of a clinical trial require a rigorous selection of treatment options that may work in humans. It is therefore important to standardise non-clinical testing procedures at this stage. This helps prioritise the most promising treatments and avoids duplication of effort.

TREAT-NMD approached this problem by searching for consensus on the most appropriate animal model for DMD, for which several are available. Then guidelines for animal (mouse) care and experimental setups were discussed and standardised. This was done in collaboration with international experts, to reduce the variability of results across laboratories. For preclinical experiments, the suggestion was that the most important endpoints were those that measure disease-relevant pathology and reflect similar results in humans. Finally, standard operating procedures were compiled by groups of researchers to assess such endpoints in animal models of DMD, SMA and MDC1A (a congenital muscle dystrophy). They were made available online, discussed and presented at several meetings and published in scientific journals. The aim was to increase awareness on the urgent need to use common procedures in the evaluation of efficacy in the preclinical phase.

The generation of the animal model SOPs has been an outstanding example of international collaboration. The TREAT-NMD website is the major route for their dissemination. The SOP pages received almost 2,000 hits in the last year; an average of 118 pdf downloads every month. The website provides a sophisticated store of SOPs, enabling ease of reference, promoting standardisation and allowing systematic updates. The website is crucial for the extension, maintenance and distribution of these tools.

Biobanking

The EuroBioBank (EBB) network (www.eurobiobank.org) is an active network of biobanks in Europe. It is the first to provide human DNA, cell and tissue samples as a service to the scientific community conducting research on rare diseases. The EBB was established in 2001 to allow access to biospecimens and associated data. It obtained funding from the European Commission in 2002 (5th framework programme) and started operation in 2003. The set-up phase, during the EC funding period 2003-2006, established the basis for running the network. The following consolidation phase has seen the growth of the network by new partners joining, better network cohesion, better coordination of activities, and the development of a quality control system.

During this phase, the network took part in the TREAT-NMD programme. It was involved in the planning of the European Biobanking and Biomolecular Resources Research Infrastructure. Recently, EBB became a partner of RD-Connect. This is an FP7 EU program aimed at linking rare disease biobanks, registries and bioinformatic data.[22] Within RD-Connect, EBB contributes expertise and promotes high professional standards and best practices in rare disease biobanking. It integrates rare disease patient registries and 'omics' data, thus countering the fragmentation of international cooperation in this area.

From 2012, the Fondazione Telethon – a partner of TREAT-NMD – took on the responsibility for EBB. This was as a 3-year commitment within the newly established TREAT-NMD Alliance. Fondazione Telethon had already been supporting genetic biobanks across Italy since 1993. The web-based EBB catalogue (www.eurobiobank.org/en/services/CatalogueHome.html) makes it possible to search for biological samples by type of biological material and disease:

- 111,000 samples were available at the end of 2013;
- 188,400 new samples were collected from 2003-2013;
- 73,400 samples were distributed over the same period.

On average, 18,800 samples are collected and 7,000 samples distributed each year. Of these, 5,700 and 3,000 samples respectively are collected and distributed for neuromuscular disease (NMD).[23]

Outcome measure validation and harmonisation

The development of medicinal products to treat rare diseases is a research area that has attracted a lot of attention over the past few years. For the stakeholders in the field, including the regulatory agencies, the area of translational research and drug development for rare diseases is still fairly new and holds plenty of challenges.[24,25] There has been a lot of progress over the past decades in diagnostic approaches for rare genetic diseases. However, developing therapies for clinical application in patients has lagged behind. Some of the major stumbling blocks for conducting clinical trials in rare diseases were and continue to be:

- The lack of standardised patient cohorts;
- Limited knowledge about the natural history of disease;
- Lack of validated outcome measures;
- The dearth of validated biomarkers; and
- The difficulty to recruit patients.[26]

There has been an effort to finish the work on new outcome measures proposed in the last few years.[26] While reviewing the existing scales, it has become increasingly obvious that there are a number of activities that are not captured by them. Most notably, the assessment of upper limb function was scarcely represented in the existing scales. The need for dedicated assessments has been highlighted both in type 2 SMA and non-ambulant DMD boys and in all the other disorders with non-ambulant patients. Several activities have been promoted by TREAT-NMD to address this issue in different diseases, in collaboration with other groups.

Natural history data allow us to follow possible changes over time in patients affected by a given disorder. These data are strongly needed at the time of designing a trial, in order to be able to power the study and establish how a treatment would be different from what is expected. This is particularly true for progressive disorders, such as DMD, when the rate of progression is different at different age points. Staging of the disease and description of the impact of changes in each stage is important for milestone/event analysis in trials. TREAT-NMD has supported and organised a number of meetings and workshops to enable this work and to coordinate these efforts internationally.

In recent years MRI has become more widely used in patients with genetic muscle diseases. The extent and localisation of muscle pathology obtained can provide useful information for the patient's diagnosis. In a number of diseases the pattern of muscle pathology detected by MRI can almost be indicative for a specific disease and can therefore guide genetic testing. Various groups have now reported their experience with muscle MRI in defined patient cohorts and have started to outline specific patterns of muscle pathology. TREAT-NMD ran a workshop aimed to increase collaboration and data collection from different groups. It gave an opportunity to share expertise about the use of muscle MRI and has led to a number of publications and grants from FP7 to further support this work.

Supporting therapeutic development

We created the TREAT-NMD Advisory Committee for Therapeutics (TACT) for the neuromuscular community.[27] TACT evaluates novel and existing compounds that have been suggested as potential therapies. It does so in a comprehensive, consistent and unbiased manner. This committee includes internationally renowned experts who cover preclinical data analysis and clinical development. They also cover ethical and regulatory requirements and commercial considerations. The aim of TACT is to provide objective, transparent and consistent guidance to the neuromuscular community. It provides education and direction context, on the readiness of drugs and/or therapeutic targets for clinical trials in neuromuscular diseases. This evaluation will also be helpful for preparing funding applications and investigational drug applications. It will serve as an unbiased appraisal to be published for the wider neuromuscular community.

To date, TACT has held 10 review meetings and reviewed 29 program applications in several rare neuromuscular diseases. Of the 29 programs reviewed:

- 19 were from industry;
- 10 were from academia;
- 15 were for novel compounds;
- 14 were for repurposed drugs;
- 16 were small molecules;
- 13 were biologics;
- 14 were preclinical stage applications;
- 15 were clinical stage applications;
- 3 had received Orphan drug designation from the European Medicines Agency and 3 from the Food and Drug Administration.

A number of recurrent themes emerged over the course of the reviews. We found that applicants frequently need advice and education on issues dealing with:

- preclinical standard operating procedures;
- interactions with regulatory agencies;
- formulation;
- repurposing;
- clinical trial design;
- manufacturing; and
- ethics.[27]

Training and education

The training and education programme was developed as part of the network. It was designed to complement and streamline those programmes already offered to the neuromuscular community. The courses were integrated to offer a full and comprehensive programme for continuing education. This was in the form of summer schools, workshops and symposia. The training programme supported the mobility of individuals through exchange programmes and short-term visits. These programmes covered many of the important topics that were identified as priorities, such as:

- Diagnosis of NMDs;
- Standards of care and management;
- Outcome measures and clinical trial design;
- Patient registries.

These programmes were specifically targeted to Central and Eastern European countries. They were very successful in disseminating important information about these diseases, especially the standards of care.

The current situation

The TREAT-NMD Alliance has shown that survival beyond a limited funding period is possible. It is now an international network for rare inherited neuromuscular disorders (NMDs). It has a significant track record and reputation in the field. Its mission is still to provide an infrastructure to support and increase collaboration and knowledge between clinicians, scientists, and patients. TREAT-NMD accelerates therapy development for these incurable conditions. It improves patient care through publication and spread of agreed best-practice guidelines. It provides reliable information for patients and professionals.[28] Although NMDs are individually rare, TREAT-NMD activities address ~200,000 patients in the EU, and ~3 million worldwide. TREAT-NMD has become a model for rare disease collaboration, and has helped to increase the profile of European NMD research and healthcare globally.

Its critical mass of expertise focusses on:

- The publication of consensus guidelines;
- Standards covering basic research (eg. standards for animal model assessment);
- Standards for translational research (outcome measures validation/protocol harmonisation);
- Standards for care (international consensus guidelines for NMD care).

These are all vital prerequisites for progress that can only be achieved by collaboration. TREAT-NMD has also become a significant catalyst for new research projects, which take advantage of the translational research platform offered by the Alliance (Figure 2).

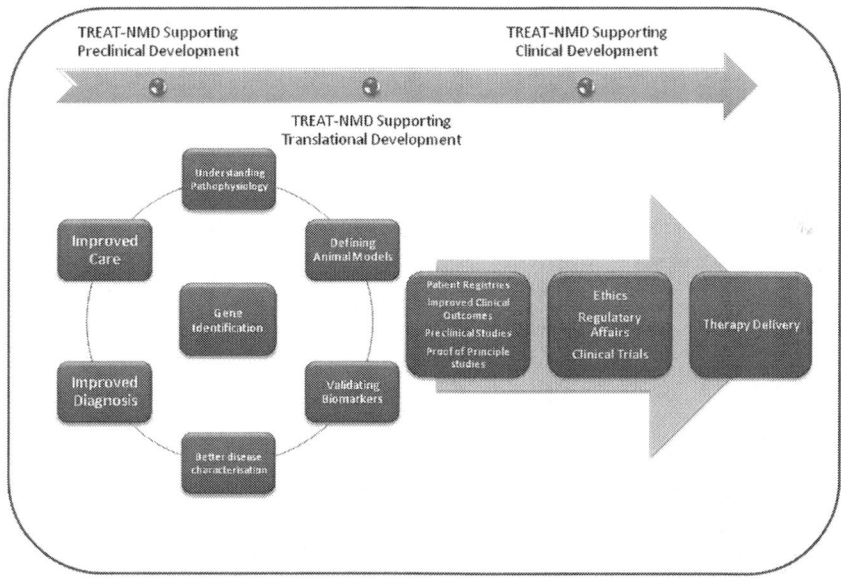

Figure 2. The translational pipeline and how TREAT-NMD has supported this from preclinical to clinical, and on to therapy delivery for NMDs

TREAT-NMD brings together leading specialists in the neuromuscular field. It is a natural partner for biotech and pharmaceutical companies developing new therapeutics. The unique tools, services and expertise available within the network can support, simplify and accelerate clinical studies. Through TREAT-NMD, companies receive advisory support from leading neuromuscular experts. They also receive assistance in locating the centres of expertise for clinical trials and find support with recruiting patients. The network offers consultancy in all aspects of neuromuscular trial planning. This ranges from the set-up of a full scientific advisory board for protocol development, to advice on the selection of neuromuscular experts with relevant expertise. The latter can include preclinical, clinical, clinical evaluator, biostatistical or regulatory experts.

TREAT-NMD has set-up and maintained the global patient registries for the collection of natural history data and post marketing surveillance. It plans to extend these, as well as the current activities on identifying and recruiting patients into clinical trials. It will make the information available to patients. Through the TGDOC we have given assistance, governance and oversight to the neuromuscular patient registries. This ensures the best legal and ethical practice according to the registries charter. It also ensures effective use of data for clinical research while safe-guarding patients and their families. The networking aspect of these registries has been clearly seen as an advantage. They maintain and further develop contacts with a number of relevant international initiatives in rare disease registries (EPIRARE, IRDiRC, PARENT Joint Action, RD-CONNECT, EUCERD Joint Action, etc.).

The TREAT-NMD Alliance addresses the aims of the International Rare Disease Research Consortium (IRDiRC) as they apply to NMDs. It does this through its synergies with FP7 projects, such as RD-Connect and Neuromics. TREAT-NMD also contributes to other funded projects, such as BIO-NMD, NMD-Chip, SKIP-NMD, RARE-Bestpractices, OPTIMISTIC, and SCOPE-DMD. Within the Second Health Programme, TREAT-NMD supports and provides exemplar information for the EUCERD Joint Action (2012-2015). It does this as part of the integration activities within the Joint Action. In addition, the TREAT-NMD Alliance contributes to the Horizon 2020 strategy through its activities and delivery of sustainable productivity and social cohesion for the NMD community.

The European Reference Networks (ERNs) are mandated in Directive 2011/24/EU (Directive on the application of patients' rights in cross-border healthcare). Their set up also acknowledges the unique potential of ERNs for the rare disease field. In this Directive, the European Commission (EC) pledges to "support the development of European Reference Networks between healthcare providers and Centres of Expertise in Member States, in particular in the area of rare diseases" (Article 12). It also dedicates a separate Article to rare diseases (Article 13). TREAT-NMD has developed strong collaborations across the neuromuscular community. It has engaged researchers and organisations worldwide, with its various tools, resources and infrastructure. TREAT-NMD is therefore in a strong position to provide a major contribution in the establishment of an ERN. It is an ERN that can integrate existing structures and participating health systems thus giving added value in the delivery of care to neuromuscular patients.[29]

Learning points

A global approach from both a research and care perspective is needed to address translational research and drug development for rare diseases. This is not only to drive international efforts towards the development of therapies. It also takes advantage of current best practice to prevent significant morbidity, avoidable premature mortality and to improve quality of life and socioeconomic potential. Substantial synergy can be won by tackling rare diseases in networks that harness the whole body of researchers, clinicians, and patient groups. Financing such

initiatives is a challenge. The TREAT-NMD network was fortunate in having funding via the FP6 funding programme. This
allowed it to put together a vital partnership of key opinion
leaders from academic institutions, patient organisations and
industry. They worked on establishing the key tools and resources of the network. Sustaining these tools and resources
currently relies on a patchwork of funding from grants, patient
organisations and other groups. There is potential for support
for some of these activities through the future European Reference Networks for rare diseases. This offers the chance of
new ways to remain sustainable. Key learning points from our
experience to date include:

1. Identify a clear and necessary aim for the consortium.
    It can diverge from this later if it grows and is success-
    ful, but it is good to demonstrate success in a defined
    area relatively early in order to gain traction.
2. At the very least, a network needs 'glue money' to stim-
    ulate communication and collaboration: Plan face to
    face meeting time as well as telephone and online com-
    munication.
3. A consortium needs to be truly multi-stakeholder:
    d. Engage the key opinion leaders in the field and en-
        sure that they have the resources to work towards
        the aims of the consortium.
    e. Ensure that patient organisations are central to the
        work of the consortium at all levels and that they
        are happy with the level of their involvement.
    f. Engage with industry and work with them to ensure
        that your aims are aligned.
    g. Establish a mechanism for communication with reg-
        ulatory authorities.
4. Establish a clear identity and strong web presence.

With these principles in mind, networking can provide a strong impetus to collaboration in rare disease drug
development.

References

1 Emery AE. Population frequencies of inherited neuromuscular diseases—a world survey. Neuromuscul Disord. 1991; 1(1):19-29.

2 Emery AE. The muscular dystrophies. Lancet. 2002 359(9307):687-695.

3 Bushby K. Neuromuscular diseases: milestones in development of treatments. Lancet Neurol. 2011 Jan; 10(1):11-3.

4 Bushby K, Lochmuller H, Lynn S, Straub V. Interventions for muscular dystrophy: molecular medicines entering the clinic. Lancet. 2009 Nov 28; 374(9704):1849-56.

5 Braun S. Gene-based therapies of neuromuscular disorders: an update and the pivotal role of patient organisations in their discovery and implementation. J Gene Med. 2013; 15:397-413.

6 Bushby K, Lynn S, Straub V. Collaborating to bring new therapies to the patient—the TREAT-NMD model. Acta Myol. 2009 Jul; 28(1):12-5.

7 Sejerson T, Bushby K. Standards of care for Duchenne muscular dystrophy: brief TREAT-NMD recommendations. Adv Exp Med Biol. 2009 65213-21.

8 Bushby K, Finkel R, Birnkrant DJ, Case LE, Clemens PR, Cripe L, Kaul A, Kinnett K, McDonald C, Pandya S, Poysky J, Shapiro F, Tomezsko J, Constantin C. Diagnosis and management of Duchenne muscular dystrophy, part 1: diagnosis, and pharmacological and psychosocial management. Lancet Neurol. 2010 Jan; 9(1):77-93.

9 Bushby K, Finkel R, Birnkrant DJ, Case LE, Clemens PR, Cripe L, Kaul A, Kinnett K, McDonald C, Pandya S, Poysky J, Shapiro F, Tomezsko J, Constantin C. Diagnosis and management of Duchenne muscular dystrophy, part 2: implementation of multidisciplinary care. Lancet Neurol. 2010

Feb; 9(2):177-89.

10 McCormack P, Woods S, Aartsma-Rus A, Hagger L, Herczegfalvi A, Heslop E, Irwin J, Kirschner J, Moeschen P, Muntoni F, Ouillade MC, Rahbek J, Rehmann-Sutter C, Rouault F, Sejersen T, Vroom E, Straub V, Bushby K, Ferlini A. Guidance in social and ethical issues related to clinical, diagnostic care and novel therapies for hereditary neuromuscular rare diseases: "translating" the translational. PLoS Curr. 2013 5.

11 Rodger S, Lochmuller H, Tassoni A, Gramsch K, Konig K, Bushby K, Straub V, Korinthenberg R, Kirschner J. The TREAT-NMD care and trial site registry: an online registry to facilitate clinical research for neuromuscular diseases. Orphanet J Rare Dis. 2013 8171.

12 Sarkozy A, Bushby K, Beroud C, Lochmuller H. 157th ENMC International Workshop: patient registries for rare, inherited muscular disorders 25-27 January 2008 Naarden, The Netherlands. Neuromuscul Disord. 2008 Dec; 18(12):997-1001.

13 Muntoni F, Bushby KD, van Ommen G. 149th ENMC International Workshop and 1st TREAT-NMD Workshop on: "planning phase i/ii clinical trials using systemically delivered antisense oligonucleotides in duchenne muscular dystrophy". Neuromuscul Disord. 2008 Mar; 18(3):268-75.

14 Mercuri E, Mayhew A, Muntoni F, Messina S, Straub V, Van Ommen GJ, Voit T, Bertini E, Bushby K. Towards harmonisation of outcome measures for DMD and SMA within TREAT-NMD; report of three expert workshops: TREAT-NMD/ENMC workshop on outcome measures, 12th—13th May 2007, Naarden, The Netherlands; TREAT-NMD workshop on outcome measures in experimental trials for DMD, 30th June—1st July 2007, Naarden, The Netherlands; conjoint Institute of Myology TREAT-NMD meeting on physical activity monitoring in neuromuscular disorders,

11th July 2007, Paris, France. Neuromuscul Disord. 2008 Nov; 18(11):894-903.

15 Bladen CL1, Salgado D, Monges S, Foncuberta ME, Kekou K, Kosma K, Dawkins H, Lamont L, Roy AJ, Chamova T, Guergueltcheva V, Chan S, Korngut L, Campbell C, Dai Y, Wang J, Barišiᵒ N, Brabec P, Lahdetie J, Walter MC, Schreiber-Katz O, Karcagi V, Garami M, Viswanathan V, Bayat F, Buccella F, Kimura E, Koeks Z, van den Bergen JC, Rodrigues M, Roxburgh R, Lusakowska A, Kostera-Pruszczyk A, Zimowski J, Santos R, Neagu E, Artemieva S, Rasic VM, Vojinovic D, Posada M, Bloetzer C, Jeannet PY, Joncourt F, Díaz-Manera J, Gallardo E, Karaduman AA, Topaloᵒlu H, Sherif RE, Stringer A, Shatillo AV, Martin AS, Peay HL, Bellgard MI, Kirschner J, Flanigan KM, Straub V, Bushby K, Verschuuren J, Aartsma-Rus A, Beroud C, Lochmüller H. The TREAT-NMD DMD Global database: Analysis of More Than 7000 Duchenne Muscular Dystrophy Mutations. Hum Mutat. 2015 Jan 21.

16 Landfeldt E, Lindgren P, Bell CF, Schmitt C, Guglieri M, Straub V, Lochmuller H, Bushby K. The burden of Duchenne muscular dystrophy: An international, cross-sectional study. Neurology. 2014 Jul 2.

17 Bladen CL, Rafferty K, Straub V, Monges S, Moresco A, Dawkins H, Roy A, Chamova T, Guergueltcheva V, Korngut L, Campbell C, Dai Y, Barisic N, Kos T, Brabec P, Rahbek J, Lahdetie J, Tuffery-Giraud S, Claustres M, Leturcq F, Ben Yaou R, Walter MC, Schreiber O, Karcagi V, Herczegfalvi A, Viswanathan V, Bayat F, de la Caridad Guerrero Sarmiento I, Ambrosini A, Ceradini F, Kimura E, van den Bergen JC, Rodrigues M, Roxburgh R, Lusakowska A, Oliveira J, Santos R, Neagu E, Butoianu N, Artemieva S, Rasic VM, Posada M, Palau F, Lindvall B, Bloetzer C, Karaduman A, Topaloglu H, Inal S, Oflazer P, Stringer A, Shatillo AV, Martin AS, Peay H, Flanigan KM, Salgado D, von Rekowski B, Lynn S, Heslop E, Gainotti S, Taruscio D, Kirschner

J, Verschuuren J, Bushby K, Beroud C, Lochmuller H. The TREAT-NMD Duchenne muscular dystrophy registries: conception, design, and utilization by industry and academia. Hum Mutat. 2013 Nov; 34(11):1449-57.

18 Bladen CL, Thompson R, Jackson JM, Garland C, Wegel C, Ambrosini A, Pisano P, Walter MC, Schreiber O, Lusakowska A, Jedrzejowska M, Kostera-Pruszczyk A, van der Pol L, Wadman RI, Gredal O, Karaduman A, Topaloglu H, Yilmaz O, Matyushenko V, Rasic VM, Kosac A, Karcagi V, Garami M, Herczegfalvi A, Monges S, Moresco A, Chertkoff L, Chamova T, Guergueltcheva V, Butoianu N, Craiu D, Korngut L, Campbell C, Haberlova J, Strenkova J, Alejandro M, Jimenez A, Ortiz GG, Enriquez GV, Rodrigues M, Roxburgh R, Dawkins H, Youngs L, Lahdetie J, Angelkova N, Saugier-Veber P, Cuisset JM, Bloetzer C, Jeannet PY, Klein A, Nascimento A, Tizzano E, Salgado D, Mercuri E, Sejersen T, Kirschner J, Rafferty K, Straub V, Bushby K, Verschuuren J, Beroud C, Lochmuller H. Mapping the differences in care for 5,000 spinal muscular atrophy patients, a survey of 24 national registries in North America, Australasia and Europe. J Neurol. 2014 Jan; 261(1):152-63.

19 Nagaraju K, Willmann R; TREAT-NMD Network and the Wellstone Muscular Dystrophy Cooperative Research Network. Developing standard procedures for murine and canine efficacy studies of DMD therapeutics: report of two expert workshops on "Pre-clinical testing for Duchenne dystrophy": Washington DC, October 27th-28th 2007 and Zürich, June 30th-July 1st 2008. Neuromuscul Disord. 2009 Jul;19(7):502-6.

20 Willmann R, Dubach J, Chen K; TREAT-NMD Neuromuscular Network. Developing standard procedures for pre-clinical efficacy studies in mouse models of spinal muscular atrophy: report of the expert workshop "Pre-clinical testing for SMA", Zürich, March 29-30th 2010. Neuromuscul Disord. 2011 Jan;21(1):74-7.

21 Willmann R, De Luca A, Benatar M, Grounds M, Dubach J, Raymackers JM, Nagaraju K; TREAT-NMD Neuromuscular Network. Enhancing translation: guidelines for standard pre-clinical experiments in mdx mice. Neuromuscul Disord. 2012 Jan;22(1):43-9.

22 Thompson R, Johnston L, Taruscio D, Monaco L, Beroud C, Gut IG, Hansson MG, t Hoen PB, Patrinos GP, Dawkins H, Ensini M, Zatloukal K, Koubi D, Heslop E, Paschall JE, Posada M, Robinson PN, Bushby K, Lochmuller H. RD-Connect: an integrated platform connecting databases, registries, biobanks and clinical bioinformatics for rare disease research. J Gen Intern Med. 2014 Aug; 29 Suppl 3S780-7.

23 Mora M, Angelini C, Bignami F, Bodin AM, Crimi M, Di Donato JH, Felice A, Jaeger C, Karcagi V, LeCam Y, Lynn S, Meznaric M, Moggio M, Monaco L, Politano L, de la Paz MP, Saker S, Schneiderat P, Ensini M, Garavaglia B, Gurwitz D, Johnson D, Muntoni F, Puymirat J, Reza M, Voit T, Baldo C, Bricarelli FD, Goldwurm S, Merla G, Pegoraro E, Renieri A, Zatloukal K, Filocamo M, Lochmüller H. The EuroBioBank Network: 10 years of hands-on experience of collaborative, transnational biobanking for rare diseases. Eur J Hum Genet. 2014 Dec 24.

24 Bushby K, Connor E. Clinical outcome measures for trials in Duchenne muscular dystrophy: report from International Working Group meetings. Clin Investig (Lond). 2011 Sep; 1(9):1217-35.

25 Aartsma-Rus A, Ferlini A, Goemans N, Pasmooij AM, Wells DJ, Bushby K, Vroom E, Balabanov P. Translational and regulatory challenges for exon skipping therapies. Hum Gene Ther. 2014 Oct; 25(10):885-92.

26 Lynn S, Aartsma-Rus A, Bushby K, Furlong P, Goemans N, De Luca A, Mayhew A, McDonald C, Mercuri E, Muntoni F, Pohlschmidt M, Verschuuren J, Voit T, Vroom E, Wells

DJ, Straub V. Measuring clinical effectiveness of medicinal products for the treatment of Duchenne muscular dystrophy. Neuromuscul Disord. 2014 Sep 11.

27 Heslop E, Csimma C, Straub V, McCall JM, Kanneboyina N, Wagner K, Caizergues D, Korinthenberg R, Flanigan K, Kaufmann P, McNeill E, Mendell J, Hesterlee S, Wells D, Bushby K. TREAT-NMD TACT: An innovative de-risking model to foster orphan drug development. Orphanet Journal of Rare Diseases. 2015 (in press).

28 Bushby K. The value of collaboration in improving knowledge on rare diseases. Can J Neurol Sci. 2011 May; 38(3):387.

29 Evangelista T, van Engelen B, Bushby K. 200th ENMC International Workshop "European reference networks: recommendations and criteria in the neuromuscular field", 18-20 October 2013, Naarden, The Netherlands. Neuromuscul Disord. 2014 Jun; 24(6):537-45.

Chapter 4

How to Promote Basic Research: An Excellent Model of the Human Disease

Craig M Keenan, Hazel Sutherland , Andrew J Preston, Peter J Wilson, George Bou-Gharios, Lakshminarayan R Ranganath, James A Gallagher
University of Liverpool

Jonathan C Jarvis
Liverpool John Moores University

The AKU Mouse

Alkaptonuria (AKU) is a good example of those many rare diseases in which the pathological mechanisms are not yet completely understood. This is even though the symptoms, genetic basis, and metabolic changes are well documented. The study of the disease in humans is limited because it requires harvesting and analysis of tissue samples. However, the only tissues are those that become available at joint replacement or other surgery, when the disease is very advanced. An animal model is therefore highly valuable if it shows the same pathological mechanism as the human disease. If the alteration in metabolism is genuinely similar in an animal model, then such models are also helpful in developing and testing new therapies.

The laws concerning the use of animals in medical research are governed by the following principle: The potential benefits must be weighed against the potential cost to the animals' welfare. The ideal animal model of a human disease is therefore one which has the same mechanism that causes pain and distress in human sufferers, but where the animals do not suffer painful or debilitating symptoms.

The alkaptonuric mouse is an example of such a model (Figure 1).

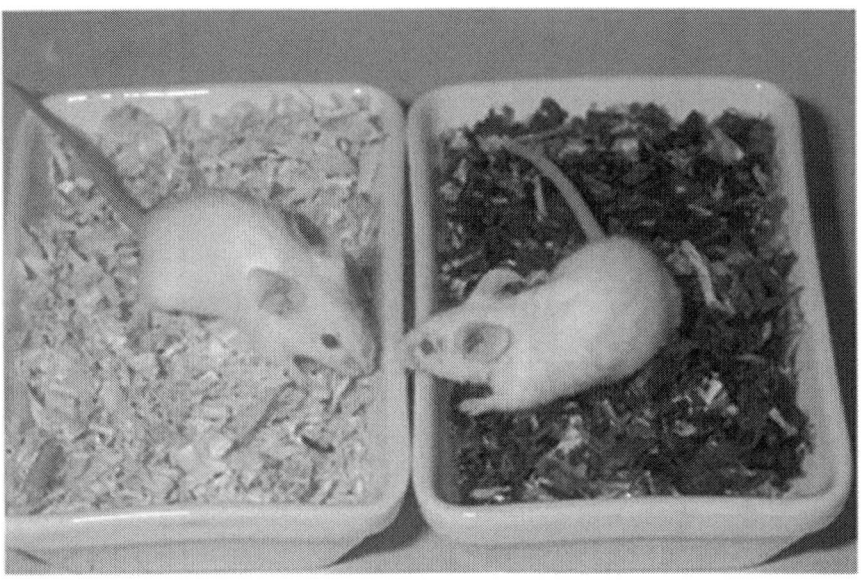

Figure 1. The photograph shows a wildtype (unaffected) mouse on the left and an AKU mouse on the right. AKU mice can be easily identified by darkened bedding resulting from high levels of HGA in their urine. Darkening of urine is a characteristic sign of AKU in humans. Picture used with the permission of Dr Jean Louis Guenet.

Moran and colleagues made an early attempt to induce AKU in an animal model.[1] They injected homogentisic acid (HGA) into rabbits over a period of 5 days. Animals which had HGA injected into their joints (intra-articular) showed a darkening of their urine and developed joint damage. Animals which had HGA injected into the peritoneum (the abdomen) or into their veins did not show any signs of the classical colouring of tissues (known as ochronosis) seen in AKU patients. This model was not suitable for larger scale studies on AKU, because the animals did not have the genetic mutation leading to AKU. However it did show the damaging effects of HGA, particularly when applied close to the cartilage coating the joints (known as articular cartilage). Another attempt to cause ochronosis in animals was made by Blivaiss *et al*, by feeding rats a diet of 8% L-tyrosine for at least 9 months.[2] The study appeared to show that a diet high in tyrosine led to the development of ochronosis and osteoarthropathy (damage to the bones and joints). Again, like the rabbit model of ochronosis, the rat model was unsuitable for long terms studies on AKU, due to the way the ochronosis was induced.

The first murine (mouse) model of AKU was created by Montagutelli and colleagues at the Pasteur Institute, Paris.[3] Eight week old mice, from an inbred stock carrying seven recessive mutations, were given a single injection of ethylnitrosourea to cause mutation. Diagnosis of AKU in the mice was confirmed by darkening of the urine when pipetted onto filter paper soaked with 0.5M sodium hydroxide. Mice with the AKU mutation (Hgd-/-) were backcrossed with mice that had BALB/cByJ and C57/BL/6J backgrounds. Although Hgd-/- mice excreted high levels of HGA in their urine, histological studies showed no signs of ochronosis in any of the tissues examined (knee, hip, ankle, spine, liver, kidneys and tail) at 18 months of age.[3] One hypothesis to explain this was that natural production of vitamin C (ascorbic acid) in the mice acted as an antioxidant, preventing ochronosis.[3] Other theories were suggested for the absence of pigmentation. These included: a better kidney function in the mice, which might prevent the build-up of HGA in plasma, due to passing high volumes of urine; and low mechanical loading of joints, because of the low mass of the mice and the sharing of weight over four limbs.

Manning and colleagues developed a modified mouse model of AKU.[4] They were working with mice which contained the tyrosinemia type 1 (HT1) mutation (FAH-/-). The FAH-/- mice were crossed with mice carrying the AKU mutation (Hgd-/- mice, see above) for several generations. Mice containing one normal and one mutant Hgd (Hgd+/-), but the full FAH-/- mutation, normally have to be treated with nitisinone from birth, to prevent the development of HT1. However, Manning and co-workers found that some mice survived if the nitisinone was removed. This was due to a spontaneous mutation which resulted in some of their liver cells having two copies of the mutant Hgd gene, resulting in mice with a Hgd-/-, FAH-/- genotype. In effect development of AKU rescued the mice from HT1. Careful examination subsequently revealed signs of ochronosis in the knees and kidneys.[5] However it was not seen as a practical model of AKU as the development of ochronosis was caused by a spontaneous and therefore unpredictable mutation and clonal growth of the mutant liver cells. Furthermore, the mutation was also associated with severe kidney damage. To fully understand the manner and development of AKU, a mouse model that replicated the natural history and pathology of AKU in humans was required.

Recent research by Tinti *et al*, showed that you could identify even low levels of ochronotic pigment in tissues by using Schmorl's stain.[6] By carefully studying AKU (Hgd-/-) mouse tissues treated with Schmorl's stain under the microscope, it was possible for the first time to detect the presence of ochronotic pigment (Figure 2).[7] The importance of observing ochronosis in mice with the same genetic mutation as AKU patients should not be underestimated. For the first time it provided an insight into the pathogenesis of AKU throughout the entire lifespan. The deposition of ochronotic pigment could be detected very early on in life, and followed as it became progressively worse with increasing age. The progression of ochronotic pigment deposition in AKU mice appeared very similar to that previously described in human AKU tissue.[8] Once pigmentation had reached a certain stage, osteoarthritic changes in the knee joint were also noticeable. These were also very similar to the AKU phenotype observed in humans. The mechanistic link between pigmentation and osteoarthritis is, however, still not fully understood and further studies are required in this model. The appearance of ochronosis, and the associated osteoarthritic changes, in AKU mice further highlighted the similarities in disease between the mouse and human model of AKU. The discovery of ochronosis in Hgd-/- mice is important. It provides a robust model in which to evaluate new novel therapies for the treatment of AKU while also providing a new model of experimental osteoarthritis.

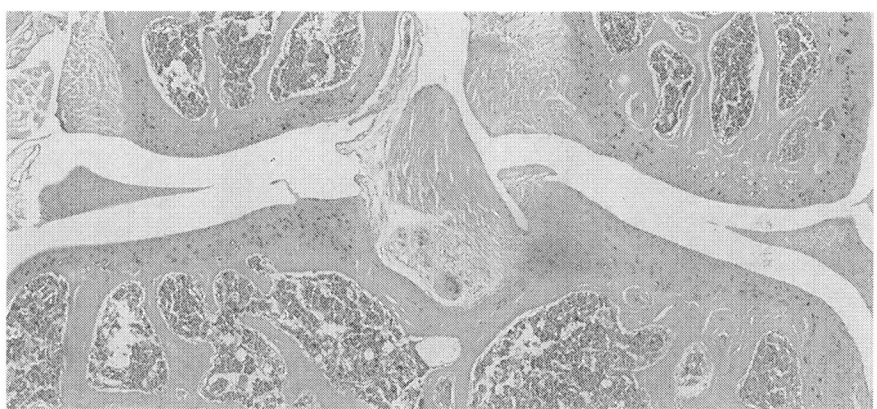

Figure 2. A panoramic photomicrograph of an aged AKU mouse showing extensive ochronotic pigmentation throughout the knee joint. Each individual blue dot represents a pigmented cell.

There are no practical treatment options currently available to AKU sufferers. As a result, AKU patients suffer severe pain prior to joint replacement surgery. The identification of ochronosis in AKU mice has provided a robust model in which to test therapeutics to treat AKU. Nitisinone was originally developed as a herbicide and subsequently used in the treatment of HT1. Nitisinone acts on the tyrosine catabolic pathway and has been a major success in alleviating the fatal effects of HT1.[9] Nitisinone can also prevent the formation of HGA through inhibition of a key enzyme involved in AKU.

Following the identification of ochronosis in AKU mice, nitisinone was administered to the mice to determine its efficacy in treating AKU. Two studies were undertaken in which nitisinone was administered to AKU mice. Treatment was either over their lifetime or starting at mid-life, when ochronosis was known to be established. Lifetime treatment with nitisinone was shown to prevent any pigment deposition in the mice. This was the first time that nitisinone had been shown to prevent ochronosis. There was no evidence from the mid-life intervention study that nitisinone therapy could reverse previously laid down pigment, however it did prevent any further deposition of pigment. Thus it might prevent or slow down progression of the disease in patients with established ochronosis.[10] The results collected from the studies clearly showed that nitisinone is an effective treatment for AKU, and provides real hope for both young and elderly AKU patients alike.

Induced random point mutations, such as in the AKU mouse, can be very useful as we have described. However, their discovery requires the laborious process of screening and selecting for interesting phenotypes. Furthermore, the mutation that confers analogy with a human disease may be accompanied by additional mutations. They may also influence the similarity between the mouse mutant and the human condition. Developments in genetics mean that it is now possible to create models of human and animal disease by targeted editing of the genetic sequence. Animal models can be generated which mirror the human specific mutations as closely as possible.

These genetically engineered mouse models will be immensely valuable for testing new therapies that may be transferred directly to humans. For example, in AKU there are many different disease-causing mutations in the Hgd gene. It is likely that one type of therapy will not work for all patients, it will depend on which mutations they carry. Therefore, having the technology to recreate the human mutations in animals is a roadmap for effective, personalised medicine in rare diseases governed by one gene.

Every research team that wishes to make use of an animal model of their disease of interest must negotiate some practical challenges. First, use of animals is subject to ethical approval and licensing processes. In the UK, for example:

- All researchers must demonstrate an understanding of the relevant law.
- They must show practical competence and be trained in animal husbandry and welfare relating to the relevant species.
- The principal investigator will be required to seek specific permission with scientific justification for every proposed experimental procedure. This is a significant task.

Last but not least, the breeding and maintenance of animals in specialist facilities is expensive.

However, without access to a practical mouse model of AKU; one which shows very similar pathogenesis to AKU observed in humans, it would not have been possible to demonstrate the beneficial effects nitisinone therapy can provide. It is essential that animal models of disease are produced and closely studied. They provide answers to questions which otherwise cannot be answered. This is particularly evident in the case of AKU where the progress that has been made simply would not have been possible without the use of the mouse model.

Finally, what are the practical lessons that can be learnt from the progress made in AKU research for other groups striving to promote research on rare diseases? Aside from the major hurdle of raising funds for research, it is important early on to develop links with scientists who are interested in researching their disease. The best way to find potential scientific partners is to use a combination of general search engines, such as Google, and academic search engines, particularly PubMed (http://www.ncbi. nlm.nih.gov/pubmed). PubMed is a free service maintained by the National Institutes of Health. With these tools it should be possible to identify existing and potential researchers in the relevant disease area.

Once potential partnerships with researchers have been established, the next step is to consider the proposed experimental approaches. As outlined in this chapter, good animal models can make a major contribution to understanding disease mechanisms and to developing effective therapies. There are many online resources that can be used to identify whether appropriate animal models already exist, as listed below:-

- http://www.har.mrc.ac.uk/
- http://jaxmice.jax.org/index.html
- http://www.nih.gov/science/models/mouse/deltagen-lexicon/list.html
- http://www.taconic.com/find-your-model/gems/knock-out-repository
- http://www.tigm.org/
- http://www.mousephenotype.org/martsearch_ikmc_project/about/eucomm

Some organisations encourage the sharing of tissues from animal models. For example ShARM is a not for profit organisation, open to scientific investigators, aiming to accelerate research into ageing by facilitating the sharing of resources. ShARM provides cost effective access to aged mouse models and their tissue through a biorepository and database of live ageing colonies. ShARM also promotes the networking of researchers and the dissemination of knowledge through its online collaborative environment: MICEspace (http://www.sharmuk.org).

There are also excellent online resources that provide advice on the welfare and regulatory aspects of animal experiments:

- http://www.rspca.org.uk/adviceandwelfare/laboratory
- https://www.gov.uk/research-and-testing-using-animals

We are fortunate enough to work in the UK, where there is robust (and time-consuming) statutory regulation of work on animal models. There is also a wealth of expertise in animal husbandry and good animal science that is easy to access for groups wanting to investigate mechanisms in rare diseases.

Acknowledgements

We would like to thank Dr Jean Louis Guenet for allowing us to use the image featured in Figure 1 and Jane Dillon for advice on the manuscript.

Contacts

Craig M Keenan, Hazel Sutherland, Jonathan C Jarvis: School of Sport and Exercise Sciences, Liverpool John Moores University, Tom Reilly Building, Byrom Street, Liverpool, L3 3AF, UK.

Hazel Sutherland, Peter J Wilson, George Bou-Gharios, Lakshminarayan R Ranganath and James A Gallagher: Department of Musculoskeletal Biology, Institute of Ageing and Chronic Disease, University of Liverpool, Sherrington Buildings, Ashton Street, Liverpool, L69 3GE, UK.

Andrew J Preston: Developmental Immunology, Paediatrics, Weatherall Institute of Molecular Medicine, University of Oxford, John Radcliffe Hospital, Oxford, OX3 9DS, UK.

Lakshminarayan R Ranganath: Department of Clinical Biochemistry and Metabolism, Royal Liverpool University Hospital, Prescot Street, Liverpool, L7 8XP, UK.

References

1 Moran TJ, Yunis EJ: Studies on ochronosis. 2. Effects of injection of homogentisic acid and ochronotic pigment in experimental animals. The American Journal of Pathology 1962, 40:359-369.

2 Blivaiss BB, Rosenberg EF, Kutuzov H et al: Experimental ochronosis. Induction in rats by long-term feeding with L-tyrosine. Archives of Pathology 1966, 82(1):45-53.

3 Montagutelli X, Lalouette A, Coude M et al: aku, a mu-

tation of the mouse homologous to human alkaptonuria, maps to chromosome 16. Genomics 1994, 19(1):9-11.

4 Manning K, Al-Dhalimy M, Finegold M et al: In vivo suppressor mutations correct a murine model of hereditary tyrosinemia type I. Proceedings of the National Academy of Sciences of the United States of America 1999, 96(21):11928-11933.

5 Taylor AM, Preston AJ, Paulk NK et al: Ochronosis in a murine model of alkaptonuria is synonymous to that in the human condition. Osteoarthritis & Cartilage 2012, 20(8):880-886.

6 Tinti L, Taylor AM, Santucci A et al: Development of an in vitro model to investigate joint ochronosis in alkaptonuria. Rheumatology 2011, 50(2):271-277.

7 Preston AJ, Keenan CM, Sutherland H et al: Ochronotic osteoarthropathy in a mouse model of alkaptonuria, and its inhibition by nitisinone. Annals of the Rheumatic Diseases 2014, 73(1):284-289.

8 Taylor AM, Boyde A, Wilson PJ et al: The role of calcified cartilage and subchondral bone in the initiation and progression of ochronotic arthropathy in alkaptonuria. Arthritis & Rheumatism 2011, 63(12):3887-3896.

9 McKiernan PJ: Nitisinone in the treatment of hereditary tyrosinaemia type 1. Drugs 2006, 66(6):743-750.

10 Keenan CM, Preston AJ, Sutherland H et al: Nitisinone arrests but does not reverse ochronosis in alkaptonuric mice. Journal of Inherited Metabolic Disease Reports 2015. 437:1-6.

Chapter 5

How to Engage with Academia for Drug Discovery: An Academic's Perspective

Anil Mehta
University of Dundee

Introduction

What is the nature of the problem? Let us suppose you or your child, your friend or your relative has a rare disease, and you want to help. The agencies you need to think about are Government/Health systems, patient organisations dedicated to the disease and researchers in pharmaceutical companies or scientists and doctors in university or research institutes, who are funded to discover cures. Many such diseases may be inherited and over 80% of all rare diseases fall into this category; the rest are acquired from external agencies such as viruses or, have a genetic propensity that remains unknown. Usually it is a combination of factors. To cope with this variation and uncertainty, the UK government is undertaking a multimillion pound experiment – the 100,000 genomes project – as a pilot to find out whether sequencing the DNA of those without a gene diagnosis will be helpful or not.[1] The interpretation of the results requires an interaction with universities and industry as follows:

The technology needed to 'discover the mutation' in the normal DNA code of a given patient is not as simple as it seems for the following reasons:

- The method used has to be reliable; many such methods exist.

- When repeated sampling is undertaken at different hospitals/universities/industrial sites with different technologies, the DNA results should not change.
- The computer code used to analyse the billions of bits of DNA data (algorithm) must be robust (must give the same answer at different sites).
- Defining what is normal is a big task, because we are all different as we look at our own 'normal' codes, which change roughly every 300 DNA base pairs as we walk along the DNA. These are called single nucleotide polymorphisms (SNPs).
- What happens if an accidental (incidental) finding of a potentially damaging, 'high risk' mutant gene, unrelated to the rare disease, is discovered when looking for the rare disease causing gene? In some countries it is forbidden to disclose this incidental discovery, in others it is mandatory!

The UK pilot will address these issues through interactions with many universities working as a consortium.

What Happens in Practice

Architects' Plans and Genetic Mutations: Imagine that the rare disease has a genetic basis, a diagnosis is made, and when sequenced, a genetic mutation has been independently confirmed by at least two technologies. This is not as big an advance as first appears, because a mutant gene does not exist in isolation. It is part of a network of other genes and their encoded proteins. Imagine an architect's design board, say a school. Is it part of a community? Who goes there? When is it open? What subjects are taught? What is the focus; academic subjects or sports, or both? Which teachers teach there? How well trained are they? Is there a sports field on site or is travel needed? *Defective genes are only the architect's drawing of the school – not the functioning school or community*. It is the outputs from the school – the quality of its graduates – that is the key. Genes and their mutations do not measure outputs, they are only plans not actions. For the real school, the design must cope with the fact that many hundreds of pupils go in and as many go out. So, if one child interacts with the school differently, is it the building or the child or both that causes the problem? In the cell, the proteins coded for by these 'diseased' genes are not just objects on a drawing, they are the real school and its pupils, constructed not with bricks and mortar, but with proteins, sugars and fat (just like a cake). These gene encoded proteins lie in networks and in the rare disease, something is very wrong with a key point in the school's essential functions, its pupils and its teachers etc... or, in cake terms, a key ingredient is too old, making the taste very poor. For example, in the genetic disease cystic fibrosis (CF), it is common for the same mutation in the causal gene to produce different disease severity even amongst siblings from the same family. The genetic defect is like repeatedly dropping a stone into a pond, but the effect of the ripples on the pond life differs between ponds.

Why should anyone help me? Universities have staff that can only focus on one or more nodes in such networks. Because they are mostly scientists, they do not know about your disease for the most part, but they are likely to help if they can use the defect to understand their network dysfunction. Unfortunately, the node experts, who have dedicated many years of their lives to the discovery of their nodes (control points) in such protein networks linked to the gene of interest, may not be willing to engage with the person who has a particular rare disease that is located within such a network. It is vital to remember that they are very unlikely to be medical doctors at all. Each node expert has become an expert not by chance, but by focussing on a process (PhD and beyond) and during that intellectual route to discovery (curiosity driven science, 'post-doctoral studies') they have become one of only a few experts in that process (principal investigators, PI). *They publish or they perish and they are very often starved of resources.*

How should I approach such node experts? The key to engagement with such communities of PI node experts is to understand their motivation – survival against their peers; very Darwinian – because money is limited and they only survive by grants. The reality is, that the university provides all or some of their salary to teach and they do their research using external grants. They need money to understand their pathways; never forget that they have their own career aspirations, and you need a cure. *These are very different needs and can cause much misunderstanding. The goal is to create an alliance, thereby creating a win-win playing field as a key to success.* This 'transformational approach' requires the rare disease patient to engage someone with the patient skills (doctor), who also has the science skills (academic, PhD etc). Since it takes 20 years to acquire both sets of skills, such people are scarce and very busy doing teaching, research and seeing patients. Not every country trains such people, they are common in some and absent in others.

Step 1: You need help and a very recently retired person is a very good choice as your advocate, and it does not matter that they have worked in an unrelated area of science for the skills are generic, independent of whether they are cell biologists or engineers or from other sciences. They should ideally have chaired groups of scientists in other fields and should be willing to dedicate significant time to the work.

Step 2: Thus a good place to start is to raise the funds to support the travel costs of such a person for a meeting and then to establish an electronic e-meeting schedule via the internet for a small fee (Skype, myglobalconference, others that might be free from larger suppliers of internet services).

Step 3: Existing communities of scientists within the EURORDIS, or other groupings such as Findacure, can be useful sources of advice, such as Adam Jolly's publication 'Working with Universities.[2] In chapter 6, Jolly advises that *specifying the question* is the key to getting the answer you need and that requires project management skills.

- In essence you need to undertake a systems analysis of the problem (computer scientists and logistic experts) but the role is best undertaken by a logical, ordered individual who can break down the key issues into component parts. This type of person may be costly, but they are cost-effective. Ideally, they will need a life science skill (biochemistry, molecular biology, physiology etc and a PhD/Masters is always a good start, but a degree in another discipline such as philosophy or logistics is also an excellent choice. Precision thinking is key.
- The key skill is framing the question, not the technical details.
- The first task is to ask such a person to undertake a *literature search* asking what is known about the network of genes and or proteins and or fats and or sugars controlled by the gene in question. This is the cake mix question – what is the composition of the cake? Has the cake been the same for millions of years? If it has, the approach will be very different because of something called tractability, where simple organisms such as yeasts can be used to find out which network the mutation belongs to.
- The next question is how to summarise the parts and bring them into a common theme. This essential step requires attendance at the nearest conference on the network components, where the node experts often meet up and create societies. These are very useful.
- Getting access to funds from those seeking to translate science to better treatment is an essential step and regional governments often have support networks to support such schemes with small sums. Finding a company with related products used in different parts of the network is also a useful approach, especially if they can partner the university.
- The good news is, that universities are now much better at engaging with communities to perform their charita-

ble roles according to their charters. The bad news is, that the costs are very high to do the groundwork.

Hurdles to be overcome

1. Academic priorities are a fact of life (publish, get grants, supervise students, or perish) but choosing the right network of academics (and funding them) is *insufficient for success.*
2. Tight project management is the key.
3. Milestones, and paying in arrears on those milestones is a tough discipline that will pay dividends.
4. This requires a match between the academic, your specification of the question, the university's need for funding that is realistic, within the aims, tied to deadlines and regular project plan meetings in place. The UK voice of manufacturing illustrates the problems with collaborating successfully: In 'New light on innovation' (Adam Jolly, 2011: Chapter 7),2 they advise: find the right partner (marriage); understand your own business (personality; you will not get a cure easily, but disease-arrest may be possible); manage the costs (bi-directional solvency: universities do not have reserves to bail you out and will likely sue for non-payment); manage the relationship (who is the go-between?); imagine what happens to new ideas and ask yourself: Who owns them? The key is the contract between parties – what happens if your funding source dries up? What is the exit strategy for both parties?

Getting started

Expert finding is usually simple via a general search engine, but often the specialist Public Library of Medicine directory of scientific peer-reviewed publications is a good 'no-cost' place to start.[3] The problem is that you may need to pay for access to many of the papers in the directory (this is how the journal publisher makes a profit) and, to make things worse, when downloaded, they are usually difficult to interpret. Hence, the search terms need to be carefully refined to add reviews of the field of the science to the search list. A local university library is a good place to refine the search, as their staff are used to helping students with literature review problems. **Searching international conferences on the topic is a very good idea and attending such conferences is the best approach.** It is as much about who you know as what you know.

However, before embarking on this route, getting up to speed through a good high school text book on bio-science will help. Learning a little cell biology (how a cell works), biochemistry (what it is made of), physiology (how it talks to the body and other cells) and pharmacology (how drugs act on cells and how cells act on drugs) pays dividends.

If the disease is genetic, then jargon words such as stop codon, splice variant, open reading frame, nonsense mutant, in frame deletion, enhancer, silencer and tissue specific knockout are important to master as short-hand that scientists use to communicate with each other, making lay comprehension very difficult.

As a young doctor, learning science, this author spent six months on the basic science vocabulary during his Master's programme and many thousands of words are needed for a full grasp (I am still learning; microRNA did not exist in my day). For example, before such deep neo-word acquisition, Vitamin D just meant rickets to me, even after Med School; but after reading some cell biology, I was able to group this vitamin into an über-group classified by actions that related to its peer group of look alikes. When my wife became Vit D deficient, I wondered what type of structure this molecule was attached to in the cell. Pubmed showed me that it controlled blood clotting, bruising, the immune system and many other processes by binding to DNA at something called an open reading frame to help unzip DNA. This explained why she had suddenly bruised so easily, having never done so before. When deficient, my new understanding of this rare vitamin disease was that the children's bone disease rickets was just the extreme manifestation of one role that this steroid like molecule undertakes (tip of the iceberg; fundamental disease or sentinel disease). Thus, my new reading showed that in each cell of the body, Vitamin D controls around 200 genes – a true 'power steroid'. Further searching showed that a very rare genetic disease exists that stops the body from processing and then synthesising the highly active form of the vitamin (the natural form found in egg yolks for example is not very potent). It means that patients have a dud form of the vitamin and interestingly, most with this very rare condition have a high incidence of multiple sclerosis. Thus a rare disease informs a common disease, just as cystic fibrosis informs us how cigarettes cause lung damage. But care is needed, carrying matches is linked to lung cancer, but is not causal. Accidental associations (as coined by Aristotle) are called confounders and they complicate interpretation.

How should we think about diseases and working with universities? Let us suppose that a rare genetic disease is present and the mutation is known in the DNA. This usually means that the malfunctioning DNA miscodes for a mutant protein that is abnormal in some cell-toxic way, and the nature of the DNA defect determines the strategy, that in turn directs the manner of the proposed 'work-around' therapy. The key issue is that the normal versions of such proteins normally work in groups (networks) and the disease in the patient is a manifestation of network dysfunction. This has many implications for working with universities and the commonly held assumption is, that there is a 'single defect' in the protein that is wrong. Proteins have many roles that depend on the cell context. Many defects can occur if the protein is missing (it may not be made at all and the baby can only survive by accessing a bypass in the network), or the protein may be made in a toxic way (preventing the network from using its normal route) and combinations of these processes commonly occur. These issues colour the interaction with universities. Nothing happens quickly; it can take 20 years to get to an answer as to whether a cure is possible.

Worked Example and Conclusions

If a small molecule therapy is found, the next problem is making the molecule to pharmaceutical standards. This task is not trivial as kilos of the drug need to be made. This requires a close interaction with an academic led Pharma group in the first instance. For example, in our recent paper, my collaborators from Italy and France and I report preliminary data on a potential therapy for cystic fibrosis developed purely by academics (de Stefano et al. 2014)[4]. This has taken over 100 years of combined investigator effort to discard defunct hypotheses and find two chemicals from millions that might be useful. The path to that discovery is long and complex. It involves five different disciplines (Physics, Maths, Biology, Chemistry and Medicine) all working in a consortium without preconceived notions. This required tight hypotheses, a lot of luck, much 'chance favouring the prepared mind' and people with the disease raising millions. It all began with a barn dance in Forfar Scotland, by one mother and father who raised £3000 for the author in 1995. Now we have a candidate therapy in 2015. Persistence, patience, passion and people are the key.

Good luck with your journey.

References

1 The 100,000 Genomes Project FAQs. 2015. Genomics England Ltd (Accessed 10 July 2015). http://www.genomicsengland.co.uk/the-100000-genomes-project/faqs/.

2 Jolly, A. 2013 Working with Universities. 2nd edition. Crimson Publishing. (ISBN9781780591346).

3 Pubmed. National Center for Biotechnology Information. US National Library of Medicine. (Accessed July 2015). http://www.ncbi.nlm.nih.gov/pubmed.

4 de Stefano, D. et al. 2014. Restoration of CFTR function in patients with cystic fibrosis carrying the F508del-CFTR mutation. Autophagy. 2014; 10(11):2053-74. doi: 10.4161/15548627.2014.973737.

Chapter 6

How to Engage with Industry

Dr Mark Edwards
Ethical Medicines Industry Group

Introduction

This is not an easy chapter to write! NHS, industry and patient groups often find it difficult to work together because they assume they should be and have not asked the fundamental questions:

- Should we be working together?
- If so, why?

Asking these questions will help those involved to identify what they could do together for patient or mutual benefit. Do not forget, we either are a patient, or are closely related to one.

I believe that while there are many benefits for patient groups, charities and the industry to work together in a more cohesive way, there is no single script or set of instructions to tell you how to do it! Neither is it possible to write one. What I do know however, is that effective collaborations ie. those that produce high value outcomes for everyone involved, are the result of true partnerships that have been built with time, and the development of trust between all parties. There should be only one, transparent agenda. In turn, what is critical to the establishment of these strong foundations is, firstly, to take due time to understand your 'could be' partners; in terms of who they are, what they do, how they do it and why. The 'why' (above) critically involves getting to a collective understanding of each other's drivers and constraints. If this understanding can be achieved, then the common ground, the common cause and the shared goals will be identified and agreed. Everything else stems from this.

Much of this chapter will focus on providing a high level 'what, why and how' of the industry.

What is 'The Industry'?

First of all, what constitutes 'the industry'? Fundamental to the Life Sciences Industry is the application of biology. It comprises a highly diverse set of commercial organisations whose work covers, broadly, medical devices, medical diagnostics and pharmaceuticals. Similar to the mistake that is often made when thinking about the NHS in England as being a single organisation, when it is, in fact, a federation of several thousand independently-operating organisations, it is also incorrect to regard 'the industry' as a single entity. Even within one of its three broad domains there are many different types of company. They vary greatly in size, degree of establishment, business model, areas of specialty and operation, to name but a few differentiating factors. While this adds to the complexity of engagement, there is one inescapable and unifying factor; they are all commercial organisations, which need to make a return on their investment. They are not charities and they are not universities. This is not 'bad' however. Wealth creation, after all, is job creation and as it is the pharmaceutical sector of this commercially-based industry, in which, I've spent most of my career as a research doctor, this is the sector whose work I will focus on. First and foremost, it should be noted that without the pharmaceutical industry, over 90% of the world's medicines in use today would not have been invented.

A brief history of the pharmaceutical industry

The foundations of what is today's modern pharmaceutical industry were laid in the late 19th and early 20th centuries. Many, like my industrial '*alma mater*', Pfizer, started out as chemical companies. Pfizer's founders were cousins and German émigrés to the United States; Charles Pfizer and Charles Erhardt. One was a chemist, the other a confectioner. Their first piece of intellectual property (IP) centred on how to sugar-coat bitter-tasting medicines! Pfizer's first 'big product' was citric acid, which it was able to produce on a commercial scale due to its investment in the technology for the 'deep fermentation' of molasses. This investment then had hugely relevant human application following the discovery of the anti-microbial properties of penicillin. This required the deep fermentation technology to enable its mass production, which of course was life-saving during the Second World War. Pfizer's leadership in this area then enabled the company to innovate in other anti-infective areas after the war, firstly to develop a new class of antibiotics, the tetracyclines. For many decades afterwards, Pfizer continued to invest and innovate in this area, with major medicines such as the anti-fungal agent, fluconazole , being approved for human use in the 1980s and voriconazole for deep-seated (eg. cerebral), life-threatening fungal infections similarly in the Noughties.[1]

Incidentally, with reference to penicillin; what was most important, its discovery per se, or the discovery of what it could be used for in humans? Both are important of course, but while 3 scientists shared the Nobel Prize for its discovery, history generally only remembers the work of Alexander Fleming. He discovered the in-vitro antimicrobial properties of penicillin in 1930. But, it was a decade later that a collaboration between Ernst Chain and Howard Florey led to the first human clinical trials of penicillin which showed its therapeutic application. This was real 'translational research' in action – a term much highlighted in importance today, and quite rightly so, but in fact something that has been around for a long time![2]

The Pfizer story illustrates a few pertinent facts about the operation of the industry – eg. investment in research, need for appropriate IP cover to protect your inventions, the importance of 'institutional memory' to enable future discoveries and that much value-added innovation is the result of incremental (step-wise) improvement over what's gone before. Many other long-established pharmaceutical firms have followed a similar evolutionary course.

The industry really began to develop at 'full throttle' in the 1950s, due to the introduction of 'systems' approaches to drug discovery and development, coupled with an ever-increasing understanding of biology and the introduction of better manufacturing techniques.

Many new drugs were discovered, developed, manufactured and marketed during this time. They included the first oral contraceptive pill, corticosteroids, anti-hypertensives, anti-depressants, minor and major tranquillizers. Examples of these medicines are still in use today. Knowing what we know now however, I suspect that if some were investigational medicines today, especially those that helped introduce the era of psychiatric medicine 'for all', such as diazepam (Valium), they would not be approved for use by the regulatory authorities They might, instead, be licensed for use in highly restricted clinical indications. With Valium and medicines like it (the benzodiazepine class), the issue has been the recognition with time of the significant levels of dependency and habituation associated with its use. I mention this only to highlight the fact that all medicines can be poisons, but, unlike outright poisons they also have a therapeutic benefit. Determining the ratio of a medicine's 'benefit' to 'risk' is a cornerstone of good therapeutic development, but it's a fact that the true nature and indeed scope of this ratio can often only be established after many years of 'real world' use. For example, it is often said that aspirin would never be approved for use as a painkiller if it were an investigational drug today. This is probably correct, given its propensity to cause bleeding if used chronically at 'painkiller dose' and also the fact that one dose pretty much anti-coagulates you (in terms of stopping platelet aggregation) for about a week. However, in recent years, the benefits of aspirin's anti-platelet action have been recognised and, now, much lower doses than those to treat a headache are frequently used as a means to prevent strokes and heart attacks in patients who are at risk. So, if it were an investigational medicine today, it would probably have a very different regulatory indication!

The other issue that the Valium example highlights and which remains as an 'elephant in the room' today, is the tension that exists between the pharmaceutical industry and many parts of society that simply don't believe that profit should be made out of medicines. Excessively aggressive sales and marketing practices, being 'only about the profit' and accusations of bribery and corruption are rife amongst industry's detractors. Do they have a point? Yes, in part. Spurred on by, for example, the craze for benzodiazepines as an apparent cure for the stresses of modern life, the market knew no bounds. Put clever human beings in an environment where commercial know-how and advances in 'underpinning' scientific understanding of disease can maximise monetary return, then, in some circumstances we do risk catastrophe and that is something that all of us engaged in the life sciences should strive to avoid.

Yet, in the sections that follow, I shall attempt to describe why it is currently only a commercially based industry that can invent the medicines of today and tomorrow in large and consistent number. As such, is it not right, just as it is for any other commercial industry, for the inventors to be able to market their products and achieve a return on investment? I believe yes, most definitely. But, doing this fairly, morally and in a manner that safeguards (as far as is possible) patient safety is what is critical.

It is for these reasons that the modern pharmaceutical industry has become one of the most highly regulated industries in the world, and I would suggest quite rightly so. Regulatory legislation of some type has been present since the foundation of the very first firms, but has hugely intensified since the 1960s, especially when the thalidomide tragedy came to light. Here, the use of this new anti-emetic in pregnant women caused severe birth defects. This extremely sad happening put the foundations in place for what are now the modern world-wide regulatory systems for the approval of research involving investigational new drugs, their subsequent review, approval for use in patients and post-marketing surveillance.

In 1964, the World Medical Association issued the Declaration of Helsinki,[3] which sets standards for clinical research and demanded that subjects give their informed consent before enrolling in an experiment. Subsequent amendments and 'evolutions' of the Declaration included the introduction of ethics committees in 1975, the World Health Organisation's 'international ethical guidelines for biomedical research involving human subjects' in 1982 and perhaps, most significantly, the formation in 1990 of the 'International Congress on Harmonisation'. This on-going project brings together the major regulatory agencies (US, Europe, Japan) and representatives of the pharmaceutical industry to discuss the key scientific and technical aspects of pharmaceutical product development and registration. Within its outputs, 'ICH Good Clinical Practice (GCP)' is now the accepted set of standards worldwide for the design, conduct and reporting of clinical research in humans.

It is perhaps interesting to note that, in terms of processes and standards, what most of us now take as 'given' for ethical drug development, has not in fact been around for that long!

Perhaps penned back by the safety concerns emanating in the 1960s, the industry overall, did not expand again quickly until the 1970s. The development of new cancer therapies began to be a major focus for many firms. The mid-1980s saw the advent of the era of corporate buyouts, consequent to smaller firms finding it difficult to survive and therefore needing a merger with, or acquisition (M&A) by a larger company. In particular, pharmaceutical manufacturing of any level of business significance became the territory of a relatively small number of large companies. This is because of the magnitude of the investment in infrastructure and skills needed to develop and manufacture pharmaceutical formulations to meet the rigorous set of quality standards and controls required by the regulators. Having a specific manufacturing capability became a major catalyst for M&A activities, sometimes for a single product.

The 1980s also saw new areas of focus for industrial research and development, eg. in cardiovascular disease and the then new and devastating disease of AIDS.

In the 1990s, the environment for M&As intensified, and compound 'licensing deals' started to become the trademark activity between firms it is today. All this, maybe paradoxically, stemmed as a consequence of increases in the scientific understanding of diseases and emerging new technologies eg. in genetics, creating more opportunities for drug discovery. These created many more, new investigational medicines, often from small and medium sized enterprises (SMEs), as well as the traditional large companies. Research 'pipelines' of companies expanded and started to overlap one with another, driving competition. New technologies, larger pipelines and the continuing increase in regulatory requirements for new medicines began substantially to drive up Research and Development (R&D) costs. The concomitant increase in corporate R&D investment needed prudent management to justify it to investors. 'Portfolio review and prioritisation' activities by the executive management of companies became commonplace. Smaller companies, while being highly inventive scientifically, might simply not have the funds or infrastructure to develop an investigational medicine fully. This, coupled with pipeline interest from larger firms, collectively drove the M&A/licensing environment that so strongly is still a feature of today's industry.

The focus on R&D costs also catalysed the era of 'outsourcing'. Companies began to look closely at all aspects of their R&D business operations. What activities were truly critical to keep in-house ie. what was a company's core 'essence', versus, what might make better sense to outsource to external providers? One consequence of this, for example, was the dramatic increase in the use of contract research organizations for clinical development. Today, a large 'hinterland' of highly skilled and regulated service providers exists to support all aspects of drug discovery and development, and on which the modern industry relies heavily.[4]

The global pharmaceutical industry of today is a very different beast from that of the 1950s. It is much bigger and more diverse, with approximately 80% of all its invention emanating from SMEs. But, increasing regulation, pressures from payers and the intrinsically long, complex, expensive and inherently uncertain nature of R&D has resulted in a steady decline in its productivity over the last decade or so. While M&A and licensing trends continue, the industry is changing its R&D model from one that was largely 'closed' (everything done in-house) to one that is embracing a more open dialogue and partnership with the large range of academic and allied research-based organisations that are such an important part of the life sciences community. Coupled with the era of stratified medicine, which aims to tailor medical treatment to the individual characteristics of each patient, it is hoped that through greater partnerships between all stakeholders, drug discovery and development can progress from a largely 'needle in a haystack' approach, to one that delivers greater precision and certainty around its outcome. New drug R&D is, frankly, now too difficult for any one type of organisation to do alone. So, what does it entail?

An overview of Research and Development[5]

Broadly speaking, pharmaceutical/medicinal R&D is divided into two main parts; drug **discovery** and drug **development**. It should also be noted that molecules being designed to be medicines can be divided into two classes – small and large molecules. They differ not only in terms of size, but also in how they are made, how they behave in the body and their suitability for certain drug forms. Small, chemically manufactured molecules are still the mainstay of today's medicines. However, large molecules (also known as biologics) are therapeutic proteins and are becoming an increasingly important component of the medical armamentarium.

The drug discovery and development sections, below, focus principally on the overall process for small molecules.

Drug discovery

Drugs discovery is the process by which new *candidate* (potential) medicines are discovered.

Historically, drug discovery was a random matter of serendipity, or achieved by identifying and then isolating active ingredients in traditional remedies eg. 'extracts' of willow bark and foxgloves identifying salicylic acid (aspirin) and digitalis (digoxin) respectively.

This progressed to a pharmacologically driven process whereby chemical libraries of synthetic, small molecules or extracts of natural products were screened in cells or whole organisms to identify potentially useful therapeutic effects. Traditionally, such 'classical pharmacology' has been the basis for the discovery of new drugs. With this approach, it is only after compounds with potentially useful effects have been discovered that work begins to understand what their biological targets might be. This process has accounted for a large number of first-in-class treatments in recent years.

Notwithstanding the success of the classic approach, it has now largely been superseded by 'reverse pharmacology'. With this approach, basic research, often conducted in academia, develops and tests hypotheses that a certain biological target is disease modifying. Compounds can then be screened for evidence that they modulate the activity of the target protein. 'Target-based drug discovery' has, therefore, been coined as another name for reverse pharmacology. The sequencing of the human genome has greatly enhanced the attractiveness of this strategy as it enables the rapid production of large quantities of purified proteins. As such, the 'high throughput screening' of huge numbers of prototype compounds for activity against target proteins has become commonplace. These molecules are stored in 'compound libraries', which sometimes contain many millions of these prototypes. As such, a pharmaceutical firm's compound library can be one of the most important 'crown jewels' of intellectual property it owns.

The aim of all screening strategies (classical, reverse, high throughput etc) is to identify a prototype molecule that has potentially useful activity against a target protein. These are termed 'hits'. The next stage is to 'optimise' the 'hit'. This involves using medicinal chemistry techniques and possibly also computer-aided (*in silico*) drug design to alter the structure of the molecule to increase its affinity, potency and selectivity for its biological target. Collectively, this aims to increase the predicted future efficacy of the molecule, while reducing the potential for side effects. The process also aims to increase its metabolic stability and oral bioavailability. Once a molecule has been optimised in this way, it is termed a 'lead hit' or 'lead candidate' and can then enter the phase of drug development. It is important not underestimate just how long this period of 'hit to lead optimisation' can take. A few years ago, Pfizer launched Maraviroc, a first-in-class treatment for HIV. The 'optimisation' phase of that drug's discovery took 2.5 years of solid focus on its medicinal chemistry, which included the synthesis of 965 different molecules before the one with the right balance of properties was found, and taken forward for development!

Drug development

Once a lead candidate (compound) has been identified via the process of drug discovery, it enters the phase of drug development. This takes it from pre-clinical research, which may include the use of animals, animal or human tissue models or in silico (computer) testing, through extensive human testing in clinical trials. Then, it goes on to review by regulatory agencies with, hopefully, an approval to market the drug. However, most of these investigational medicines (now known as new molecular/chemical entities – NMEs or NCEs), fail *en route*.

Pre-clinical development

When an NCE enters pre-clinical development, nothing is known with certainty about its safety or toxicity in humans, or how the human body will handle the drug in terms of its absorption, distribution to various parts of the body, metabolism and excretion. It is a key function of this phase to determine these factors prior to entering human clinical trials and also to recommend the initial dose and dose schedule to be used.

Most aspects of pre-clinical drug development are driven by the requirements set by the major regulatory agencies. Drug development is usually done on a global basis and the two principal regulatory authorities, whose requirements the industry aims to meet, are the Food and Drug Administration (FDA) in the USA and the European Medicines Agency (EMA) in Europe. The regulators will usually request tests that are designed to determine the major toxicities of a novel compound prior to first use in man. It is a legal requirement that an assessment of major organ toxicity be performed (effects on the heart and lungs, brain, kidney, liver and digestive system), as well as effects on other parts of the body that might be affected by the drug (eg. the skin, if the new drug is to be delivered through the skin). Testing for a compound's mutagenic potential is also mandatory.

Other testing is done to help predict the likely beneficial effects of an NCE in humans and to help inform the initial dose to use in human trials. But, it must be remembered that **all** of this type of research is a *prediction* of effects in humans, not a 100% certain science. If it were, then testing in humans would not be necessary. What it aims to do therefore, is to lessen the risk to human subjects who volunteer to take part in the subsequent clinical trials.

While, increasingly, these tests can be made using *in vitro* methods (eg. with isolated cells), many tests can only be made by using experimental animals, since it is often only in an intact organism that the complex interplay of metabolism and drug exposure on toxicity can be examined.

The use of animals as research tools is clearly a controversial, sensitive and emotive area. I suspect and hope that the vast majority of normal people would like to see the use of animals for all forms of biomedical research ended. I would. Do I think that's likely? No, because new scientific opportunities are always emerging needing the development of new research tools and it's simply not always possible for this to be a cell, tissue or computer model straightaway. Do I think however, that major progress can be made to reduce, refine and replace the use of animals? Yes, absolutely, because it is already happening.

Firstly, and pertinent specifically to the UK, there are stringent rules and regulations governing the use of animals in research. Every project that would use animals, every person who would conduct the research and every institution where the research would be done, has to be approved by the Home Office. Research that would duplicate research already done would not be allowed. Secondly, animals that are used for research are bred specifically for that purpose. They are born in a laboratory to live in a laboratory, and this can be for many years. Any institution that breeds, houses or uses animals for research can be audited without warning by the Home Office. This greatly helps safeguard all research animals' dignity and welfare. Indeed a personal observation during my years working at a major pharmaceutical R&D site, is that some of the most passionate and dedicated scientists are those whose responsibility it is to look after the welfare of the animals used for research.

Thirdly, in recent years, scientists from academia and industry have been working more closely together and with government bodies to pursue the 'reduction, replacement and refinement' (the 3Rs) agenda. In the UK, the National Council for the 3Rs (NC3Rs) has been a major funding catalyst for these works and is constantly producing innovative methodologies as a result.[6]

Individuals must make up their own minds about the ethics of the use of animals in research. I am personally satisfied that what is conducted by the research-led pharmaceutical industry is necessary, well-regulated and conducted to the highest animal welfare standards, while significant on-going efforts are also being made to reduce, replace and refine their use.

The other major focus of pre-clinical development is to establish the physicochemical properties of the NCE ie. its chemical makeup, stability and solubility. This is the area of pharmaceutical formulation science and is fundamental to the ultimate achievement of the quality medicinal products that we all take as 'given'. The process by which the NCE is made will be evolved, such that the small milligram quantities that are made for 'bench' research can be scaled up to be manufactured on a kilogram basis (eg. for clinical trials) and then on a tonne scale (for commercial use). Extensive research will also be done to assess how the NCE – the 'active pharmaceutical ingredient (API)' – will be best formulated for human use eg. as a tablet, capsule, injectable, inhaled etc. Sometimes, and irrespective of whether other pre-clinical research suggests that the NCE should be suitable for clinical trials, its development can be stopped simply because it proves impossible to formulate it in an appropriate way to meet the needs of the planned patient population.

When complete, the information collectively gathered from all the types of pre-clinical development is submitted to the regulatory authorities, from whom, approval is then sought to move to the clinical phases of development.

Clinical development

Fundamentally, this is about research using human volunteers. Classically it is divided into phases:

Phase 1 trials

These are usually performed in healthy volunteers, as their primary purpose is to determine the safety and pharmacokinetics ('PK' – how the body handles the drug) of the investigational medicine. Single escalating dose studies will be used to determine the 'maximum (acute) tolerated dose'. Based on this and what the preliminary PK results show, multiple dose studies may then be performed which will further evaluate safety and PK over a longer period, eg. to assess the degree to which the drug accumulates in the body.

Although efficacy determination is not a primary objective of healthy volunteer studies, it is sometimes possible to get an early idea of potential efficacy in patients from them, if a suitable study methodology or physiological parameter can be measured, eg. electrophysiological studies of heart function or bronchial airway changes, for investigational cardiac and respiratory medicines respectively.

For this type of study using people, where safety and PK are the primary objectives, it is important to have study volunteers who do not have existing illnesses, or requirements for other drugs that could confound the results or, very importantly, add risk. Hence, the usual need for healthy volunteers. However, some new drugs would, by the nature of the disease they are intended to treat, eg. cancers, be too toxic to evaluate ethically in healthy volunteers. In these instances, phase 1 studies will use patients and early indicators of efficacy are therefore commonly sought, eg. tumour size regression in cancer studies.

Phase 2 trials

These trials use small numbers of patients with the disease under study to explore the efficacy and safety of the investigational medicine. Sometimes they are split into parts 'a' and 'b'. Phase 2a trials are 'proof of concept (PoC)' studies, where often the maximally tolerated dose from phase 1 is assessed against a placebo. The studies are short and usually measure a 'surrogate effect'. This is a measurable marker of a disease or disease process that is known to relate to the long-term outcomes of the disease process. An example is bone density that is a surrogate marker for osteoporotic bone fracture.

Assuming PoC is demonstrated, Phase 2b studies explore the relationship of dose to response. Drug development always has at its centre, the need to describe the benefit/risk ratio of a new medicine. Key to this is to define the lowest dose that produces the maximum response and, as such, phase 2b studies are often known as 'dose-ranging' trials as they explore a number of dose levels. They will therefore need larger numbers of patients, but are still usually fairly short-term in nature and measure surrogate outcomes.

Sadly, a large number of drugs fail in this phase of development. Most usually this is because they simply do not show any sign of the desired efficacy, despite perhaps the many years of 'positive' research that have preceded. They might also fail because of unexpected 'off-target' pharmacological effects that cause toxicities and adverse events. Reducing this so-called 'attrition' has been a major focus for the industry in recent years. I think it is fair to say that there is a long way to go! Fundamental to achieving this are to better understand:

1. how a biological target relates to the human disease;
2. in which specific patient disease sub-populations this is relevant;
3. how to measure accurately the effects of altering the target's function.

The various scientific approaches contained in the increasing number of evolving global initiatives in translational research, disease stratification and personalised medicine are central to improving this problem.

Phase 3 trials

If phase 2 studies are 'exploratory' in nature, then those that follow in phase 3 are often termed 'confirmatory'. 'Pivotal' is also another word used to describe this type of trial, as they are the major source of clinical data to support the registration of a new medicine for use in humans. Usually phase 3 trials test the best dose (or sometimes the two best doses) found during phase 2 trials and often this involves comparing their effects against a drug already available as a treatment, instead of comparing against a placebo.

Their confirmatory nature also means that instead of measuring 'surrogate' endpoints, they will usually assess the effect of the investigational medicine on a clinical outcome that is known to represent accurately, an important feature of the disease, eg. slowing of actual disease progression in rheumatoid arthritis. Additionally, regulatory authorities usually want to see the safety and efficacy of new medicines replicated in more than one pivotal trial to ensure that a first set of positive results did not happen by chance.

For all these reasons, phase 3 trials are therefore usually very large, often involving many hundreds, sometimes thousands of patients and are conducted in many centres worldwide. They are also often much longer than phase 2 trials and may take several years to complete. The cost to a company of designing, conducting and reporting a phase 3 programme can therefore be huge – maybe hundreds of millions of dollars. Regrettably, drug failures still happen at this stage, which again points to the critical need for the 'right drug to be assessed in the right patient, at the right dose and at the right time'. Plus, it is critical to ensure that all clinical trials are designed with utmost statistical rigour and conducted with detailed attention to all the methods described in the clinical protocol. This will help reduce the risk that sources of bias are introduced into the study that can lead to false-negative or false-positive results, or unclear 'don't know' answers.

Phase 4 trials

These are also known as post-marketing surveillance studies, wherein a key feature is safety assessment or 'pharmacovigilance'. This is because phase 3 trials, even though they may be very large and long, cannot determine a drug's full safety profile, as rare but important adverse events may only come to light once the drug is on the market and being taken by many thousands of patients all over the world. Phase 4 trials are therefore often required by regulatory authorities, as conditions of approval ie. are a 'post-approval commitment'. Such requirements can also include studies to 'fill in the data gaps' that phase 3 could not answer, eg. how the new drug compares in terms of safety and efficacy against existing medicines, or in key patient populations not studied in the phase 3 programme.

In some cases, the outcomes of safety surveillance trials, or observations from the 'real world' use of medicines, may lead to the withdrawal of a medicine from the market, as happened a few years ago with rofecoxib (Vioxx), or perhaps to a more restricted license of use.

Phase 4 studies may also be undertaken by the company for direct competitive reasons. These may, *inter alia*, include investigating the drug against others on the market, or testing the drug in additional indications to expand its market potential.

Key points for biological drug discovery and development

Biologics (or biopharmaceuticals) are a class of drugs based on proteins that have a therapeutic effect. They are large protein molecules, which are essentially copies or enhanced versions of endogenous human proteins.

Biologics bind to specific cell receptors that are associated with the disease process. For example, a 'monoclonal antibody' will target a very specific structure on a cell surface. This means that when used in cancer therapy, it will bind very selectively to a target receptor, thereby making it possible to kill the abnormal cells, while usually leaving untouched the healthy cells that do not express the receptor.

Biopharmaceuticals are administered by injection or infusion because, if taken orally, they would (like other proteins) be digested in the stomach and intestines, and therefore be rendered ineffective.

They are produced in biotechnological processes via genetically modified cells of micro-organisms such as bacteria, or yeasts or in mammalian cell lines. Over 1,000 process steps may be necessary to assemble and optimise a complex protein.

There are many areas of overlap between small and large molecule development, eg. the use of high throughput screening techniques and much of the clinical development process.

Largely because they are medicines based on human proteins, they are much less likely to fail in development than small molecules. However, their manufacture is more complicated and therefore more costly than small molecules, which makes the resultant biological medicine usually extremely expensive.

Candidate success rate in drug development

I mentioned 'attrition' above. It is the major Achilles' heel for the R&D side of industry. Candidates for a new drug to treat a disease might theoretically include from 5,000 to 10,000 chemical compounds. On average about 250 of these will show sufficient promise for further evaluation using laboratory tests, mice and other test animals. Typically, about ten of these will qualify for tests on humans. Of these, maybe only a couple will make it through the development and regulatory processes and be approved for marketing. So, you can see that compound attrition is enormous and extremely costly. Part of it is driven by the inherent uncertainty of drug discovery, part by the increasing need to maximise benefit/risk and differentiate new from existing medicines, while other aspects can perhaps be mitigated by an ever greater focus on translational/personalised sciences and clinical trial design elements mentioned above. However, greater open collaboration between all parties involved in life sciences research must underpin all of these efforts.

The cost of drug development

The full cost of bringing a new drug to market, ie. from discovery through clinical trials to approval, – is complex and not without controversy. It is complex because the figure can include:

1. the direct expenses of a drug's development;
2. the estimated capital costs incurred over the 10-12 year development period;
3. a figure to account for the same elements for all the investigational medicines that have undergone attrition en-route, while the successful drug was being developed.

However, it is not always clear which of these factors have been taken into account by the manufacturer. Additionally, all cost estimates are based on confidential information released voluntarily by companies. So, there is in fact no mechanism to validate their accuracy.

Controversy arises because companies use the costs of development to justify a high price to payers for their innovation. Are they right to do this? I would suggest sometimes yes, but by no means always, especially when the benefits seem to be marginal.

A study published by Steve Paul *et al.* in 2010[7] compares many of the studies of drug development costs. They provided both capitalised and out-of-pocket estimated costs for each to give a range of $870 – $1800 million. Whichever way you look at it, the truth is likely to be a big figure! Couple this with the fact that only around 30% of approved medicines ever recoup their R&D costs, and you can perhaps see why every company needs to have at least one or two products that 'win big' for them.

However, some medicines are too highly priced for what they deliver in return. Every healthcare system in the world has a finite budget for medicines, so it is frankly pointless for companies to carry on trying to charge the Earth for every new medicine they invent. They simply will not be adopted by healthcare payers if they are too costly or do not deliver the value required by the system. Companies could do themselves and patients a big favour by engaging actively, not just with regulatory agencies during drug development, but also with payer bodies, such as the National Institute for Health and Care Excellence (NICE) in England and the Scottish Medicines Consortium (SMC) in Scotland. Listen to what they ask for and do this at a time that allows you to start incorporating their requests into pre-registration clinical development plans. The outcome might well be a better quality product, at least in the eyes of the payers, that is more likely to be bought by healthcare systems. Additionally, there is no medicine that has 100% of the world market. As there is a price/volume relationship for every commercial commodity, perhaps it would make sense for companies to look at charging less to gain on volume.

Looking to the 2020 horizon, and in addition to doing everything possible to speed up the drug development process, drug pricing and 'value return' are the next big issues requiring pan-stakeholder agreement, in order to ensure that patients get timely access to the new medicines they deserve.

Ideas to enable engagement with the industry

I said at the top of this chapter that 'how to engage with industry' *per se* would be virtually impossible to write, at least without prefacing it with a high level explanation of its 'what, why and how'. I have tried to do this from an R&D perspective and also include some of the industry's challenges and controversies, which are partly of its own making, but where others are consequent to a public lack of understanding or misperceptions about what the industry does.

What I do know, however, is that drug discovery and development is a lengthy, uncertain and hugely costly enterprise. It is now far too difficult for any one type of organisation to do alone. At the commercial end of the process, and specifically, where a payer organisation such as NICE has recommended or issued guidance for the use of a new medicine, it is often the case that the healthcare system still does not readily adopt and diffuse it throughout. Consistent patient access to such medicines is therefore not always present.

These are two key areas where greater engagement between industry, patient organisations and charities could bring dividends for all. However, such engagement needs to bear in mind the governance of the industry's relationship with its stakeholders and in particular, the fact that the advertisement and direct promotion of prescription-only medicines to the public by companies is forbidden by UK and EU law. Such advertisement and promotion activities can be hidden, purposely or inadvertently, within other seemingly unconnected activities, such as simply holding a meeting with patient groups.

For these reasons, there are two key 'codes of practice' in the UK:

The first is the Association of the British Pharmaceutical Industry's (ABPI) code, which is administered by the Prescription Medicines Code of Practice Authority (PMCPA). A summary of the code for patient groups is available from their website.[8]

The second is the Medicines and Healthcare Products Regulatory Agency's (MHRA) 'Blue Guide'. A copy can be found on their website.[9]

All companies are subject to the Blue Guide, which sets out the law for the advertising and promotion of prescription-only medicines in the UK, but companies can opt in or out of the ABPI Code of Practice. Neither the ABPI nor MHRA codes state that companies *cannot* engage with patient groups. However, companies need to be very careful how they plan and conduct such meetings, as the risk of a complaint being made alleging attempts at promotion are always there. It is therefore recommended that companies establish a signed 'memorandum of understanding' (MOU) with prospective patient stakeholders, as the plans for a joint meeting are formulated. The MOU would set out the meeting objectives, desired outcomes and topics for discussion. Company lawyers would often also be involved, to approve any materials intended for presentation.

From my personal R&D perspective, this is all a bit sad and is a situation made worse by the fact that many companies over-interpret the stipulations in the codes, to the point that little, if any direct contact with patient groups is made. I remember being asked to host a visit of a patient group to Pfizer's Sandwich laboratories, during which they would meet scientists, see what they do and learn something about the medicinal R&D process. However, we would have had to do it without ever mentioning any medicine that might have been the end result of many years of R&D. 'Dry' or what? The meeting did not take place and an opportunity to engage and inform was lost.

Time for a new start? I think so. There is just so much to gain for everyone. If, for example, you consider just three key stakeholder groups in life sciences research – academia, industry and charities (research funders and patient groups), what would they collectively bring to the table for discussion if the objective were to do better R&D?

Academia would bring knowledge and expertise in disease mechanisms, new targets & biomarkers, clinical practice expertise & skills training. But, there has to be the understanding that they're not companies and do not operate in the same way.

Industry would bring medicinal discovery, drug development and commercial expertise. But, the honest caveat is, that it will always ultimately need to derive a return on its investment and to its investors.

Charities and patient groups would bring access to patients for dialogue and research participation, the best possible understanding of patients' needs in a disease area, access to academia and potentially research funding. But, they have a duty consistently to focus solely on their charitable objectives.

Are these various drivers and constraints a barrier to doing great work together? Not at all, if everyone takes due time to understand each other's objectives and challenges. By so doing you can then work effectively to enhance patient outcomes, add value to the healthcare system and indeed, create wealth for the nation.

So, firstly, look at your own objectives and challenges. In this instance, how can better engagement with industry specifically help you? What areas of expertise do you have which you think would be of help to industry? Then, you need to identify your potential industry partners. These will often be completely unknown at this stage and even when a company is identified, finding the right person to approach in that company can be difficult.

However, our world works and is made small because of networks. There is clearly nothing to beat using existing industry contacts to try and help identify the right companies, and people within them, to approach. However, you should also ask the various membership organisations for advice and direction. They should be able to help with the initial 'match-making' and also potentially the brokerage of an initial meeting. UK examples are:

The Association of Medical Research Charities (AMRC)
http://www.amrc.org.uk/
The AMRC is the national membership organisation of leading medical and health research charities. It has a strong interest to help foster more and better quality research-driven partnerships between charities and industry.

The Association of the British Pharmaceutical Industry (ABPI)
http://www.abpi.org.uk/Pages/default.aspx
The ABPI represents principally the large pharmaceutical company sector, eg. AZ, GSK, Merck, Novartis, Pfizer, Sanofi.

The Bioindustry Association (BIA)
http://www.bioindustry.org
The BIA represents principally the biopharmaceutical technology sector and within this, especially the smaller biotechnology firms for whom the funding of research is often a key issue.

The Ethical Medicines Industry Group (EMIG)
http://www.emig.org.uk
EMIG represents principally small and mid-sized pharmaceutical companies, eg. Gentium, Genzyme, Nordic, Prostrakan, SOBI, Teva.

The three pharmaceutical organisations cited here do not represent the totality of industry membership organisations. There are others that, for example, have the manufacturers of generic medicines or pre-sales (emerging R&D) companies as members. You might reasonably ask why are there so many for just one part of the life sciences industry? My personal answer to this is that the biopharmaceutical industry is extremely diverse in its make-up, consisting of companies of all shapes and sizes, varying types of business interest and business model, and stages of corporate development. They therefore have different needs. For me, it follows that no single membership organisation can adequately, or fairly, represent the views and needs of all the industry and this has driven the establishment of a variety of membership organisation, each with its own unique core identity.

Once your industry partners (and you might well have more than one for a specific challenge) have been identified, then the crucial next step is simply to get together around a table and talk. Talk about 'who you are and what you do'. Talk about your individual visions, opportunities and challenges. From this, the common ground will be identified and, in turn, lead to the development of collaborative approaches with the delivery of solutions.

Summary thoughts

In this chapter, I have attempted to provide a summary 'what, why and how' of, and personal reflections on, the very diverse, complex and global industry in which I have spent the major part of my career as a medically-qualified doctor. I know for sure that the industry has benefited human health and healthcare enormously. I also know, however, that it is an industry often blighted, fairly or unfairly, by controversy. What will undoubtedly strengthen the former and weaken the latter is the development of more, and better-quality, honest, open and transparent dialogues and partnerships between all stakeholders involved in the research and delivery of healthcare technologies. Accordingly, I would be very glad to assist any reader who wishes to establish a link with industry. Please do not hesitate to get in touch.

Dr Mark Edwards BSc (hons) MB BS FRCA FSB
E-mail: mark.edwards@emig.org.uk
Mobile: +44 (0)7887 831942

References

1 A Pioneering Spirit on the Frontiers of Medicine. 2015. Pfizer. (Accessed 14 July 2015). http://www.pfizer.com/about/history/timeline

2 Howard Florey: the story. Maker of the miracle mould. 1998. Australian Broadcasting Corporation. (Accessed 14 July 2015). http://www.abc.net.au/science/slab/florey/story.htm

3 Ethical Principles for Medical Research Involving Human Subjects. 2008. World Medical Association. (Accessed 14 July 2015). http://www.wma.net/en/30publications/10policies/b3/17c.pdf

4 For further information about the history of the pharmaceutical industry, go to: http://www.britannica.com/EBchecked/topic/1357082/pharmaceutical-industry

5 See also; http://www.phrma.org/sites/default/files/pdf/rd_brochure_022307.pdf

6 National Centre for the Replacement, Refinement and Reduction of Animals in Research. (Accessed 14 July 2015). http://www.nc3rs.org.uk

7 Steve Paul et al. 2010. Nature Reviews: Drug Discovery. (Accessed 14 July 2015). http://www.nature.com/nrd/journal/v9/n3/abs/nrd3078.html

8 The Prescription Medicines Code of Practice Authority. (Accessed 14 July 2015). http://www.pmcpa.org.uk

9 The Medicines and Healthcare products Regulatory Agency. (Accessed 14 July 2015). https://www.gov.uk/government/organisations/medicines-and-healthcare-products-regulatory-agency/about

Chapter 7

How to Set up a Centre of Excellence: Alström Syndrome UK's Experience

Kay Parkinson, LLB (Hons) Dip Legal Practice
Director and Founder, Alström Syndrome UK (ASUK)

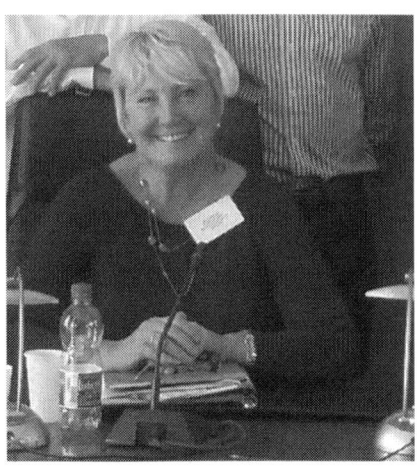

Introduction

Alström Syndrome UK (ASUK) became aware of the possibility of NHS Commissioning following a talk by Alastair Kent at our Family Conference in 2005.

Alström Syndrome is a life-limiting disease which, in my two children's case, caused childhood blindness, hearing loss, heart failure , diabetes type two, kidney failure, bladder dysfunction and many associated problems. Matthew died aged

25 following heart transplant surgery in 2003 and Charlotte following heart and kidney transplantation in 2010 aged 29.

I founded Alström Syndrome UK charity in 1998, following the late diagnosis of my two children, Matthew was 18 and Charlotte was 15. They had years of mis-diagnosis at my local hospital, before finally being asked to attend Great Ormond Street Hospital, as a doctor was looking into their latest diagnosis. I had studied Law at Exeter University as a mature student, primarily because I was having to fight so many issues for my children and fortunately, also specialised in Charity Law.

I informed the Consultant who made the diagnosis that I wanted to start a charity for the condition and she contacted 12 other families she knew with the condition and invited them to our first family conference in 1998. Seven families attended and it soon became clear that even those with a diagnosis were not having all aspects of the disease identified. The following year, we invited physicians who were working with my own two children from Torbay Hospital to attend. Although we did not realise at the time, this was the beginning of our multi-disciplinary clinics. In a hotel in Brixham, Devon, audiology tests took place in the bedrooms, families gathered round a cardiologist, an endocrinologist and dietician and ad hoc consultations took place wherever a spare room in the hotel could be found. The unmet needs of these families were clear, as were the needs of the physicians to see more patients, gain more experience and learn more about the disease. ASUK united families to meet in one place and facilitated and funded this development through applications to grant making trusts. Our first grant was from Awards for All, shortly followed by a Jeans for Genes grant and a BBC Children in Need grant.

The family conference/clinic progressed on these lines for a number of years. As our numbers grew it became increasingly difficult for families to travel to Torbay and back in a weekend. I was already in touch with Birmingham Children's Hospital and it was agreed that we could use their facilities at the weekend of our family conference. All was still on an ad hoc voluntary basis, with doctors giving freely of their time at the weekends to examine our Alström patients, and Alström Syndrome UK charity organising and funding the family conference and the clinic lists and developing a UK wide database of affected patients. Our web site (www.alstrom.org.uk) was key to diagnosed patients finding the support and expertise we could offer.

Next steps

Following Alastair's talk, Torbay Hospital, Birmingham Children's Hospital and ASUK decided that we would apply for NHS Commissioning to fund the clinical service on a more professional basis. We were pleased we had developed the clinics, as the NHS would only fund a clinic if it was already in place. In 2006, the NHS Commissioning Team for Highly Specialised Services agreed to fund 4 clinics for children at the Birmingham Children's Hospital yearly and 4 adult clinics at Torbay Hospital. Two outreach clinics in Leeds were also arranged. However, the NHS said at that time that they did not fund charities.

Fortunately, my legal training equipped me with the skills to challenge this decision and I set about tracking the legal basis to do this. The COMPACT document, signed by Tony Blair when Prime Minister, laid out the principles of how the public sector should work with the voluntary sector. Reading the document it became clear that there were a number of breaches in our dealings with the NHS. The NCVO had COMPACT officers, funded by the Big Lottery, who took up our case. When the breaches were pointed out to the NHS Commissioners, ASUK was invited to meet with them. The outcome was that we were to be funded as equal partners, with the two hospitals we worked with in delivering the Alström clinical service that we had initiated, funded and developed.

The NHS-commissioned clinics have gone from strength to strength since we started. Our numbers have doubled since we incorporated an Asian Mentoring Scheme; the Alström gene has been found to be present in a number of families in the Leeds, Bradford area. The addition of an NHS-funded, Asian mentoring worker proved very successful, with in-roads being made into this often hard to reach community. This resulted in the doubling of numbers over a 3 year period. In 2012 we successfully moved the adult clinic from Torbay Hospital to the brand new, state of the art Queen Elizabeth Hospital in Birmingham. It had become clear that the needs of our adults could not be met at a district hospital and, although thankful to Torbay for their initial help with setting up the clinics, it was time to move on. The Queen Elizabeth Hospital Birmingham is the largest hospital in Europe and their state of the art services can offer transplantation of all major organs. Transplantation is often needed for Alström patients, so to have clinics here with doctors familiar with our patients is a real privilege.

Peer to peer support is the backbone of the services ASUK provides. Newly diagnosed families, as well as attending the multi-disciplinary clinics, are eager to talk with other mums or dads with affected children or adults and hear how they cope. Older patients know they have someone to turn to. Activity holidays have not only helped with an enjoyable way of weight control and exercise, but have helped formed friendships for patients who are often isolated. The clinics now also offer professionals from across the world the chance to meet and discuss developments.

Funding & partnerships

On the back of the success of the clinics, ASUK applied for, and was successful in gaining, a Big Lottery Medical and Scientific grant to develop research into the condition through taking skin samples from consenting patients and starting a research database. Cambridge University partnered with ASUK and were commissioned to generate pluripotent stem cells that will be differentiated into cell types. Birmingham and Torbay Hospitals were commissioned to take the skin samples and develop a research database.

Six months prior to the completion of the grant, when ASUK were expecting to be able to review the database, Torbay Hospital announced that ASUK could not have access to it for ethical reasons. As we were not NHS "employees", it was unethical for us to have access and, as our patient numbers were so small, we would still be able to recognise anonymised data. The fact that we see un-anonymised patient information, as part of our role as a partner in the NHS England, National Specialised Commissioned Alström Clinical Service was ignored. The fact that we owned the database was ignored. This information, announced at such a late date in the project, put the grant and ASUK into jeopardy. If the Big Lottery were to call back in the grant, ASUK would be ruined. Our members had believed that when they consented to the database that ASUK would, as owners of the database, have access to it.

ASUK kept the Lottery closely informed of discussions and an emergency meeting was held between partners.

The outcome was thought to be that the Database would move to the Queen Elizabeth Hospital, Birmingham and all patients will be re-consented to the database, explicitly stating that they allow ASUK access. ASUK will now add further consents to the form, allowing the data to be shared with EU and International databases.

We have now had discussions with doctors at Cambridge and Birmingham Children's Hospital and another project, EU-WABB, has ethics in place which will cover the Big Lottery grant. All this has taken a great deal of time, which patients with life-limiting conditions can ill-afford. We do have a pharmaceutical firm, interested in developing an anti-fibrosis treatment, who have requested the samples, but at the time of writing they have not yet been sent.

In April 2014, the London School of Economics (LSE) MSc students who, as part of their degree had worked with ASUK, provided a report on a "Cost benefit analysis" of multi-disciplinary clinics (available in the annexe). This independent report has been hailed as much needed evidence of multi-disciplinary working for rare diseases. The report was produced as part of our Horizon 2020 bid, PHC 26 "Patient Empowerment through M health". In this bid, we hope to extend our role-model clinics "virtually", to reach professionals working with Alström patients across Europe. Patients will be connected to medical devices, which will monitor their condition in "real" time through M health applications. We are delighted that Orange Healthcare have partnered with us in this bid.

Conclusion

In June 2014, Torbay Hospital awarded me the Blue Shield Partnership Award for setting up the multi-disciplinary clinics and developing research into Alström Syndrome.

Alström Syndrome is an ultra-rare condition; the vast majority of patients have been found through the infrastructure and services that I have developed over the years. I instigated, pioneered and fought for the first Alström Syndrome multi-disciplinary clinics in the UK and started the first research through the Big Lottery grant. The multi-disciplinary clinics have now been used as a role-model for both Bardet Biedl syndrome and Wolfram Syndrome. A Ciliopathy Service has also been requested using this model. EURORDIS, the European Patient Organisation, awarded Alström Syndrome UK, Patient Organisation of the Year 2013 for outstanding services to Alström patients. This has led to the opportunity to speak at many conferences for Rare Diseases and Orphan drugs across the EU and USA on how the Alström Service has developed.

I hope our story helps other groups be more prepared for issues which can arise when working with the NHS and helps avoid some of the problems we encountered.

Patient groups have patient interests at heart. The solutions for rare diseases will only come by all parties to their care bringing down the barriers that prevent collaborative working.

With such a complex condition as Alström, it is only the patient groups, families and patients who have lived with all the multiple manifestations of the disease and managed them on a daily basis. We cannot "lock out" their valuable experience and expertise. Patient groups deserve and need better recognition.

My case study demonstrates how a mother can effectively drive services which are truly patient centred and the difference a correct, timely, diagnosis makes to affected individuals' lives.

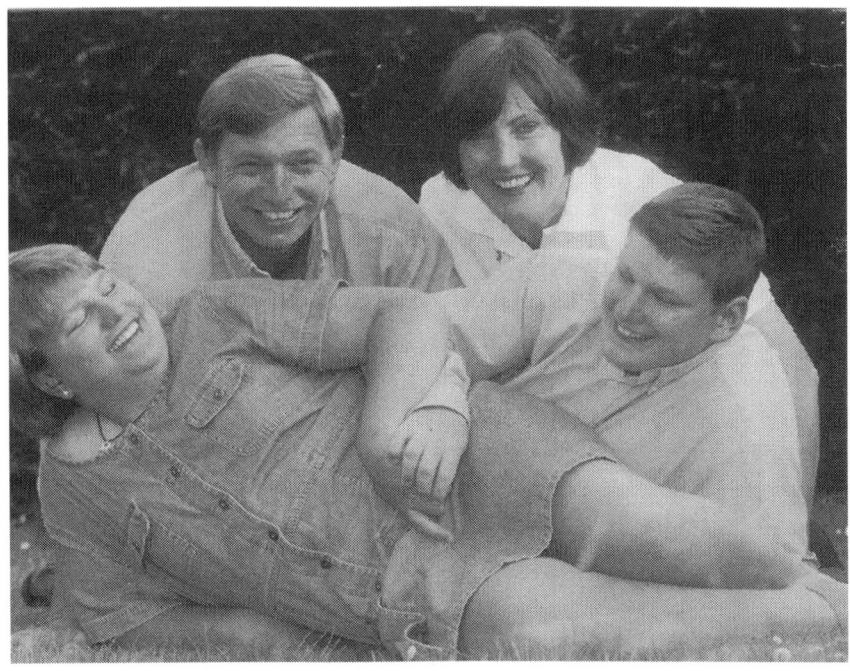

Mathew Parkinson (9.2.1978–11.5.2003) and
Charlotte Parkinson (11.4.1981 – 29.4.2010)
The picture was taken in 1998 shortly after diagnosis by Great Ormond Street Hospital. We are flying to the USA – the only country at that time with any knowledge of the disease. Local press took the photo as we were about to depart.

HOW TO CREATE A NATIONAL RARE DISEASE CENTRE

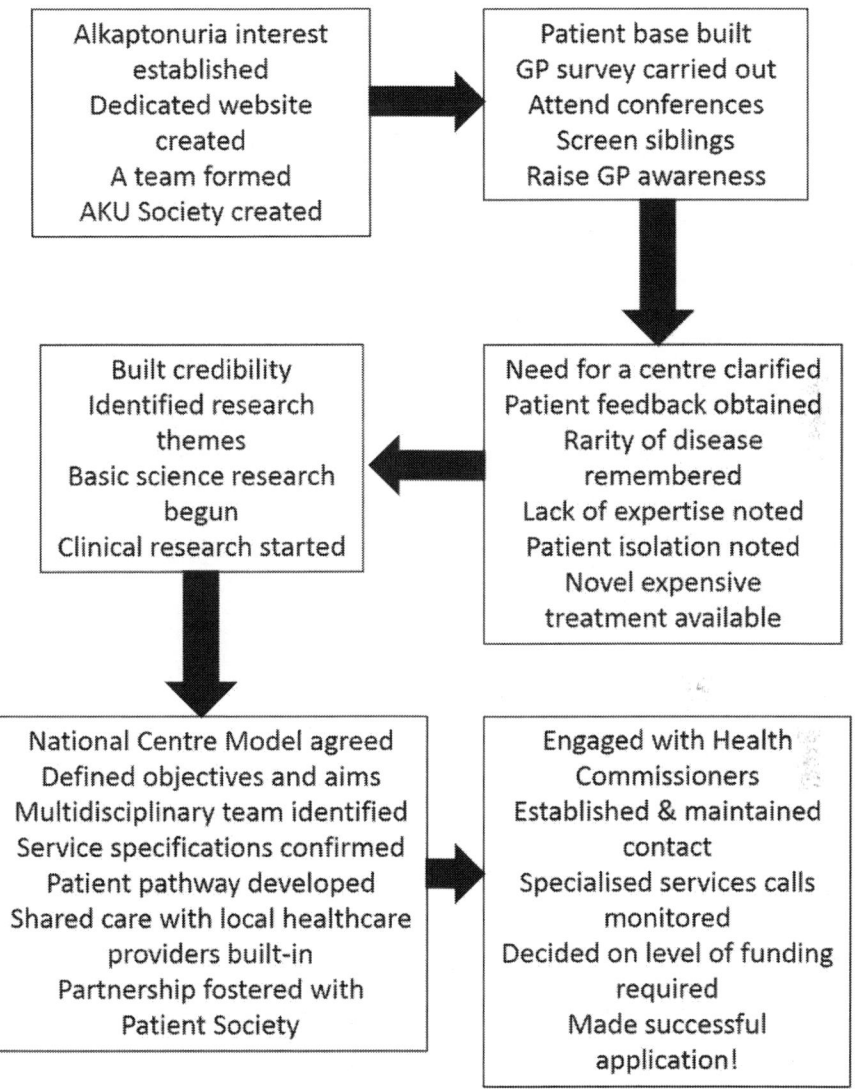

How to create a national rare disease centre. Lakshminarayan Ranganath, 2015

Chapter 8

New Funding Strategies for Clinical Research – Social Finance

Bruce Bloom
Cures Within Reach

Social Impact Bonds and other Social Finance funding of medical research

What is Social Finance?

Social finance is any financial investment method that delivers both a social dividend and an economic return. Social finance can include a wide variety of investing methods. Examples are:

- Community investing;
- Microfinance;
- Social enterprise lending;
- Social enterprise investment;
- Social impact bonds.

Philanthropic grants and program-related investments are sometimes lumped into social finance. Based on outcomes, they can also be referred to as venture philanthropy.

Social finance is designed to create social and financial returns for both investors and for the public. Examples of social returns might be:

- A reduction in homelessness;
- An increase in educational levels;

- Better health;
- Lower healthcare costs;
- Reduced pollution;
- Non-violent resolution of gang disagreements; or
- Less drug use among teenagers.

Examples of public financial returns have historically been:

- Direct reduction in government costs;
- Improvement in conditions or skills that allow individuals to be more productive and actually pay taxes to the government, or to be less reliant on future government programs;
- Elimination of the need for costly programs; or
- Consolidation of programs that reduce costs.

Government has historically tackled many of these social issues. It spends taxpayer dollars up front in an effort to create social returns. Sometimes government does very well with these initiatives, and sometimes not. Whether government does well or not, these programs tend to be very expensive. Often they do not provide the public financial return to offset the government investment made by taxpayers.

Sometimes the government does not collect the data necessary to record the public financial return. This makes the major long-term expense difficult to continue, even if the program gives the needed social return.

Many for-profit and non-profit organizations already create the combination of social and financial return. They do this in many ways, such as for-profit childhood education companies,[1] for-profit prisons,[2] and non-profit water treatment projects in developing countries.[3] In the for-profit sector, these businesses can make a corporate financial return. They simply charge a consumer, a business or a governmental entity a fee for the service that is greater than their cost for delivering it. In the non-profit world, these organizations flourish by raising philanthropic dollars which are then spent on the programs. The program's success can then raise future philanthropic dollars. These organizations succeed through either capitalism or philanthropy. They are not working under a social finance model since they are not generating and documenting public financial return, and getting paid from that financial return.

Social finance is necessary when for-profit or non-profit organizations are not creating enough social and public financial returns using the capitalism or philanthropy models, and when the government is not able to raise the funds or create the social impact. In these cases, government or some other 'success payer' can work together with the for-profit and/or non-profit organizations. Together, they create a social finance model that is designed to provide the desired combination of social and financial return. "With government budgets increasingly tight, this could be a major innovation," says Sir Ronald Cohen.[4] A financier, he began chairing the global Social Investment Task Force of the G8 in 2013. He also chaired the charity-backed commission that proposed the creation of the non-profit called Social Finance.

Social Impact Bonds

The Social Impact Bond (SIB) is a method of social finance that seems most appropriate for creating treatments and cures through medical research. A SIB is an arrangement between one or more government agencies, or other 'pay for success' guarantors, and an external organization, called a Social Impact Bonding Organization (SIBO).

In a SIB, the 'pay for success' guarantor specifies a social outcome it desires and promises to pay the SIBO a pre-agreed sum if the SIBO is able to accomplish it. The SIBO then solicits private investors to provide the necessary upfront capital to the SIBO so that the SIBO can select and pay service providers to perform the required services to achieve the social outcome. The investors agree to provide this funding in exchange for a potential share of the government payments, if and when the social outcome performance targets are met. Figure 1 provides a visual of this Social Impact Bond scenario.

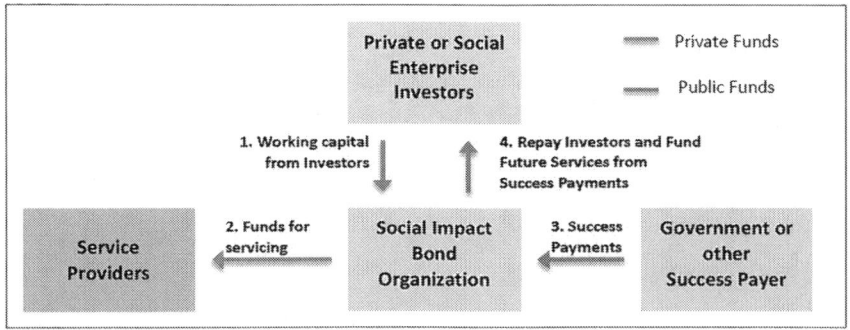

Figure 1. Social Impact Bond Scenario

One huge advantage to a Social Impact Bond is that the government or other 'Success Payer' has little or no upfront financial risk. While there can be considerable costs in the development of a SIB, any actual 'pay for success' payments are made only after the social outcome is achieved, and only for the agreed amount. This provides government or other 'Success Payers' the luxury of creating the opportunity for social impact without either the huge upfront costs or the infrastructure investment in a system that might ultimately fail to create the desired social outcome. Social Impact Bonds shift much of the financial risk from the government or 'Success Payers' to the SIB investors. The social return risk still exists for the government.

There are several key factors to the creation and success of a SIB. In order to create a SIB there must be a solvable social need. There must also be service providers that have either demonstrated the ability to create the desired social outcome, or have a new technique that appears likely to achieve the social outcome. Once those are in place, the first key to the success of a SIB is to have a 'Success Payer' that promises to pay for the achievement of the social outcome, and has the ability to make those payments. While this seems obvious, it is often more challenging to find a 'Success Payer' than might be expected, considering the 'Success Payer' has no upfront expense and often cannot afford any other way to achieve the social outcome. Governments are often reluctant to try anything new, and sometimes factions of the government cannot agree on enough common ground to create something like a SIB. In a situation like treatments and cures created through medical research, governments have worried that they will bear the expense even though patients in other countries or covered by other payment systems will reap the benefits. They feel it is not fair for them to 'pay for success' when other governments or payers do not have to pay.

In the treatment and cure SIB, the argument to the government is that, while a treatment or cure might benefit other countries and their patients, the payment for success is only related to the actual patients helped in the country sponsoring the SIB. Therefore, there is actual value created in the country sponsoring the SIB equal to, or greater than, the actual payment. The benefit outside the country is philanthropic, but not relevant to the pay for success arrangement.

Once the government or other 'Success Payer' is in place, the social outcome is specified, and the service providers are vetted. Then the SIBO has all of the necessary ingredients to entice investors to participate. This process can last as little as 6 months, or as long as several years. During the process, additional 'Success Payers' can join, and the SIB can grow geographically, topically and financially.

A second key to a successful SIB is to set clear performance measures, so that service providers and the outcomes within the SIB can be tracked and documented. The creation of these clear performance measures is the responsibility of the SIBO, in concert with the service providers. The government or other 'Success Payers' will scrutinize these performance measures to make certain that achievement will return the desired social outcome. Investors will scrutinize these performance measures to make certain that they are achievable, so that the investors will receive their return on investment.

Let's look at a real life example of a Social Impact Bond. The first Social Impact Bond, launched in September 2010 by the organization Social Finance UK (the SIBO), is a six-year

Social Impact Bond to reduce recidivism (reoffending) for prisoners.[5] The SIB service providers will provide intensive interventions, both in prison and in the community, for nearly 3,000 short-term prisoners from Peterborough prison. Private investors provided the funds to pay for the services, which will be delivered by service providers with a proven track-record of working with offenders. If reoffending is reduced by at least 7.5%, the investors will receive their return on investment from the government (the pay for success guarantor).

Late in 2014, the first report was issued about this 'Peterborough Social Impact Bond' to reduce recidivism. The service providers generated data that recidivism was reduced by 8.4%, which was better than the benchmark of 7.5%. The trigger for an initial success payment was 10%, so no initial payment was made to the SIBO, but if the reduction continues to exceed 7.5%, a payment will be generated in 2016.[6]

As of 2014, there was considerable Social Impact Bond activity around the globe. See Figure 2 below, taken from information in the Wikipedia article on Social Impact Bonds and from other sources.

Social Impact Bonds and Repurposing

Disease specific non-profits and other interested parties may be able to create Medical Research SIBs to find treatments and cures for the diseases and patients they care about the most. They can also further a government's dual mission to improve the health of its citizens and reduce the healthcare costs to the government. New drug development is often done through the capitalism method, repaying the investment in drug development through future sales of the approved drug. However, this capitalism method does not often succeed for the repurposing of safe, widely available and inexpensive generic drugs and devices.

A Medical Repurposing Research SIB could provide the economic engine for these repurposing projects using a 'pay for success' model. Government or another 'Success Payer' would

Country	Locale	Social Issue	Investment	Date	Active/ Planned
AU	NSW	Recidivism	Unknown	2012	Planned
AU	NSW	Foster Care	Unknown	2012	Active
AU	NSW	Childhood	Unknown	2012	Active
AU	NSW	Youth Justice	Unknown	2012	Active
Israel	Israel	Recidivism	Unknown	2014	Planned
Israel	Israel	Employment	Unknown	2014	Planned
Israel	Israel	Health	Unknown	2014	Planned
Israel	Israel	Education	Unknown	2014	Planned
UK	Peterborough	Recidivism	$8M	2010	Active
UK	London	Homelessness	Unknown	2012	Active
UK	Manchester	Foster Care	Unknown	2012	Active
UK	UK	Community	Unknown	2013	Planned
UK	Leeds	Elderly	Unknown	2013	Planned
UK	Bradford	Community	Unknown	2013	Planned
US	NY State	Recidivism	$12M	2012	Active
US	MA	Recidivism	$3M	2012	Active
US	MA	Homelessness	Unknown	2012	Active
US	NYC	Recidivism	$9.6M	2012	Active
US	DOT	Various	$300M	2013	Active
US	HUD	Infrastructure	$5B	2013	Active
US	UT	Childhood	$7M	2013	Active

Figure 2. Table showing global SIB activity

guarantee payment to investors for the improvement of healthcare outcomes and the reduction in healthcare costs created by the repurposed therapies. Investors would provide the initial resources to fund these repurposing research projects, and they could see significant ROI from receiving a percentage of the healthcare cost savings realized by the government. The ROI could begin within 2-4 years of the completion of a clinical trial that provided proof of the utility of a repurposed therapy. The remaining 'pay for success' funds paid by the government to the SIBO would be used to fund additional Medical Research SIB projects. This would create a self-sustaining system that lowers costs and saves lives.

Figure 3 provides an example of a Disease Agnostic Medical Repurposing Research SIB. It is being organized by the non-profit Cures Within Reach. Any disease-specific non-profit could organize a similar Medical Repurposing Research SIB in its disease of interest.

Features of the SIB

- Testing a repurposed drug is, at worst, like testing a new drug compound in a Phase II study; both have been tested on humans and found to be 'safe', and both have some preliminary data and/or science information that predicts efficacy.
- Depending on the time period studied, Phase II success rates to get to Phase III range from 32-39%. Phase III to an NDA are 60-68%, and NDA to approval are 83-86% (same study). When you do that math, you get a range of 16-23% from Phase II to approval.[7]
- Some drugs in Phase II fail for safety or toxicity, which is less likely to happen with already approved drugs, so that increases the likelihood of success for repurposing.
- Some newly approved drugs are withdrawn for later toxicity or drug-drug interactions, which is unlikely to happen with repurposed drugs that have been used for many years by millions of patients, so that increases the likelihood of long term success for repurposing.

There are thousands of safe, generic drug, device and combination Repurposing Research projects waiting to help patients when funding is available. Between 10-30% of these projects are estimated to yield a 'new' treatment that helps at least one patient population reduce or eliminate the symptoms of their disease and significantly reduce their healthcare costs. The rate-limiting step of creating treatments and cures for these repurposed compounds is the upfront funding to pay for the preclinical and clinical research.

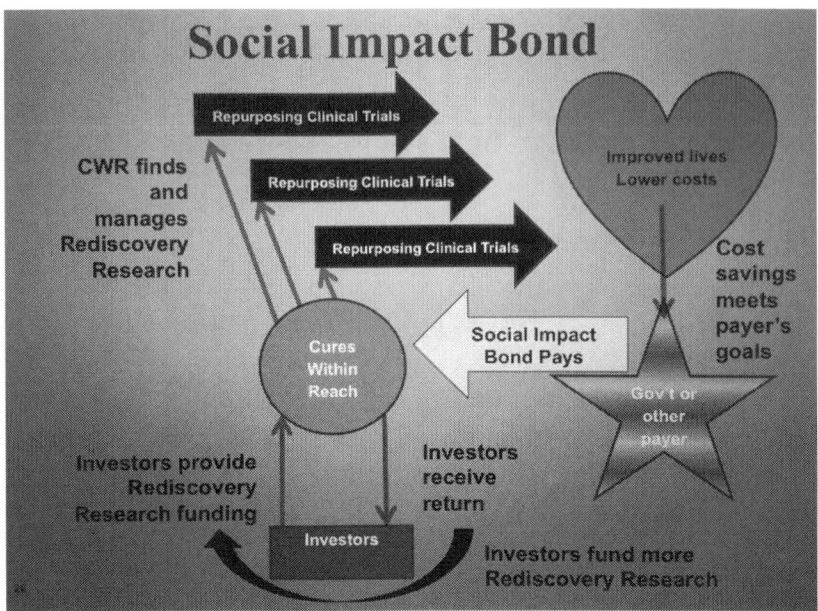

Figure 3. Example of a Disease Agnostic Medical Repurposing Research SIB
Copyright 2015, Cures Within Reach. Used with permission.

The average cost of a Repurposing Research pilot clinical trial project is under $250,000 US. This is based on data collected over the past five years from the non-profit Cures Within Reach. The average time for initiation of that project to patient availability through off-label use is 36 months. Almost all successful Repurposing Research projects save significant healthcare dollars. This is much faster and much cheaper than the costs ($2.6bn+) and timeline (12-19 years) for New Drug Discovery Research,[8] and New Drug Discovery Research almost always increases healthcare costs.

The Cures Within Reach project that successfully repurposed the generic drug sirolimus is an example of a Repurposing Research success that might come out of a Medical Repurposing Research SIB. It is for Autoimmune Lymphoproliferative Syndrome (ALPS), the deadly childhood disease. There are about 600-1000 children in the US with this disease. This is too small a patient population for industry to create a brand new treatment. Cures Within Reach funded a physician researcher and his team at the Children's Hospital of Philadelphia. In less than 30 months they first created a mouse model of the disease and cured the mice. They then conducted a pilot human clinical trial that proved that this drug significantly reduced – or eliminated – symptoms of ALPS in over 85% of the test subjects.[9] All this for less than $200,000. Within 90 days of publication of the results, physicians from around the globe began to contact the researcher for dosing instructions.

A few years later, this drug regimen is considered the off-label standard of care for patients with ALPS.

On average, the sirolimus treatment eliminates most hospitalization, and reduces or eliminates all other expensive forms of treatment. This results in average healthcare cost savings of over $100,000 per patient per year for patients reporting data to Cures Within Reach. While the treatment itself might not be a covered medical expense, since it is not FDA approved for this indication, the annual cost for this treatment is under $4000. It generates an average net saving per patient of about $96,000 per year. If all ALPS patients were using this treatment and 85% of them were eliminating all symptoms, the total annual healthcare cost saving in the US alone would be more than $40m. If even 10% of the patients had this result, it would still generate an annual saving of $4m on a total investment of $200,000.

Repurposing such as this can create huge positive healthcare impact for patients, a significant ROI opportunity for investors, and a measurable and substantial impact for the government that would justify creating a Repurposing Research SIB.

A Repurposing Research SIB supported by the efforts of a variety of disease-specific non-profits might raise as much as $50m US over 5 years to fund 200 or more Repurposing Research projects. It also covers the costs for managing the Repurposing Research process. Based on past experience, it is likely that 10-30% of these Repurposing Research projects would yield 'new' treatments that would reduce patient suffering and healthcare costs. These 20-60 successes could achieve healthcare cost saving totaling $50m per year or more.

Figure 4 provides examples of potential cost savings for various scenarios.

Number of proof of concept clinical trials	Average cost per clinical trial	Total Repurposing Research Costs	Potential success rate	Number of "new" treatments created	Number of patients who have one disease with a "new" treatment	Projected annual healthcare $ saved/ average patient	Total potential 5 year savings for all patients with these diseases	% patients actually using the "new" treatments	healthcare $ saved on this sub-population of patients AFTER repaying investors
200	$250,000	$50,000,000	10%	20	500	$2,500	$125,000,000	50%	$12,500,000
200	$250,000	$50,000,000	10%	20	1000	$5,000	$500,000,000	15%	$25,000,000
200	$250,000	$50,000,000	10%	20	3000	$10,000	$3,000,000,000	10%	$250,000,000
200	$250,000	$50,000,000	20%	40	3000	$10,000	$6,000,000,000	25%	$1,450,000,000
200	$250,000	$50,000,000	20%	40	3000	$30,000	$18,000,000,000	10%	$1,750,000,000
200	$250,000	$50,000,000	25%	50	1000	$40,000	$10,000,000,000	20%	$1,950,000,000
200	$250,000	$50,000,000	30%	60	500	$50,000	$7,500,000,000	80%	$5,950,000,000

Figure 4. Potential cost savings for various scenarios
Copyright 2015, Cures Within Reach. Used with permission.

Even a repurposed treatment can still generate a significant return on investment while improving the lives of patients who would have no other hope of getting an effective treatment. This is the case, even if it only generates a couple of thousand dollars of cost savings for a small population of patients, a minority of which are covered by the government or other 'Success Payers' involved in the Social Impact Bond. This Repurposing Research SIB could target some large patient populations, with very expensive diseases. Their lives could be improved through repurposing, and those successes could create a significant ROI.

There are thousands of repurposing opportunities and thousands of diseases with unmet needs.

Disease-specific non-profits around the globe have partnerships with enough researchers and academic medical centers to generate many of these Repurposing Research ideas. They would create inexpensive and potentially successful projects each year. Organizations like Cures Within Reach, Findacure, Global Cures, and the AntiCancer Fund have the expertise and the experience. They can inspire, identify, validate, select, and manage these life-saving Repurposing Research projects. The only thing keeping Repurposing Research from saving lives and reducing healthcare costs is the funding to get the projects started. A Repurposing Research SIB would be an ideal method to fuel a 'Repurposing Revolution.'

What challenges must we overcome?

First, we must secure government and other funders (heath care insurers, foundations, WHO, etc.) to agree to provide payment for success. There are many ways for this to happen. It could happen because a large number of disease-specific non-profits work together to convince a government or other payer to participate. Often, it is the aggregation of many voices that can create change such as this. In other cases, someone already associated with a government or other payer has a personal or political or profit motive for wanting their entity to participate.

Second, for a Medical Repurposing Research SIB to be effective, there needs to be an easy, valid and reproducible measurement of success. This can happen using ICD codes (International Classification of Diseases, now in its ninth and soon to be tenth iteration). They are a vital part of global health care operations. Health care facilities worldwide use ICD codes for workload and length-of-stay tracking, as well as to assess quality of care.[10] The US Veterans Health Administration uses ICD codes to set capitation rates and allocate resources to medical centers caring for its 6 million beneficiaries. Medical research uses ICD codes to study patterns of disease, patterns of care, and outcomes of disease.[11] Health services researchers use the codes to study risk-adjusted, cross-sectional, and temporal variations in access to care, quality of care, costs of care, and effectiveness of care. Health care payers use these codes to make healthcare payments to providers.

These codes could serve as the basis for tracking patients around the globe who are using and benefitting from the use of a 'new' Repurposing Research treatment. And since each patient is tracked individually in most countries, each patient can serve as his or her own 'cost comparison'. They can use historical costs for patient care compared to new costs after the patients begin using the Repurposing Research treatment. This provides the Medical Repurposing Research SIB with the outcome tracking vital to its success.

Third, there needs to be a consideration of 'off label' use[12] and other regulatory issues. The cost effectiveness of Repurposing Research stems from its ability to re-use drugs, devices and nutriceuticals that are already proven safe for human use. They are often very inexpensive to produce and purchase, and are widely available. This repurposing creates both a problem and an opportunity. The problem is that this low cost of manufacture and sales makes it challenging to recoup the cost of research required for regulatory approval. In many countries this can be in the tens or hundreds of millions of dollars. Without regulatory approval, no company can market the therapy for the repurposed indication. For a small patient population using a very inexpensive repurposed therapy, few companies could ever expect to recoup a multi-million dollar investment to get regulatory marketing approval. This can limit the testing, and therefore the use of the repurposed therapy. This is either because physicians are unaware of the repurposed use, or they are afraid to use it without regulatory approval, even though in many countries a physician or other healthcare worker can prescribe the drug, device or nutriceutical for an off label use.

As part of the implementation of a Medical Repurposing Research SIB, there would need to be some legal, or other changes. They would support the off label use of the repurposed therapies. In addition, there would need to be a concerted effort to create awareness among both patients and physicians about the repurposed therapies.

This lack of regulatory approval also creates potential reimbursement issues. In many countries, healthcare payers, whether government or private, are not required to reimburse patients for the expense of treatments that are not approved by the regulatory authorities. This is true even if the repurposed therapy reduces the cost to the healthcare payer by eliminating other expenses and approved therapies. Again, as part of implementing of a Medical Repurposing Research SIB, there might need to be some legal or other changes that would deal with this potential issue.

However, all of these issues can be overcome. Physicians in many countries already prescribe drugs for off label use. In the US, it is estimated that 20% of all prescribing is off label. This is much higher in pediatrics and mental health.[13] Non-profits that have no vested financial interest in the sale of these repurposed therapies can help spread the information once a repurposed use is proven through a pilot clinical trial.

Conclusion

There are more than 7000 diseases without a universally effective therapy. Social finance methods like Social Impact Bonds are an exceptional way to provide the financing to bring 'new' repurposed therapies to patients, especially for the small and acute diseases.

Social Impact Bonds are being used in the public sector to create solutions for other social issues. The social issue of disease has many advantages that make it ideal for a Social Impact Bond. There is already a system of tracking individual patients by disease and treatment. There are many medical research 'service providers' (clinicians and scientists) who already know how to conduct the types of clinical trials necessary to validate a Repurposing Research treatment.

The costs of untreated disease are high and growing. The cost of repurposed therapies is low and the therapies are widely available. There is a network available through peer reviewed journals and professional conferences to broadly disseminate information on new treatments.

If we all work together, we can create many repurposed therapies. We can create improved healthcare outcomes for patients and reduced healthcare costs for all.

References

1 Valerie Strauss, The failures of for-profit K-12 schools, The Washington Post. (Accessed March 13, 2015). http://www.washingtonpost.com/blogs/answer-sheet/wp/2013/10/04/the-failures-of-for-profit-k-12-schools/

2 Wikipedia, Private prison. (Accessed March 15, 2015). http://en.wikipedia.org/wiki/Private_prison

3 Soft Investment, How Social Finance Helps To Increase Online Banking. (Accessed March 14, 2015). http://softinvestment.net/how-social-finance-helps-to-increase-online-banking/

4 The Economist. Financial innovation and the poor: A place in society. 9/25/2009. http://www.economist.com/node/14493098

5 Darrick Jolliffe and Carol Hedderman. Peterborough Social Impact Bond: Final Report on Cohort 1 Analysis. QinetiQ Ltd, 8/7/2014. https://www.gov.uk/government/uploads/system/uploads/attachment_data/file/341684/peterborough-social-impact-bond-report.pdf.

6 The Rockefeller Foundation. The Success of the Peterborough Social Impact Bond: Impact Investing and Innovative Finance, 8/8/2014. https://www.rockefellerfoundation.org/blog/success-peterborough-social-impact/

7 Hay, M. et al. Clinical development success rates for investigational drugs. Nature Biotechnology 32. 40–51 (2014) doi:10.1038/nbt.2786 http://www.nature.com/nbt/journal/v32/n1/full/nbt.2786.html and Supplementary Materials: http://www.nature.com/nbt/journal/v32/n1/extref/nbt.2786-S1.pdf

8 Rick Mullin, Scientific American, 11/24/2014, Cost to Develop New Pharmaceutical Drug Now Exceeds $2.5B, "http://www.scientificamerican.com/article/cost-to-develop-

new-pharmaceutical-drug-now-exceeds-2-5b/"

9 Teachey DT, Greiner R, Seif A, et al. Treatment with sirolimus results in complete responses in patients with autoimmune lymphoproliferative syndrome. Br J Haematol. 2009. Apr:145(1):101-6.

10 World Health Organization, 2015, International Classification of Diseases. http://www.who.int/classifications/icd/en/

11 Centers for Disease Control and Prevention, 2015, International Classification of Diseases, (ICD-10-CM/PCS) Transition. http://www.cdc.gov/nchs/icd/icd10cm_pcs_background.htm

12 Wikipedia. Off-label Use. http://en.wikipedia.org/wiki/Off-label_use

13 David C. Radley, MPH; Stan N. Finkelstein, MD; Randall S. Stafford, MD, PhD. Off-label Prescribing Among Office-Based Physicians. JAMA Internal Medicine. http://archinte.jamanetwork.com/article.aspx?articleid=410250

Chapter 9

Raising Funds for Clinical Research: Statutory Investment Funding

Liz Philpot
Association of Medical Research Charities (AMRC)

The government recognises the importance of clinical research, by providing a number of funding streams. Each has a specific focus, and so, can support clinical research in many ways. This section describes these funds, who can apply and how rare disease charities can ensure that their disease area is being supported.

Medical Research Council

The Medical Research Council (MRC) receives money from the Department for Business, Innovation and Skills (BIS) to support medical research – from basic research that tells us how cells work, to studies that look at the underlying causes of disease, or develop new potential treatments. Academic researchers from across the UK can apply for funds from the MRC.

Areas of funding for clinical research include:

- Clinical research fellowships[1] – to allow doctors to develop their research skills and take a stronger role in research;
- Project grants[2] – looking at causes of disease, or method of action of a potential treatment;

- Pre-clinical development and early clinical testing of new drugs, devices and diagnostics,[3] – to show proof of concept;
- Experimental medicine studies[4] – investigations in humans to identify the cause of disease and to test the validity and importance of new discoveries and treatments.

Patient groups can get involved in MRC funded research number of different ways:

- Funding pilot studies to allow researchers to collect evidence for a full grant;
- Co-funding a clinical research fellowship – to encourage more clinical research in your disease area;[5]
- Telling researchers about these funds and offer in-kind support for research (access to patient registries to allow researchers to gain information or tissue from patients with the condition, to carry out 'basic' research).

National Institute of Health Research

NIHR received almost £1bn from the Department of Health to support clinical research both by direct grants and infrastructure. Researchers in England, Wales and Northern Ireland can apply for funds to carry out a wide range of clinical research projects from clinical trials of new diagnostics or treatments, to examining how a proven treatment can be adopted by the NHS and made available to patients in all parts of the NHS. Some of the research funded by NIHR is driven by researchers defining what they want to work on (response mode); other studies are commissioned by the NIHR, to ensure that the research is answering a relevant clinical question, and that the results can be incorporated into clinical practice.

Areas of funding include:

- Programme grants[6] – funding for a series of related projects, including clinical trials, in an area of priority or need for the NHS;
- Research for Patient Benefit (RfPB[7]) – research into everyday practice in the health service, decided by regional competitions;
- Invention for Innovation (i4i) Programme[8] – funding for the development of medical product prototypes between at least two partners from industry, NHS organisations and universities;
- Health Technology Assessment trials[9] – designed to produce research information about the effectiveness, costs, and broader impact of health technologies for those who use, manage and provide care in the NHS;
- Public Health Research (PHR[10]) – looks at the benefits, costs and acceptability of public health interventions (for example prevention of obesity in children and speed humps for the prevention of road traffic accidents).

As well as providing direct funding for research, the NIHR also helps make the NHS a great environment for clinical research. Many NIHR funding streams are based on the priorities and questions that patients, carers and their representatives have identified in Priority Setting Partnerships.[11] All NIHR funded research needs to include 'All NIHresearchers are encouraged to include patients in the design of their research, to ensure it will be practical for patients to take part, and that the outcomes being assessed are relevant to patients. The NIHR Clinical Research Network,[12] allows research to take place in all NHS trusts with minimal delays.

Patient groups can get involved in a number of different ways:

- As patient representatives in the PPI activities related to a research project;[13,14]
- By telling their patient group that a study is open to recruitment (eg Asthma UK[15] or MND Association[16]);
- By taking part in a priority setting partnership,[17] or sending in research questions to feed into the research commissioning process.[18]

Technology Strategy Board

The Technology Strategy Board was set up in 2004 to support the translation of research ideas generated in universities into new products by working closely with industry. As well as funding alone, the Technology Strategy Board works with the Medical Research Council on a number of funding streams.

Areas of funding include:

- Biomedical Catalyst and feasibility funds[19] – allows companies to investigate the feasibility of new ideas and prove the concept;
- Collaborative grants[20] – theme specific funding for partnerships between business and academia, to reduce financial and technical risk and encourage the exchange of knowledge;
- Smart scheme[21] – mco-funding for UK-based small companies to carry out R&D projects which could lead to successful new products, processes and services.

The Technology Strategy Board also funds not-for profit centres that help specific aspects of the translation and adoption of research. For example, the cell therapy catapult,[22] centre is working with academic and commercial organisations to develop new cell therapies that are safe, effective and cost-effective to manufacture.

The **Assisted Living Platform**[23] helps businesses to deliver new technologies and services for independent living. This includes Dallas – the Delivering Assisted Living Lifestyles at Scale programme.

Patient groups can get involved in a number of different ways:

Patient groups can interact with The Technology Strategy Board via their links with academic researchers and with commercial organisations. Patient organisations can be partners in applications for funding.

Engineering and Physical Science Research Council

The Engineering and Physical Science Research Council (EPSRC) is interested in the basic research that underpins the healthcare and life sciences sectors by creating new techniques and technologies. The 'Healthcare Technologies'[24] theme aims to accelerate translation of funded research through to products and practices and is focused on developing new treatments and technologies including diagnosis.

Patient groups can get involved in a EPSRC funded research by:

- Encouraging researchers by identifying areas of unmet need where technological research can make a difference.

Statutory funding outside the UK

Research is an international endeavor, particularly in rare conditions, where patient populations are small, and expertise is widely spread. Patient groups should also be aware of the European and US statutory funding streams that may be relevant to them or their researchers (see chapter about large scale (public) funding for clinical trials).

European IMI funding

The Innovative Medicines Initiative (IMI) was set up in 2007 and is jointly funded by the European Union and the European pharmaceutical industry (EFPIA). It aims to speed up the development of better and safer medicines by encouraging broad collaboration between networks of pharmaceutical companies, small- and medium-sized enterprises, patient organisations, regulatory agencies, and academics.

Now in its second phase, IMI funding[25,26] is focusing on increasing the success rate of medicines insclinical trials and developing new and approvedof medicines ins, and 11 disease areas including arthritis, cancer, diabetes, auto immune, respiratory, neurological, orphan and neurodegenerative diseases.

Calls for proposals are published on the IMI website,[27] where all interested parties from academia, small- and medium-sized enterprises (SMEs), patient organisations, regulatory agencies, large non-EFPIA companies etc. are invited to form consortia and to submit an Expression of Interest in response to the call.

What charities can do:

Charities can take part in consortia,[28] or bring groups together to develop a consortium.

References

1 http://www.mrc.ac.uk/skills-careers/fellowships/

2 http://www.mrc.ac.uk/funding/how-we-fund-research/research-grant/

3 http://www.mrc.ac.uk/funding/browse/developmental-pathway-funding-scheme/

4 http://www.mrc.ac.uk/research/initiatives/experimental-medicine/

5 http://www.mrc.ac.uk/skills-careers/fellowships/clinical-fel-

lowships/jointly-funded-clinical-research-training-fellow-ship/

6 http://www.ccf.nihr.ac.uk/PGfAR/Pages/Home.aspx

7 http://www.ccf.nihr.ac.uk/RfPB/Pages/home.aspx

8 http://www.ccf.nihr.ac.uk/i4i/Pages/Home.aspx/

9 http://www.nets.nihr.ac.uk/programmes/hta

10 http://www.nets.nihr.ac.uk/programmes/phr

11 http://www.lindalliance.org/Priority%20Setting%20Members.asp

12 http://www.crn.nihr.ac.uk

13 http://www.peopleinresearch.org/view-opportunities/

14 http://www.ccf.nihr.ac.uk/RfPB/PPI/Pages/PatientsandPublic.aspx

15 http://www.asthma.org.uk/volunteer-help-us-with-our-research

16 http://www.mndassociation.org/research/MND+research+and+you/Get+involved+in+research

17 http://www.lindalliance.org/Priority%20Setting%20Members.asp

18 http://www.nets.nihr.ac.uk/identifying-research/make-a-suggestion

19 https://www.innovateuk.org/-/biomedical-catalyst

20 https://www.innovateuk.org/-/collaborative-r-d

21 https://www.innovateuk.org/-/smart

22 https://ct.catapult.org.uk/

23 https://connect.innovateuk.org/web/assisted-living-innovation-platform-alip

24 http://www.epsrc.ac.uk/research/ourportfolio/themes/

healthcaretechnologies/

25 http://www.imi.europa.eu/content/imi-2

26 https://www.youtube.com/playlist?list=PLvrEEDAAI_
jFF0fSLckLaTAgXVww8AKEt

27 http://www.imi.europa.eu/content/future-topics

28 http://www.imi.europa.eu/content/partner-search

Chapter 10

Fund a Cure: Crowdfunding for Rare Diseases

Barry James
The Crowdfunding Centre

Flóra Raffai
Findacure

Oliver Timmis
AKU Society

Olivier Menzel
BLACKSWAN Foundation

Introduction

New Economic Model – Huge Potential… Changing What's Possible

Crowdfunding is an exciting new way for people to come together to get things done – often important things that would just not have been possible before. This can be a community project, launching a new business, or funding a cause or objective. If you can find enough people prepared to contribute then you can get the funds you need for your project – and more.

It is a 'child' of social media, with its core online. This makes it easier to keep in touch, foster the interest of your crowd, and get them engaged enough to contribute and become a part of what you are doing. Because crowdfunding, as you will discover later in this chapter, is just as much about the crowd as it is about the funding.

It is about working with the small group of supporters you have, nurturing and growing that crowd by engaging them. Generating more and more interest and, through and with them, reaching out to their circle of friends and engaging their interest – growing your crowd.

This is a resurgence of a natural process of community that has been submerged by our busy and fragmented lives, where these days, families and communities are often spread over many cities or countries. Social media allows closer, more frequent, contact to be re-established and is a natural way for people to keep up to date with what is going on in each other's lives.

A crowdfunding campaign adds a focus that encourages and enables people to come together around a clear, shared, objective and so helps create and bolster a sense of shared endeavour and community.

Which is why it is such a powerful new approach, and a natural fit for those who care about rare diseases and those who suffer from them.

It is a powerful counterbalance too. Over recent decades as corporate forces have made medicine and the global pharma industry more commercially focused, thinking and planning have been increasingly driven by 'best use' of capital employed and ROI (Return on Investment). Those suffering from rarer diseases have too often been left aside, or behind, when treatments are inevitably viewed as less profitable and therefore less viable in this highly competitive, financially driven, environment.

Crowdfunding brings a different, more diverse, economic model, better suited here because it can successfully fund anything that enough people care about. It does not need to create larger and larger 'markets' for fewer and fewer behemoths to 'compete' over. Instead, it can build small but thriving communities around a need or an idea.

This is why crowdfunding (specifically 'rewards' crowdfunding) is revolutionising innovation more generally. A brief look at the projects past and present on thecrowdfundingcentre.com is more than enough to convince the most hardened of cynics that we are now seeing an explosion of new ideas, embodied in new products, becoming real and viable. The vast majority of which would never have been created in a corporate environment. Those that made it out of the lab would probably never have made it to market, past the intensive, competitive selection processes governed by corporate priorities.

Crowdfunding throws open the doors and puts the initiative back with people who care enough to act. With communities that can come together to do the things that matter to *them*.

Which is why we were excited to play a small part in the campaigns documented on the following pages. And why we are yet more excited by the myriad possibilities they offer to others. They are truly pioneers, trail-blazers, proving this new model in a new way and showing the way forward. There is much yet to explore and discover – much that can change the way patients are treated, research is commissioned and done, treatments created and marketed, and carers supported and involved – and probably much else.

We will hear from three ground-breaking projects. Firstly Flóra, who works at Findacure, a charity building the fundamental disease community to accelerate research and develop treatments. She will explain the preparation that went into the "Fundamental Disease: It's Time to Care" Indiegogo campaign. Oliver from a patient group, the AKU Society, will discuss how to maintain a campaign, with examples from their "Help Us Cure Black Bone Disease" campaign. Then, we will hear from Olivier, who created the BLACKSWAN Foundation, who will explain new methods of crowdfunding being pioneered with their RE(ACT) Community.

But, as the old Chinese proverb has it, 'the journey of a thousand miles starts with but a single step'. So it is with your project. The experience and advice you find here will, I think, open new ways for many a journey to happen and will help make the early steps surer and more rewarding. They are practical – and will give you the chance to think more deeply about your own needs, those of your community and those they support and care for.

They will also, I believe, open up a whole new way for caring, support, research, invention, innovation, treatments and much more to be supported and funded. The next step is yours.

Planning Your Campaign

Flóra Raffai
Findacure

On April 28th 2014, we launched our crowdfunding campaign "Fundamental Diseases: It's Time To Care" on the Indiegogo platform, with the aim of raising $25,000 in 53 days. The money was to go towards developing training workshops and an online toolkit covering information about important issues for fundamental disease patients and patient groups. We managed to beat our target and raise $29,200 from 182 donations from 15 countries.

While the campaign itself lasted just over seven weeks, planning for the campaign started back in November 2013. During these five months, we learned a lot of lessons on how to successfully prepare a crowdfunding campaign.

Pick the right project

It is important to distinguish between community fundraising and crowdfunding. In community fundraising, supporters donate to the charity and to the idea that charity represents, whether it be curing a type of cancer or helping children in a war-torn country. In crowdfunding, supporters donate to people and to a specific project. There needs to be a concrete project where supporters can see their donations directly helping and making a real difference. General appeals are usually not successful, there needs to be a proof of concept, proof that the organisation has put in work to get to the stage where they need a final push of funding to fully launch.

Part of deciding on the project is setting your funding target. While it may seem appealing to set the target as high as possible, this would not be wise. Instead, it is better to set a target amount lower than the amount needed to completely fund your project. This target can be achieved earlier in the campaign, making your campaign appear highly successful and strongly supported. People will continue to give, at which point you can set a 'stretch' target which can be the total amount needed to fund your project.

Build a strong team

Crowdfunding campaigns consume a lot of time and require a lot of creativity to appeal to supporters in new ways. The team needs to include individuals with different backgrounds to channel new ideas and approach the campaign from different angles. Additionally, research has shown that campaigns with more than two team members usually raise more funds as potential supporters are reassured by a team backing an idea rather than just a few individuals.[1]

Do your research

The number of crowdfunding platforms in existence has rapidly increased over the past few years, with several interest-specific platforms forming. A critical step in the planning of a campaign is picking the platform on which to run it. Multi-interest platforms, like Kickstarter and Indiegogo, are good for reaching large crowds, but there is a lot of competition for the attention for that crowd. Smaller, interest specific platforms may not draw as many people to your campaign, but you have a higher chance that those who do come across your campaign will donate. Test each platform by finding campaigns similar to yours to see how successful the ideas have been in generating support.

Another aspect to consider in choosing your platform are their stance on rewards and flexible funding. Many crowdfunding platforms are rewards-based, where supporters receive a 'perk' in exchange for donations. These rewards can be quite costly and remove a large portion of your final fundraised total. If you decide to launch a campaign that gives rewards, be sure to budget out the cost of each reward and set your fundraising target accordingly. The other policy that should be checked before choosing a platform is their policy on flexible funding; whether they allow you to keep what you have raised, regardless of your target or if it is an 'all-or-nothing' system. Although flexible funding options come with higher fees if you do not reach your target, it is useful to have this in place as you still get some money for your efforts, instead of losing it all, even if you only needed one more pound to get to your target.

Nail your video

The next step is developing a strong message for your campaign, and the best way to convey this message is through a campaign video. It has been shown that campaigns that have a video are 147% more likely to achieve their target than those that do not have a video.[2] The best videos are those that begin with an emotive and heartfelt story, which then branches into a narrative about the project itself. It is important that this video is not treated like a general TV advert. It has to be direct and involve a personal appeal to those on the platform. You need to hone your message to fit within two to three minutes, grabbing the attention of the viewer in the first 30 seconds.[3]

As the video is such a crucial part of a campaign, many decide to hire a professional filming team to develop it for them. While this does have its benefits, it comes with a high price tag. For the Findacure campaign, we decided to take an alternative route and purchase our own camera equipment. We reasoned that not only would we be able to film the main video, we would then be able to create interesting updates throughout the campaign, and use the equipment for other charity functions. Using a bit of free editing equipment, we were able to create a professional looking video for a fraction of the cost that hiring a team would have entailed.

Time it

Crowdfunding is all about a sense of urgency, that you have a limited time to raise a lot of money for a great project. Therefore you need to pick a period of time that allows you to convey this sense of urgency, but still allows you to generate donations. Schedule your campaign for less than 30 days, and you will not have given yourself enough time to create momentum. Schedule it any longer than 60 days, and people will stop paying interest.

Additionally, when deciding on the period for your campaign to run, arrange it around key dates that are important to your project. As the Findacure campaign was crowdfunding to run patient workshops, we made sure to time it around one of our patient workshops to demonstrate our ability to deliver our campaign project. We also planned the campaign dates to coincide with conferences such as the European Conference on Rare Diseases and Orphan Products 2014, to ensure we would be able to advertise the campaign among an interested audience. Identify similar events for your project, and time your campaign around it.

Create a clear plan of action

A key mistake made by newcomers to crowdfunding is simply launching their campaign and then leaving it on the platform, waiting for donations. This method does not work. You need to constantly push the campaign among your network, and continually update your page to make it engaging to those who are on the fence about donating.

In our campaign preparation, we created a schedule of weekly updates, delegating among the team who was going to write what, about what, and when it would be uploaded. This gave time for everyone to write and during the campaign gave the image to our followers that we were very dedicated to our campaign and constantly working on it.

Prime your network

The final step in your planning is to prime your network. To run a successful campaign, it is advisable for you to generate 30% of your donations from your existing network.[4] Make sure in the run up to the launch of your campaign, you create a buzz through engaging your social media networks with a custom hashtag and frequent messages counting down to the launch day. Each day, reveal a little bit more about your campaign, such as a reward or your logo, to get your followers talking and sharing with their extended networks. Additionally, email your core contacts, explaining the aim of the campaign and have them commit to donating on the launch day. By getting a large influx of donations in the first few days, you will create the perception that your campaign is an innovative project with lots of support, which will attract new supporters to join your crowd.

Maintaining your campaign

Oliver Timmis
AKU Society

In the last section, Flóra explained how at Findacure, she planned a crowdfunding campaign. It is vital to be prepared for the work ahead, and in this section, I will cover how to maintain your campaign.

Why crowdfunding was right for AKU

In 2013, my charity, the AKU Society launched an Indiegogo campaign called "Help Us Cure Black Bone Disease". We needed the funding to enable us to support ongoing clinical trials called DevelopAKUre. These trials may offer the best hope for treatment of AKU patients. The clinical aspects of the trials are funded by the European Commission. However, as the patient group involved, we lead on the patient support and so needed funding to help us pay for patient travel, patient workshops, communications with patients (especially for translations to allow us to speak to foreign patients), and help setting up new sister societies. A great example of the work the funding allowed us to do was to form better links with the clinical site in Slovakia, find a band of enthusiastic patients and supporters who wanted to do more, and help them form the brand new AKU Society Slovakia. This group is now providing local support to more than 30 Slovak patients. We hope that this level of care will ensure that our trials have the best chances of success.

This chapter will look at the methods we used to make sure that the campaign, once launched, gained and grew in momentum to eventually hit our target.

Updates

Updates are by far the most important tool a crowdfunding campaign has to ensure success. And it amazes me how many campaigns completely ignore them! A recent article published by Charity Comms explained that 'Campaigns that update at least three times on Indiegogo raise on average 239% more than campaigns that update twice or less'.[5] The AKU Campaign lasted 44 days (31 August 2013 – 20 October 2013)[6] and over that time we sent out 30 updates, with a couple more after the campaign ended.

I would recommend sending at least two to three updates per week. They are key for motivating people to donate:

1. To turn 'watchers' into donors: Most campaigns will have 'watchers'; people that will follow the campaign sometimes for weeks and only donate when they see it is worthwhile. This can be useful, as often it means a campaign will get a surge of donations in the last few days when the watchers are encouraged to donate before time runs out. However, as

a campaign organiser, it is your job to ensure they do not lose interest on the way.

2. To turn donors into campaigners: Once a supporter has donated, they are still a very useful resource. Excellent updates, with good reasons to care about the campaign can turn these donors into campaigners for you; willing to share the campaign with their family and friends and widen the network of people you can interact with.

Additionally, updates can be used to attract support from those who cannot donate. I am from a rare disease charity, and many of our patients are physically unable to work. That means that many cannot afford to donate to a crowdfunding campaign. They still wanted to be involved and so, we created the "Help Us Cure Black Bone Disease" photo competition. We made a simple poster and asked supporters to take a picture with them holding it up. It is a great way for supporters to remain involved, and we received hundreds of photos from across the world. It also directly helped the campaign, helping us spread word of the campaign and attracting more potential donors.

For the end of our campaign, we decided to increase the speed of updates. For the last 10 days, we released an update every day, with an infographic explaining a fact about the AKU Society (for example, 10: the number of years since the AKU Society launched, 7: the number of countries involved in the clinical trials, and 4: the number of diagnostic symptoms in AKU).

Media work

The key to raising donations is increasing your network of contacts. Updates are great for this, however, the most effective method we have used is working with the media. We had some contact with reporters before the campaign launched, and so primed them before starting. We prepared a press release for around a fortnight after launch.[7]

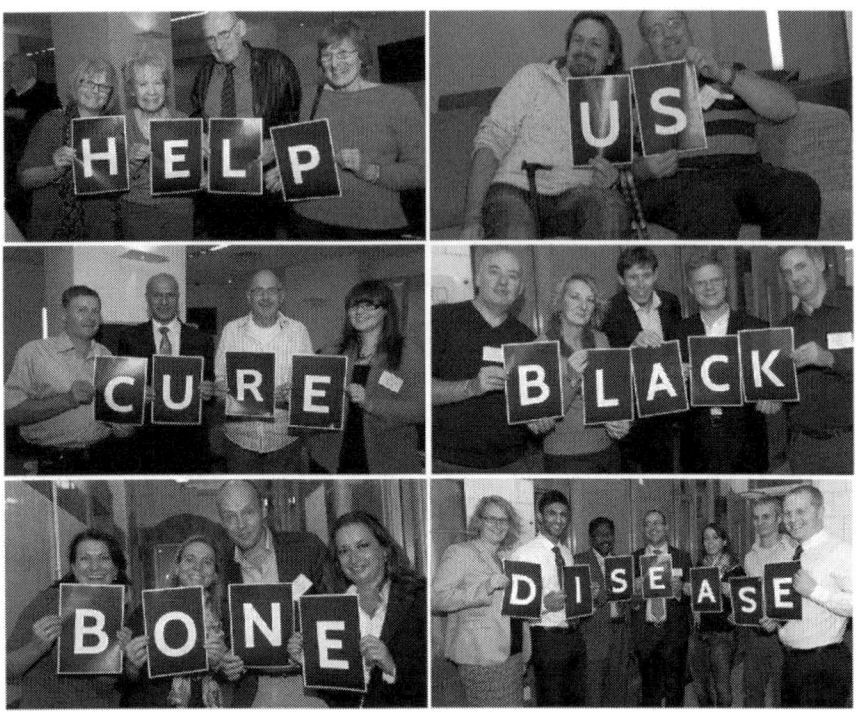

Collage of "Help Us Cure Black Bone Disease" photos

This press release led to several great promotions, including features on BBC Radio 5 Live,[8] The Daily Mail,[9] The Telegraph[10] and The Mirror.[11]

At the end of the campaign, we followed up with another press release.[12] The key is to maximise your promotion in a crowdfunding campaign. Rare disease charities have few chances to publicise, so emphasise your campaign at every opportunity.

Serendipitous

The one aspect you cannot plan for in a crowdfunding campaign is the serendipitous fundraising. A great example from the AKU campaign is from a family affected by AKU in Canada. Pam Mann is the mother of a young AKU patient and, as a high school teacher, got her whole class involved. They raised money through bake sales, volleyball game tickets, and a Delta Ice Hawks hockey game.

There are plenty of other examples, including a UK family that run a weekly curry night on a Friday with donations coming to the campaign. This kind of support is amazing, and truly helped us achieve our goal. However, it is also completely spontaneous.

Follow-up

It is important to maintain the support. Not only as a reward for supporting the campaign, but also to encourage your supporter base to retain interest if you want to move into a second campaign. Make sure that the perks (rewards) are sent out, and send out additional updates. The donors that have supported your campaign throughout, and spread word to their family and friends, will want to know if the funding was useful, and if it led to the project you aimed to fund. Give them updates, letting them know what happened next.

However, it is important to remember that crowdfunding is not just about the money. For us, and for many rare disease charities, it is also an effective way of raising awareness of your disease, and even of finding patients. The AKU campaign led to the identification of several new patients; people that may not have found the support they needed without our campaign.

The RE(ACT) Community: the first online platform for crowdfunding in rare disease research

Olivier Menzel
BLACKSWAN Foundation

The BLACKSWAN is a Swiss Foundation created to support research on rare and orphan diseases in Switzerland and worldwide. Its principal mission is to collect funds for research projects but also to improve the public awareness of rare and orphan diseases by promoting exchange of information and public campaigns.

Rare diseases (RDs) are characterised by their low prevalence (less than 1 in 2,000) and their heterogeneity. Because RD patients are a minority, there is a lack of public knowledge and these diseases do not represent a public health priority, despite the fact that taken all together, RDs affect about 30 million people in Europe. The market is so narrow for each disease, that the pharmaceutical industry is often reticent to invest in research and to develop treatments. Consequently, little research is performed and the existing research efforts are still scattered and implemented with little coordination between laboratories.

This lack of coordination is particularly detrimental to the increase of knowledge and to the delivery of new therapies, especially in this field, where the resources are very limited and the patient population is small for each disease. There is therefore an urgent need to increase international cooperation in scientific research on RDs. For this reason the BLACKSWAN Foundation promotes the RE(ACT) Initiative with the aim of boosting research and facilitating the discovery of new molecules and therapies for millions of patients.

The Initiative is structured on two main axes: The RE(ACT) Congress and the online RE(ACT) Community. Their mission is to strengthen the synergies between researchers and other stakeholders that are related to different extents with rare and orphan diseases. The RE(ACT) Congress is organized every two years and brings together world leaders and young scientists from stem cell, cell biology, gene therapy, human genetic, or therapeutic applications to present state-of-the-art research, to discuss results and to exchange ideas. The online RE(ACT) Community facilitates continuous collaboration between researchers on projects, as well as communication amongst patients and between patients and researchers; information gathering; crowdfunding for research projects; and promotes opportunities to optimize synergies between stakeholders, from patient organizations to academic institutions, centres of expertise, the health industry, regulators and policy makers.

The main and most critical factor to the success of the RE(ACT) Community is the capability of stimulating a massive engagement and participation of stakeholders from all over the world. This risk can be solved thanks to strong digital marketing and PR activity and to intensive partner's involvement and collaboration. To this extent, the BLACKSWAN Foundation has established important partnerships with rare disease organizations, like Eurordis, E-Rare, Findacure and the *Foundation Maladies Rares*. A marketing and PR plan will contribute to populate the Community thanks to the support of partners, the use of social networks, digital marketing and web monitoring.

The RE(ACT) Community (www.react-community.org) brings together all stakeholders on the same platform and gives researchers the possibility to raise funds for their projects through a crowdfunding mechanism and the use of social media. An analysis conducted through a survey shows a large interest, especially from researchers and patients, to join the RE(ACT) Community and use this innovative way to fund research. It is also evident from the survey that rare disease stakeholders are looking for effective tools to promote new funding opportunities and new partnerships for scientific collaboration. The RE(ACT) Community is the answer to their quest.

How it works:

The online RE(ACT) Community is organized around four main axes dedicated to research on rare and orphan diseases: Learn, Meet, Share and Support. Learn from the knowledge and experience of other researchers and patients; meet other researchers and facilitate the exchange of information between researchers and patients; share scientific knowledge and experience; and financially support research projects.

The majority of the interactions are developed around the "Disease Dossiers". Each Disease Dossier includes the name of the disease, a description of the disease and its symptoms, possible research projects ready for funding and prospective amount of donations received for a project, information on scientific publications and research, patients' experiences, names of researchers and patients following the disease.

Knowledge Sharing

A follower (researcher, patient or supporter) can participate in one or more Disease Dossiers and receive alerts with specific information. Every member also receives a newsletter with information on relevant studies, conferences, meetings, calls for proposals, grants, and other information related to the topic.

The RE(ACT) Community facilitates connections and knowledge sharing among researchers that are not necessarily working on the same rare disease, but that have common scientific interests. Upon registration to the Community, researchers can provide specific information that will help identify potential mutual interests with other members.

Financial support of research

The RE(ACT) Community allows three different types of donation via crowdfunding: to projects, to a disease or to the RE(ACT) Community.

Support to Projects:

Research projects declared eligible for funding by the RE(ACT) and BLACKSWAN Foundation Scientific Advisory Board are associated to a Disease Dossier. They are also visible on a specific section of the platform dedicated to crowdfunding ("Projects" page). Once the Scientific Advisory Board approves a project, another criterion is required for funding entitlement: a minimum number of followers on the Disease Dossier. This additional criterion prevents the dispersion of small donations through a large variety of research projects.

All research projects must pass though the screening of the Scientific Advisory Board, which determines the status of an "eligible project" or rejects the project application. The Scientific Advisory Board works therefore as a "guarantor" of the quality and honesty of the researcher referent.

Every project folder ready for funding contains the following information: description and expected results; team of researchers; projects milestones; distance to funding target; updates from the team of researchers; and a list of backers/supporters. By accessing the Project Folder, users can enter a donation and monitor the evolution of the project through researchers' updates and published results showing the different stages and the work in progress.

The Secretariat of the RE(ACT) Community provides the services of media relations for the promotion of the selected research projects throughout their life cycle (from the beginning of the crowdfunding to the communication of the research results).

Support to a Disease:

In the event that a "Disease Dossier" receives a donation and reaches the threshold of interest (15 followers) before there is an "eligible project" associated with the dossier, the BLACK-SWAN Foundation proceeds in the collection and selection of proposals.

Support to the RE(ACT) Community:

It is possible to donate directly to the RE(ACT) Community to support its work. Donations to the Community facilitate cooperation on rare diseases research worldwide and move research forward.

The promotion of both projects and Disease Dossiers can be facilitated by the use of social media and "social plugins". These allow a follower to sensitize his network of friends and acquaintances to improve awareness of specific research and reach more supporters.

Conclusion

Barry James
The Crowdfunding Centre

As you see, crowdfunding has many uses and advantages, helping meet needs that have proved difficult or impossible to fund or support. These include:

- Funding:
- Treatment trials
- Research
- Innovation
- Information gathering
- Community activities and events
- Bringing patients and carers together who otherwise would never meet
- Growing the crowd who care – and will contribute or act on it
- Providing a route for carers and contributors to made a difference, be and feel a part of the process

Crowdfunding fits very well with 'open innovation' and the crowdsourcing of ideas and solutions, as the RE(ACT) Community is showing. It is itself a powerful new opportunity, brought about by social media and the internet and which we have yet to learn how we might properly exploit. What is for sure is that there is a very long way to go.

These are all parts of the emerging 'sharing economy', which is driven by innovation, demand and need, rather than purely ROI and economic considerations. What has been called the 'democratisation of finance' and 'the third industrial revolution' is driven by the crowd and can support many, many, more ventures, social and commercial, charitable and non-profit, than have ever before been possible. This is good news for the 3.5 million rare disease patients in the UK and the 30 million in Europe. It is good news for those who care about them, because it means that the future – and their future – is no longer so much in the hands of those who care first, mostly or exclusively about ROI. The doors are open for entrepreneurs of all kinds to re-shape our world in many different ways, powered and guided by crowds large and small.

Pioneers, like those here, are showing the way, but from our unique vantage point at The Crowdfunding Centre, I can tell you that this is the tip of a fast-growing iceberg; growing as people like you and I start to realise the potential – and act on it.

Crowdfunding takes various forms, including:

- 'Rewards' crowdfunding (or seed crowdfunding as I prefer to call it)
- Donations crowdfunding
- Equity crowdfunding

All can and will be used to power this revolution, which is as much about collaboration, inclusion and participation as it is about financial contributions.

We no longer have to wait – or persuade governments or a huge corporate – to get things started. The pioneers are showing us that by coming together we can MAKE THINGS HAPPEN! What we have seen is just a beginning.

Someone, in a University, asked me recently of whom he must ask permission to start a crowdfund. The answer, of course, is no-one. The crowd will guide and tell you whether you are on track or not; not just by funding you but with feedback, wisdom, ideas and other support. However, it needs people like you to make a start – strike a spark.

So the doors are open. For the right ideas, the support is out there. The future belongs to the crowd and to people like you who will work with us to make good things happen.

Barry James, The Crowdfunding Centre
(Barry.James@TheCrowdfundingCentre.com)

Flóra Raffai, Findacure (flora@findacure.org.uk)

Oliver Timmis, AKU Society (oliver@akusociety.org)

Olivier Menzel, BLACKSWAN Foundation (olivier.menzel@blackswanfoundation.ch)

References

1 Indiegogo (2013). Field Guide for Campaign Owners, 8.

2 Sponsorcraft. (2013). The Crowdfunding Handbook: A guide to running your campaign. 11.

3 Outlaw, S. (2013). How to Use Video to Promote Your Crowdfunding Campaign. Entrepreneur. (Accessed 15 July 2015). http://www.entrepreneur.com/article/228547

4 Indiegogo (2013). Field Guide for Campaign Owners, 11.

5 How to run a successful crowdfunding campaign. Charity Comms (Accessed 15 July 2015). http://www.charitycomms. org.uk/articles/how-to-run-a-successful-crowdfunding-cam-paign

6 Help Us Cure Black Bone Disease. Indiegogo. (Accessed 15 July 2015) https://www.indiegogo.com/projects/ cure-black-bone-disease#activity

7 One man's fight to save his sons from a rare and debilitat-ing disease. AKU Society 11 Sept 2013. (Accessed 15 July 2015). http://www.akusociety.org/aku-in-the-news/one-man-s-fight-to-save-his-sons-from-a-rare-and-debilitating-disease

8 Dad quits job to find disease cure for two sons. BBC Radio 5 Live, 3 Oct 2013. (Accessed 15 July 2015). http://www. bbc.co.uk/news/uk-24382011

9 Father gives up job to research cure for rare disease that is turning his sons' bones, eyeballs and sweat BLACK. Daily Mail, 4 Oct 2013. (Accessed 15 July 2015). http://www. dailymail.co.uk/health/article-2443833/Father-gives-job-re-

search-cure-rare-disease-turning-sons-bones-eyeballs-sweat-BLACK.html

10 Father discovers cure for sons' rare genetic disease. The Telegraph, 3 Oct 2013. (Accessed 15 July 2015). http://www.telegraph.co.uk/health/healthnews/10352631/Father-discovers-cure-for-sons-rare-genetic-disease.html

11 Dad quits job to find cure for his two sons' rare genetic disease. The Mirror, 3 Oct 2013. (Accessed 15 July 2015). http://www.mirror.co.uk/news/uk-news/dad-nick-sireau-quits-job-2332478

12 Patient group crowdfunds $120,000 for trial to treat Black Bone Disease. AKU Society 31 Oct 2013. (Accessed 15 July 2015). http://www.akusociety.org/aku-in-the-news/patient-group-crowdfunds-120-000-for-trial-to-treat-black-bone-disease

Chapter 11

Collaborative Grants for Rare Disease Research: Practical Thinking to Win Bids

Ritchie Head*†, Christina Olsen*†, Marc van de Craen*† and Nick Rhodes‡

*Ceratium Limited, †Biotechsubsidy Group and ‡University of Liverpool

Grant Funding- Why Bother?

Research and Innovation grant funding divides opinion. Put simply, are grants a brilliant source of funding to help develop the next therapy, or a source of overwhelming administration in exchange for a modest subsidy? There are those vehemently opposed to the whole idea of accessing grants as simply too much trouble, citing hard-working colleagues swamped by reporting and regulations losing innovative zeal whilst bowing to bureaucrats. In the opposite corner are the bright-eyed evangelists with tales of great partnerships and funding that really makes things happen, translating science to therapy.

In reality the truth lies somewhere in the middle so it is important to ensure a balanced view. Applying for large grants requires hard work and, in the case of collaborative projects, the building of a highly skilled partnership. These projects can lead to excellent rewards including: new knowledge on diseases, better understanding of the safety and efficacy of therapies, opportunities to adopt good practice, new networks and long term benefits through working relationships with excellent partners.

There is of course administration linked to grant funding, but in general, a calm well organised approach and applying common sense can reduce the burden hugely.

In our experience, often the most vocal critics of grant programmes are people who have not succeeded or have not tried to win funding. In contrast, those who have been successful tend to apply for further funding, finding the positives of grant funding far outweigh the negatives.

In this chapter, we look at how grants are being used to support rare diseases research and use the European Commission's Horizon 2020 programme as a case study to provide examples of practical steps to have a successful application.

Grant funding used effectively is a catalyst for change

Globally, the small, dispersed patient populations, limited scientific understanding of many rare diseases, absence of suitable diagnostics and a lack of medical expertise and public awareness, coupled with the small market size of orphan diseases and perceived limited economic payback have hindered investment in orphan drug development by the commercial pharmaceutical sector. These challenges make rare disease research an excellent target for grant funding. Public sector bodies, many patient advocacy groups and private sector foundations provide grant funding programmes to overcome these barriers and encourage projects that will innovate and develop new interventions and better drugs. But funders also require a consensus of approach, to ensure precious financial resources are used effectively and that knowledge and skills are shared rather than duplicated. The role of a grant should be to accelerate activity to better develop therapies, especially in areas that may be important but not necessarily economically viable.

Policy driven Grant Funding Stimulating Translational Research for Rare Diseases

For the rare disease community at present the main focus is new therapies, better treatment regimens, and a deeper understanding of the disease and potential diagnostics. In Europe rare diseases are estimated to affect 30-40 million people, in the US 25-30 million Americans and globally, rare diseases are estimated to affect around 350 million people and are responsible for 35% of deaths within the first year of life.[1] Currently, 6000-8000 diseases are considered to be rare, affecting less than 5 in every 10,000 people. Most of these diseases have a genetic origin, but some are caused by infections, allergies or environmental factors.

The Rare Disease area has a strong policy background to combat these challenges. Projects funded by public bodies at National, European or International level typically need to be addressing policy priorities that have been developed to target perceived shortcomings in the availability of treatments for rare diseases.

In 2007, the European Commission's Health and Consumer Directorate-General (DG SANCO) undertook a large consultation exercise for the Commission Communication on Rare Diseases. The EC adopted the 'Communication on Rare Diseases: Europe's Challenges' in 2008 followed by a proposal for a European Council Recommendation on an action in the field of rare diseases. This was adopted in June 2009. The two documents establish a comprehensive, integrated strategy on issues including diagnosis, treatment and care for rare disease patients throughout Europe.

The US Congress enacted the Orphan Drug Act of 1983. This provides incentives to sponsors of orphan drugs including market exclusivity for 7 years. The EMA Orphan Drug Designation similarly provides 10 years market exclusivity. The EC and US administrations provide grants for drug development and supporting the rare disease communities. In the US, there is fast-track approval of drugs indicated for rare diseases and further financial incentives. These interventions appear to have been successful. In the US before 1983 only 10 new drugs for rare diseases were developed by the pharmaceutical industry (NORD 2014).[2,3] According to Fagnan et al (2015), the FDA database now indicates that 221 orphan-designated products received FDA approval over the decade ending November 2014.[4]

Following changes in legislation in recent years, the pharmaceutical industry has increased focus on rare diseases. Global incentives and the policy drivers have helped, but finding adequate funding opportunities remains a significant hurdle. Rare Disease UK reports researchers have felt there was an uneven playing field in funding for rare diseases compared to more commercially viable disease areas. Addressing the need for cohesive and high profile funding, the International Rare Disease Research Consortium (IRDiRC) (http://www.irdirc.org) was launched in 2011. This has brought international funders together within the IRDiRC collaboration to develop a programme of funding to optimise the effectiveness and efficiency of the grant funding available. The funders invest a minimum of $10 million in rare disease research programs over a period of 5 years. Consequently, the IRDiRC website is an excellent place for researchers or patient groups to identify funding opportunities for their rare disease project. Table 1 highlights some of the main funds. Ideally, the IRDiRC also brings patients and researchers together in novel rare disease projects. The highest profile objective for the IRDiRC consortium has been the global drive to deliver 200 new therapies for rare diseases by 2020 and accompanying diagnostics for most of them. The EC also co-funds E-Rare-3 to strengthen collaboration between EU countries on rare diseases.

For a rare disease where little is known about the aetiology of the disease, most research is up-stream in an academic environment needing basic research grant funding. Typically, when the molecular origin of a rare disease has been identified, the race begins to identify and develop medicines that counteract the origin of the disease. Increasingly, biotech companies have gained interest in developing rare disease therapeutics, partly due to the regulatory stimulations and subsidies governments have put in place to help bring rare disease therapeutics to the market. These reasons have encouraged some very innovative biotech companies (eg. Prosensa, apceth, ProQR Therapeutics, Unique) to target a rare disease to obtain clinical proof of concept and regulatory validation of their innovative technologies.

The EC is a major funder of such rare disease research through DG Research and Innovation. In 2015 alone €62m of grant funding was earmarked for developing new therapies for rare diseases. Under the previous Framework Programme FP7 (2007-2013) over €620m funded about 120 rare disease projects and in FP6 (2002-2006) €61m funded 18 such projects. Further downstream, between 2008 and 2013 funding from DG SANCO funded 30 rare disease projects for patients and health professionals for improved access to medical and research information, treatment centres and support groups. The third Health Programme (2014-2020) will continue to provide support on rare diseases.

Patient organisations are also active in funding promising research on their disease area. Typically these grants start with funding basic research and then progress to fund follow-on applied research. A mixed grant funding strategy can be highly effective. ReveraGen have used seed grants, project and programme grants to advance their VBP15 (Verolene) drug development using a Venture Philanthropy (VP) model.

Case Study 1–Grants in a Venture Philanthropy model to develop rare disease drugs faster and cost-effectively.

ReveraGen BioPharma uses a grant-led VP model to advance the development of the orphan drug Verolene for Duchenne Muscular Dystrophy (DMD). Support from NIH NCATS

TRND program and NIH small business grants, and funding from the US Department of Defense (CDMRP) has been complimented by financial support from 11 DMD foundations via grants and VP. They include: Foundation to Eradicate Duchenne (USA); Joining Jack (UK); Duchenne Research Fund (UK); Duchenne Children's Trust (UK); Save Our Sons (Aus); Parent Project Muscular Dystrophy (USA); Muscular Dystrophy Association (USA); Michael's Cause (USA); Pietro's Fight (USA); Alex's Wish (UK); Ryan's Quest (USA). To date $10m raised has facilitated de-risking the pipeline, preclinical studies, Phase 1 and preparation for Phase 2a clinical studies, and Verolene manufacturing optimisation.

Overall, many grant funding streams may be available for a rare disease. For example, through an extensive deskstudy, Stehr and Forkel identified 192 funding opportunities supporting research for Batten disease (Neuronal Ceroid Lipofuscinosis), and other rare diseases.[5] This highlights the need to broadly review available options and take time to identify potential grants for project development.

Are you "funding ready"?

The lure of grant funding is attractive but the scale of projects can often be 2-5 years, and the need to collaborate with multiple partners requires organisations to commit the time and resources to developing a winning bid. Preparing a project takes careful planning and considerable commitment, from identifying funding opportunities, finding partners (if collaboration is needed eg. Horizon 2020), writing the proposal, completing the necessary administration and meeting financial requirements. Decision makers must be involved early to ensure the rationale is supported. Project participation should be part of an organisation's overall strategy, with management firmly endorsing the approach and overseeing the process. An assessment of your organisation's capabilities and ambition is a useful exercise before investing time and resources in project development.

Collaborations: What is in it for us?

The rationale behind collaborative projects is that the efficient development of new products or services, for example the discovery of biomarkers, or advancing a drug development pipeline requires expertise from a range of disciplines and often the involvement of stakeholder groups and end-users. A consortium approach should show clear benefits of working together; any individual agendas need to be put aside to avoid distorting the project mission. This need for partners creates both a great opportunity and a potential barrier to participation.

Opportunity: The grant funding acts as a catalyst, bringing together experts and accelerating development through a multidisciplinary approach, combining the right skill sets with new ideas; this can also create long-term partnerships. Projects should be based on excellence, whether that is in developing infrastructures, networks, and translational pathways or more commonly scientific research and demonstration. Activities must go beyond peer review publication: this is translational and must have clear application goals to improve the quality of life of patients and offer realistic options to health care providers. The funding allows progress to be made without diluting the value of the intellectual property (IP) or existing investment.

Barriers: Working with partners is not without problems, including different working practices and culture or research interests. Simply finding partners can seem a daunting prospect for the inexperienced. Here a focus on rare disease can be an advantage, since the community is well networked and there is energy and goodwill behind the successful groups. However, the small size of a disease community can also be problematic. Competition between research groups might create barriers to cooperation, and a small group of researchers may narrow the focus of research or risk isolation. For many, finding good partners and building a really strong consortium remains challenging. This is discussed below.

Another barrier can be the perceived need to share existing IP. In fact, this should not be necessary, but access rights may be required. New IP will normally be owned by the inventor, or in the case of jointly developed IP, the ownership will be shared or an agreement reached on ownership and access rights. In Horizon 2020 projects, a Consortium Agreement is made that outlines the agreed process for managing IP, indeed this is good practice for any collaborative project. In our experience, amicable agreement between partners is normally relatively straightforward to achieve.

Find information and help available

Funding bodies typically provide online information about their grant programmes; the IRDiRC portal is a good starting point. Table 1 provides summary information of key grants. For EC Horizon 2020 and Health Programmes, this information is available from the EC Participant Portal on the Europa website. It includes:

- **Call Detail:** Topics open for funding with budget allocations; deadlines for applications;
- **Work programmes:** A description of the topic areas open for applications and the type of project structure required;
- **Guide for applicants:** Instructions for completing an application including the type of forms to be completed and the required information;
- **Evaluation Guidelines:** If funders provide a description of the evaluation process and scoring criteria, use this to guide you.

Timescales

Grant funding timescales differ. Horizon 2020 has some of the longest; normally from preparing a proposal to receiving the first payment can be 9-12 months. This funding is not a 'quick fix', although some programmes can be much quicker, three months or less. These timescales are usually acceptable since drug development pipelines require several years. The projects can often last 3-5 years co-funding key stages in the translation of a therapy from bench to clinic providing excellent opportunities to deliver advances in rare disease therapy and in some cases prevention.

Start Before the Beginning!

Funding calls come out periodically throughout the year. In Horizon 2020 there is usually one main call per year, but some areas and other funders have multiple calls or rolling programmes, that is when a call is 'always open'with various cut-off dates for evaluation (eg. H2020 SME Instrument; Eurostars; UK SMART grants). A successful grant strategy benefits from a flexible approach, the best groups are prepared to adapt and reshape their thinking to meet funder requirements. The reality of grants is that they will normally only fund part of the work required to develop a cure based on new or repurposed drugs, or undertake research to better understand the disease. Effectively, they only fund part of the jigsaw.

To be well-prepared requires that key relationships exist, most obviously between the research and clinical communities, industry and the patient groups. In addition, ideas around approaches towards a disease area should already be in a formative stage. The key benefits are:

1. Multiple organisations are looking for relevant funding options. Often University research groups are particularly well positioned to do this, supported by institutional research grants specialists or consultants;
2. When funding calls open, there is already a core group of experts in place to react quickly and begin the development of a proposal.

Developing a competitive project proposal

The application process to apply for grant funding differs between funders, reflecting their own interests, timescales and priorities. Here we use the European Commission Horizon 2020 process as a useful model, since the proposal encompasses all the main aspects a funder is likely to require from scientific and innovation excellence, to societal impact and robust management processes. Typical steps to build a strong proposal include:

STEP 1 The Idea and choice of funding

A good project starts with a great idea that is also innovative. In other words, your project needs to be doing something new such as identifying and validating novel biomarkers for diagnostics, or applying an existing technology in a new way, repurposing a drug towards a new disease for example. Ideally your innovation will create a positive change and have clear beneficiaries. Developing a new therapy for a rare disease clearly meets this criterion.

The next stage is to find suitable funding. In the realm of Rare Diseases, there is a wealth of information on funding as discussed above. But don't only look at rare disease specific calls, it may well be that other health care topic areas are also relevant and often a rare disease provides an appropriate starting point for the development of new therapeutics that have the potential for much broader applications.

STEP 2 Project idea to project plan

Funders will often have priority areas or topics that they wish to support. The challenge is to identify a grants programme suitable for your project idea. The original idea then needs to be shaped to fit precisely with a call topic area and expected impact. A well-defined topic needs to be addressed very precisely, this has the advantage that competition will be lower as fewer projects will meet the criteria. Recently the EC and others have favoured broader topic areas. This is easier to address but may also attract a greater number of competing bids. It is very important to balance the requirements of the grant call with your own requirements to ensure your ambitions are met.

STEP 3 Be the Best Consortium: Winning Friends and Influencing People

Typically, projects developing better understanding of diseases and new therapies require a range of experts that may include patient representatives, clinicians, scientists, clinical trial experts, biostatisticians, pharmacoeconomics and manufacturing specialists, and project managers. It is very important to build a strong consortium, but for many new to grant funded projects, the idea of developing such a partnership can seem very daunting. Indeed, it is cited as a key barrier to progress for new collaborative projects, but it doesn't need to be. So, where do great partners come from and how do you persuade them to work with you?

Your Networks

Begin by looking for partners from within your own organisation's networks. Patient group members often have excellent relationships with key clinicians and research hospitals, and sometimes also to research groups. Clinicians with rare disease expertise are good links to the research community, since by the nature of their role in rare disease, they are likely to have a keen professional interest in the research efforts targeting the disease. Patient Groups themselves often have a good overview of the research landscape, who the key opinion leaders are and who has progressed potential therapies. A core group forming the basis of the consortium will often emerge from these personal relationships. Ideally, this group will include some partners with grant funding experience, but most importantly each team needs a clear role and brings high quality skills and expertise. Developing a partnership in this way, using people you know or have been recommended, has the advantage that initial due diligence is achieved; you are not risking linking to some completely unknown entity.

Previous Projects

Choosing partners with a track record of success in projects is an attractive option. These teams will often be familiar with collaborative working and the culture of European and international projects. Not only do you get the technical expertise, but the partner will understand the administration required to fulfil financial and technical reporting obligations.

The EC make it relatively easy to identify previous project partners through their Europa (Cordis) website listing of Framework programme projects since 1990; Horizon 2020 projects are now being added (http://cordis.europa.eu/projects/home_en.html). Other funders also list awards on their websites, including: the National Institutes of Health (US) RePORT website (http://report.nih.gov/award/index.cfm); the Welcome Trust funded project archive (http://www.wellcome.ac.uk/Managing-a-grant/Grants-awarded/). In addition, patient advocacy groups funding projects often provide lists, eg. National Organization for Rare Disorders (NORD http://www.rarediseases.org/) in the US.

It is advisable to look at your chosen funder and see what information is available about what has already been funded as part of the 'landscape'. In addition, the Orphanet portal offers a directory of expert resources: 6600 expert clinics, 3300 medical laboratories, 20,000 professionals, ongoing research projects, clinical trials, registries, networks, technological platforms and patient organisations, in the field of rare diseases. See www.orpha.net.

Professional Networks and Associations

The Rare Disease community is extremely well served by networks. Higher profile diseases have extensive patient organisations across the globe; these can contribute to projects and will have local knowledge about clinical experts and centres of clinical knowledge. A good example is Muscular Dystrophy, where multiple groups are linked under the worldwide United Parent Projects Muscular Dystrophy (UPPMD). At the same time, TREAT-NMD, provides a more academic grouping and includes patient registries and links to centres of expertise. Many other diseases have similarly well organised and networked groups, or inspirational patient organisations that can link to partners or facilitate consortium building.

In addition to disease specific groupings, generic tools supporting networks including EURORDIS, the European alliance of patient organisations and individuals active in the field of rare diseases, and the US NORD collaboration (https://www.rareconnect.org/en) provide useful portals. These resources also provide guidance on areas such as policy that help to build a strong societal case for the research proposals.

Attend events

Funders may hold information days about a grant call, the EC run 'Health info days' close to when their calls open. One can learn about the grant programme and network with others looking at the same funding streams. This can be a useful source of new partners but be aware that other delegates are potential competitors. Academic and industry events on specific technology or disease areas can be good ways to meet academic, clinical and industry experts. Events more broadly targeting the Rare Disease community often have good representation of both patient groups, the clinical research community, funders and policy makers, providing another pool of potential partners, eg. IRDiRC conferences, the European Conference on Rare Diseases and Orphan Products; and World Orphan Drug Congresses.

Collaboration means working with partners, and in competitive research bids we need to make sure that the people within a partnership are strong and effective. We need to be clear about the qualities we want and the people to avoid.

Partner Qualities: The good, the bad and the ugly

The Good	The Bad and the Ugly
Capable and skilled expertise for project role	Unresponsive and disinterested
Demonstrate a track record	Single minded agenda not team players
Complement the other partners	Driven by grant funding not project concept
Be reliable and proactive	Mediocre skill sets
Financially stable to meet obligations	Disorganised and chaotic
Have a team work approach	Token partners – no clear role

Preparation

It is advisable to prepare for partner search activities with a clear idea of the skills and expertise you are seeking, but also with a summary of your own strengths allowing you to 'sell'your organisation as a strong partner for relevant projects. In early stage discussions it is important to be enthusiastic and offer insight into the areas and topics of interest. A 1-2 page, well thought-through project overview without giving away confidential information is an excellent way to engage potential partners. Be clear on why you are applying for the funding and how your organisation and interested parties will benefit. In the case of EC project grants there is typically a need to develop a strong pan-European consortium; the multiple countries adds complexity, but also creates a great opportunity to develop a team of international excellence and reach a larger pool of patients for trials. Even at an early stage, this can be important since the more advanced your planning the more coherent and convincing your funding proposal will be.

STEP 4 Navigating the landscape

A grant-funded project does not happen in a vacuum. It is important to understand the surrounding 'landscape'. In the case of Rare Diseases, there are multiple stakeholders, interest groups and often background research exists. In high profile rare disease areas such as Duchene Muscular Dystrophy or Cystic Fibrosis, multiple projects exist and effectively programmes of activity have developed over the years. New projects need to be clearly advancing the knowledge base and not repeating previous work. The strongest projects often have clear complementarity or synergies with existing activities, or use tools and resources developed in previous projects.

Case Study 2 – Projects to Programmes

The FP7 SCOPE-DMD project benefits from advances made in previous projects and forms part of a programme of activity contributing to advancing new therapies, clinical trials design, biomarkers and outcome measures. Overall, this advances the neuromuscular disease translational pathway.

Prosensa (NL) with leading expert centres in DMD (University of Newcastle (UK), the Institute of Myology (FR), and Leiden University Medical Centre (NL)) and industrial partner, BioSpring (DE) were awarded a grant of approximately €6 million to evaluate its exon 45-skipping drug candidate, PRO045. This project built on outcomes and exploited a translational pathway developed in the FP6 project TREAT-NMD and implemented and further validated novel biomarkers and functional outcome measures developed in TREAT-DMD and the FP7 BIO-NMD project. The project also uses Nuclear Magnetic Resonance imaging and spectroscopy (MRI and MRS) as exploratory endpoints from the FP7 project BIOIMAGE-DMD. The latter is linked to the on-going EC grant funded COST Action BM1304; 'Applications of MR imaging and spectroscopy in neuromuscular disease translational research' that shares best practice between researchers and scientists from over 16 countries.

Eurospeak

It is also important to understand the Work Programmes and funding opportunities, from not only the scientific, clinical disease focus and patient perspective, but also to have a heightened awareness of the EC policies and drivers to ensure that a project proposal addresses the political and societal priorities driving the call funding. Take time to understand and interpret this 'Eurospeak' language of the EC, and the broader context of the funding to adapt a research project if required to address the issues important to funders.

Think about where the work programme topics come from and why this topic is being funded now. There is a perception that funding is often already targeted at specific groups, and newcomers have little chance of success. In fact at the EC level, informal discussions with independent evaluators for the Framework Programmes (Horizon 2020) suggest the process is very transparent and open. When the same groups win several grants it is often because they have well-developed project ideas, can demonstrate a plan to deliver significant impact, and are in an excellent consortium. They will have made efforts to understand and address the funders' priorities, the history of the topic, if it emerged from previous project results or consultations and workshops with stakeholders or a patient and clinician lobby, and the linkage to policy background as drivers for funding. A good proposal addresses these items to a greater or lesser extent depending on the application process.

STEP 5 Writing Proposals to Win: Once upon a time....

Proposal writing has one purpose: to win funding against the competition. A winning bid tells a story that is more exciting, innovative and convincing than the opposition. Evaluators will decide they like a project within the first 2-3 pages. Writers need to **hook** the reader at this early stage by setting out clearly and concisely a very exciting and relevant programme of activity. This is best done in the final stages of writing when the project is fully worked out and an excellent summary can be constructed. Clear quantifiable specific objectives and a timescale for delivery are crucial.

Many of the grant schemes are open competitions. The level of competition and the way bids are judged differs between funding bodies. Although funders' application processes may vary, the need for research, demonstration and innovation **Excellence,** delivering state of the art results and a well-defined **Impact** to society is fundamental and requires a well-managed, cost-effective work programme delivered by high quality beneficiaries (**Implementation**). Unlike research papers this requires socioeconomic, political and scientific content supported by facts and figures to educate the evaluators. Essentially, the consortium needs to demonstrate that they have the most credibility amongst their competitors. It is not enough just to demonstrate that consortium members could deliver the research programme, but that they are the best placed to do so, and most likely to achieve the objectives.

One or Two Stages

Some funders use an expression of interest or Stage 1 proposal (eg. the EC), to identify and invite the most promising projects for a full proposal submission. In Horizon 2020, the Stage 1 proposal is a small document but writing is demanding; the consortium is required to capture the full essence of the whole project. This needs the main project parts to be worked out including the mechanisms for demonstrating that impact is delivered. Putting together large proposals is not trivial. Typically, an EC proposal can take 3-4 weeks of very hard work for the lead writers over a period of 3-6 months and may require a consortium meeting or several teleconferences to finalise the project plan. The stage 2 proposal should not differ significantly from a Stage 1 submission.

Excellent Science

The level of the science and quantity is dependent on the stage of drug or therapy development. Earlier stage projects are expected to have a high level of exciting science and innovation. This could involve cutting edge techniques using 'omics'that are allowing state of the art molecular biology to increase understanding of the cause and mode of action of a disease, and finding clever ways to interfere with disease pathways or block activity. More applied research and clinical trials should emphasise innovations but translational pathways to the clinic are key here. Writers must justify the proposed approach and convince evaluators about the power of studies, clinical relevance and robustness of design.

The Science should be written by the consortium's scientific experts, ideally overseen by a 'lead scientist', but it needs to be understandable to evaluators who may not be experts in the field. A common mistake is to present an in-depth literature review of the field and poorly explained methods, the focus should be on the advances proposed without assuming knowledge.

Impact through valorisation – how patients, science and society benefit

Understanding the impact expected of any grant funding is very important and differs depending on the priorities of the funder. Patient Foundations will have a very specific and focused priority to the disease area of interest, public bodies will also seek broader societal benefits. A strong grant proposal needs to describe the valorisation of results; indeed Horizon 2020 projects request a draft Plan for the Use and Dissemination of Foreground to do just this.

Valorisation is a term used by the EC to describe the activities of disseminating, communicating and exploiting the research data, products and outcomes of funded projects. In all cases to maximise the benefits of the money invested, any consortium needs to optimise the use of results.

Dissemination

Dissemination focuses on publicising the technical information and scientific results of a project through conferences, peer reviewed journals and technical workshops or seminars. The aim is to raise the profile of the scientific excellence and contribute directly to the scientific and technical knowledge base, ideally through open access publication routes and databases.

Communication

Communication activities should inform society and key stake-holders about the project through a strategic approach. Tools including stakeholder management, newsletters, articles, web-sites, social media, events, press releases, policy briefings, etc. will all be useful to deliver targeted project messages to well defined audiences. A range of activities should be envisaged across and beyond the project lifecycle. The recent document 'Communicating EU research and innovation guidance for project participants' (EC 2014) is a useful starting point.[6]

Communication also benefits from patient networks and expertise in marketing, event organisation and using social media. Key tasks could be awareness-raising of upcoming clinical trials to aid recruitment, communicating project aims or educating target groups for awareness and acceptance of a potential therapy.

Exploitation

Exploitation activities should look to see the use of research results in the next stage of development. Who will use the results and what is the next step? Practical plans need to be outlined showing how useful results can be transferred effectively and how the intellectual property (IP) developed in the project will be protected and managed.

For example, a project delivering positive preclinical and safety data would allow the sponsor to seek Orphan Drug Designation from the EMA, protecting the 'market position'. The next step would be to move a lead technology into clinical testing. Biomarker discovery in the project could require further validation and transfer of the technology to potential users, such as scientists or companies developing diagnostic or disease monitoring tests. An important step would be protecting the invention by patenting. For both these technologies (lead drug and biomarker) further collaboration and continuing development would be planned, endeavouring to utilise project results and practices.

Valorisation is also about continuing to build upon project results by taking them (or aspects of them) to new organisations, new sectors, new countries and new target groups in order to widen the impact of the project.

Patient group input is crucial to many projects:

Increasingly, funding agencies stimulate involvement of patients early in the Research and Development (R&D) phase of therapeutic rare disease projects. The IMI-funded EUPATI project trains patient organisations in clinical R&D processes and provides tips and tricks on how to interact in an ethical way with industry. Patient organisations understanding the R&D process and its regulatory restrictions can more effectively stimulate academia and industry to perform research on their disease.[7]

The value of patient knowledge and opinions in applied projects is recognised as a major advantage. Their unique perspective gives intelligence on activities from developing novel treatments to clinical trial design, recruitment and implementation. Patient groups can participate either directly as beneficiaries, with distinct roles and responsibilities in the project and dedicated budget, or in an advisory role that the project utilises as required. Expenses should then be allocated through a grant holder.

Effective patient group involvement at the outset can strengthen the feasibility of the project, especially if a project is undertaking clinical trials. Patient representatives provide a valid perspective on benefit/risk considerations, and can offer insights and advice on protocol design, the running and monitoring of clinical trials and may bring experience of dealing with regulatory and ethics committees. They can also contribute to the development of trial information, including informed consents leading to better recruitment and retention of subjects. Even early in the research, patient groups can bring a clear understanding of what types of research outcome are most beneficial for their disease.

Another aspect of patient group involvement is the dissemination and communication of the project to a large network of stakeholders. This could be for awareness-raising of an upcoming clinical trial for successful recruitment, communicating the project aims and educating target groups for acceptance and awareness of a potential new therapy, and supporting the development of communication material for use in newsletters, webinars, workshops and the project website.

But what about diseases without a formal patient group, for example, some of the many rare infectious diseases? To address this issue and ensure a good level of patient engagement the FP7 Orphan Drug for *Acanthamoeba* Keratitis (ODAK) project has activities and budget to develop a patient platform.

Case Study 3 – A grant-funded project helping develop a patient voice

ODAK – Orphan drug for Acanthamoeba Keratitis (AK) is an EC FP7 funded project developing a safe and effective treatment for AK, a rare infectious eye disease, which can cause severe debilitation and blindness, which predominantly affects contact lens wearers.

The ODAK project is a particularly interesting example of how patient groups can be directly formed through FP7 activities. The disease has no established patient group, although Moorfields Eye Hospital coordinates UK support for AK sufferers including patient focus meetings providing support and advice. Establishment of an active AK patient group is difficult because a) as an infectious rare disease, AK is not well-known and there is no predisposition, and b) patients are generally ephemeral. Grant funding has enabled the ODAK team to liaise with AK patients, provide disease awareness and prevention information, share patients' stories and support patient group development. Patients are now advising on protocol development for a Phase 3 clinical trial, raising the profile of a disease for faster diagnosis and preventative measures.

Implementation

In the development of a proposal, the work plan must be well designed and intermediate targets clearly defined. The Project Coordinator or a consultant generally takes overall responsibility for defining the work plan, building the consortium, proposal writing (or overseeing this) and submission. The coordinator role is often filled by the organisation with the greatest interest in the project results, for example a drug development company, but may be a partner with relevant experience in grant administration, eg. a University.

For Horizon 2020 collaborative projects, the coordinator must ensure that the project has the relevant expertise in the consortium to fulfil the project objectives and that the consortium is well structured. It is important that the project has the right people doing the right things and that the organisation is clear and sensible. The proposal should provide detailed information on the quality of the consortium, their expertise and track record, the complementarity and synergy between partners and the rationale for this project consortium. The coordinator must also ensure that the resource allocation to partners is appropriate for the work undertaken including person months, consumables, equipment and all related travel to form the budget. The coordinator is responsible for the grant distribution and management throughout the project.

An effective work plan will apportion the project work into work packages, typically managed by work package leaders with relevant technical expertise. The purpose and value of the work undertaken and the importance and efficacy of any results needs highlighting. Each work package will detail its timings, person effort, partners involved, the objectives, the tasks required to meet these objectives, the methods used (including new techniques to be developed) and the results to be achieved.

A beneficiary of the grant will need to ensure they are aware of the financial and administrative responsibilities required by a grant agreement. Partners bring a range of expertise to a project which can be utilised to strengthen the proposal, including information relating to advances in the state of the art and the impact of the project, exploitation routes and dissemination activities pertinent for their discipline, justification for their inclusion in the consortium and a clear budget for the work. This input can be overwhelming for a partner inexperienced with funding applications, but a good coordinator or consultant will address the requirements at an early stage and provide clear guidance.

There are other ways of participating in projects without being a beneficiary of the grant. External advisors are often selected to strengthen the skills of the consortium and can offer advice and assistance in specific areas. Patient groups, regulatory consultants, world leading experts or academics may be included in an advisory group to add value and expertise to the project. The advisory group should be budgeted for in the proposal and can play an important part in bringing knowledge and experience into project decision making.

Experts to help beat the competition

In any proposal, make best use of the expertise available to your consortium. It is a mistake for one person to try to write it all and an even bigger mistake for partners to let them. Many people now use consultants such as our Biotechsubsidy group to support proposal preparation and/or experienced peers, as in the case study below. In all our experience the best projects come from a team effort; each expert bringing their expertise and insight to make the proposal as strong as it can be. So put the effort in – be the best you can.

Case Study 4 – Nick Rhodes' Personal View of Scoring Top Marks

EC FP7 project DevelopAKUre (2012 – 2018):
I have had considerable experience with EC funded scientific research projects (Framework Programme proposals) over almost 20 years, from performing the scientific experiments,

contributing ideas and planning to someone else's grand idea and succeeding in having multi-partner research programmes funded. Colleagues within the University were keen to exploit a call in 2011 in the FP7 programme directly relevant to their expertise in the rare disease Alkaptonuria, but they had limited experience at constructing proposals for submission to the Commission. Below I will describe how my input helped ensure a successful conclusion.

You will have already seen in this chapter that successful EC proposals require a credible consortium of partners, fitting together in a highly synergistic manner, each being experts in their respective fields and with a breadth of experience sufficient to successfully deliver the research. In the DevelopAKUre proposal, the partners had already conducted preliminary research together, providing initial evidence and therefore considerable credibility to the consortium. Without such evidence, credibility can be difficult to establish.

Due to the increasing quality of the proposals submitted to the Commission during FP7 and the current Horizon 2020 programme, strict adherence to the requested scope of research and expected impacts is now a requisite for success. My role in perfecting the submission was to craft the introductory sections, impact statements and concluding paragraphs into a message fully in-line with these expectations. In addition, highlighting the ability of the commercial partners to fully exploit their market position in order to bring technology to clinic, to deliver high-level health impact and fulfil the EC's wider societal mission. Fortunately, the call topic was directly in-line with the research being conducted.

However, even demonstration of a highly credible consortium and an extremely relevant research programme no longer guarantees success. A wider understanding of how scientific experts, not specialist in your specific field, can fully appreciate the minutiae of the scientific arguments requires a number of different approaches. To achieve this, I was able to fully re-craft the introduction so that it made logical sense to a non-specialist expert, such as me. I used strategies in which we were able to:

- *attract and keep the attention of the reviewers;*
- *instil a high level of confidence in the reviewers;*
- *conclude the proposal in a way that had the reviewers understanding our deeper mission.*

We also used Ritchie Head (Ceratium Ltd.) as an experienced consultant at Stage 1 and Stage 2 to review the draft versions; his suggestions helped to polish the proposal. In this way, we were able achieve a perfect 15/15 score, and therefore able to negotiate the contract with no reduction in research funds.

Evaluators are human too

Each grant programme has an evaluation process. This may be a dedicated panel of external stakeholders including academics, clinicians, industrialists and patient representatives, or it may be mixed external and in-house groups such as a Scientific Board and Advisory Panel or Council (eg. NICATS). Whatever the process and approach, there are clear advantages if you make the evaluators' life easy. Write for your reader. Be clear and concise in the arguments that are put forward and ensure the proposal is easy to follow. Break the text up with sub-titles that make the text easy to navigate. Many funders are open about the evaluation criteria you will be judged against, so ensure your reader can easily identify the key text and bring out the critical points they will be most interested to review. Burying your great ideas in too much text and the curse of 'over writing', when you try to cover too many points or swamp good ideas in academic text with multiple references needs to be avoided.

The EC framework programmes have been unfairly judged to be biased; the 'grapevine' is full of rumours of the money already allocated to the 'usual suspects'. Our experience and discussions with evaluators indicates that overall the EC is run with a very independent and transparent process. They select evaluators from a pool of people like you and me. In rare diseases this can include patient groups, clinicians, academia and industry. Anyone is able to submit a CV to join the pool, and we recommend that you do. If invited as an evaluator you gain experience of:

- what winning and losing projects look like;
- how a multinational group of evaluators review and the decision making process;
- working with others in your evaluation team. This provides an excellent opportunity to network with international experts.

The evaluation process for EC funded projects

Horizon 2020 funded projects have a maximum 5-month evaluation period from call deadline to notification of funding success or failure. Each proposal is first checked by an EC administrator for admissibility (ie. readable and all requested forms complete), eligibility (ie. minimum partners/countries and call criteria met) and that it is within the scope of the call.

The proposal is then evaluated by a minimum number of three independent experts, who will follow EC guiding principles to produce an individual evaluation report. The evaluation criteria in Horizon 2020 are **Excellence, Impact,** and **Quality and Efficiency of Implementation.** The criteria are adapted to each type of action (project) and are specified in the Work Programme. Each criterion is scored between 0 and 5 (5 being excellent and 0- failing or incomplete) and the default threshold is 3 (except for first stage proposals where the threshold is 4). The total score default threshold is 10, unless specified in the Work Programme.

Individual evaluation reports are then considered by a consensus group moderated by an EC representative to find agreement on scores and comments. A consensus report is produced for the next stage – the Panel Review. This will comprise experts from the consensus groups and/or new experts to produce a final list of proposals in priority order for funding. The Commission then works down the list to allocate funding. This will primarily be based on the evaluation score, but they will also ensure that a range of research themes is covered. It is possible that if two high-scoring projects focus on the same disease area or technology, only one will be funded, and a lower scoring project in another area will also be selected to diversify the range of funded projects. This approach also demands that in developing a project, you ensure enough difference from other current or previously funded projects to convince the evaluators and EC that your project will be an excellent use of the available grant money.

Summary

Grant funded projects have many benefits for the rare disease community offering non-dilutive funding to advance our understanding of rare diseases and the development of therapies. This gives opportunities to create multidisciplinary consortia across public and private sectors, to bring together expertise and interest groups to share knowledge, expertise and know-how. Some grants, including Horizon 2020, allow crucial international cooperation that can really benefit from access to small patient populations across countries and international centres of expertise. To succeed in getting funding requires high quality proposals to be prepared by an excellent consortium. Such documents need to propose excellent, ambitious science and innovations with a clear impact aligned to funder priorities. This requires a good understanding of the funding available and careful writing. Both can seem daunting to the inexperienced; funding choices need to be selected, the correct information gathered, the proposal written and the application submitted. Engaging a consultant specialised in this area of grant funding and managing projects is one solution. Other sources of help include National Contact Points or funder helpdesks and the Rare Disease and biotechnology communities themselves run occasional grant writing and strategy workshops. Finally, successful peers will often support and advise. Key individuals can make a difference, but a team effort wins as in the *DevelopA-KUre* case study.

The following table provides a summary of some of the main funding schemes currently available in the field of rare (orphan) disease research. Many other programmes exist and the increasing focus on personalised medicines is creating more opportunities for the Rare Disease Community.

The International Rare Diseases Research Consortium (IRDiRC):
Summary: A consortium of 40 member institutions from 16 countries and EU (international, national funders, charities and industry) and invited patient groups. International and national funders. http://www.irdirc.org
Activities: Funding through national and international grants teams up researchers and organisations investing in rare diseases research and clinical trials to deliver by 2020 **200 new therapies** for rare diseases and means to **diagnose most rare diseases**. IRDiRC related calls and member funded research is listed on the website. IRDiRC also fund support activities eg. RD Connect – an integrated research platform combining clinical profiles, -omics data and biobank samples to improve effective use of RD knowledge base (http://rd-connect.eu).
European Commission Horizon 2020 European Union/ International: https://ec.europa.eu/programmes/horizon2020/
Main European Research and Innovation funding programme 2014 – 2020. An important grant funding resource for the rare disease community funding a diverse range of collaborative projects. Relevant topic areas include rare disease, chronic conditions, and personalised medicine approaches that often use a rare disease as a model condition for new therapy and research tool development. The main opportunities are under the Health, Demographic Change and Wellbeing challenge. Some unrestricted call topics are also suitable for rare disease research.

EC ERA Net Research Programme on rare Diseases–E-RARE-3 (2014-2019) http://www.erare.eu/

Annual programme of calls funding translational collaborative research in Rare Diseases. Topics and eligibility change with calls. The website lists current topics, and funders of rare disease research in partner countries and at European level.

EC – Third Health Programme http://ec.europa.eu/health/programme/policy/index_en.htm

Public health programme is designed to help implement EU Health Strategy and includes grants to support access to therapies in Europe for rare diseases. Previous initiatives have included EU-wide activities to pool scarce expertise and provide patients and health professionals with improved access to medical information, treatment centres, patient support groups and epidemiological/research data.

Wellcome Trust (Pathfinder Awards) United Kingdom: http://www.wellcome.ac.uk/Funding/Innovations/Awards/Pathfinder-Awards/index.htm

Funding of early-stage pilot projects in areas of unmet need related to Orphan and neglected diseases. Supports collaborations between academia and commercial research institutions (UK, Republic of Ireland and rest of the world).

National Institute for Health Research (NIHR) United Kingdom:

http://www.nihr.ac.uk/funding/

The last NIHR call was an example of a funder using all their programmes to target Rare Diseases in projects that support IRDiRC aims.

NIHR supports research in very rare diseases (<1/100,000 affected) using existing NIHR's research programmes: Health Technology Assessment (HTA) Programme; Efficacy and Mechanism Evaluation (EME) Programme; Research for Patient Benefit (RfPB) Programme; Health Services and Delivery Research (HSandDR) Programme; Invention for Innovation (i4i) Programme; Programme Grants for Applied Research (PGfAR) Programme.

The National Center for Advancing Translational Sciences (NCATS): http://www.ncats.nih.gov/funding-and-notices/funding.html

NCATS is one of the Institute and Centres (ICs) of the NIH (currently 21). NCATS stimulates the advancement of technology to enable more efficient disease identification and treatment. An array of collaborative grant programs and in-kind services support research projects, core facilities, and scientific resources and tools. NCATS also provides collaboration opportunities for small businesses and other partners. A large range of diseases is targeted.

The NCATS Therapeutics for Rare and Neglected Diseases (TRND) program is designed to accelerate the development of new drugs for rare and neglected diseases. TRND stimulates drug discovery and development research collaborations among NIH and academic scientists, non-profit organizations, and pharmaceutical and biotechnology companies working on rare and neglected illnesses.

The NCATS site currently provides a general listing of relevant NIH grants and some third party grants relevant to rare diseases: http://rarediseases.info.nih.gov/research/8/research-funding-resources .

US Food and Drug Administration (FDA): http://www.fda.gov/ForIndustry/DevelopingProductsforRareDiseasesConditions/WhomtoContactaboutOrphanProductDevelopment/default.htm

The goal of the Orphan Products Grants Program is to encourage clinical development of products for use in rare diseases or conditions. The products studied can be drugs, biologics, medical devices, or medical foods.

National Organization for Rare Disorders (NORD) http://www.rarediseases.org

Provides seed money in small grants to academic scientists studying new treatments or diagnostics for rare diseases. NORD is well connected to Rare Diseases Europe (EURORDIS) and Japan's patient organisation (JPA). Their grants are competitive and international. The grant selection process is unbiased and independent; awards are based solely on scientific merit, as determined by NORD's medical advisors. The review process follows NIH guidelines.

Fondation Maladies Rare: (French Foundation for Rare Diseases) France/ International http://fondation-maladiesrares.org/international3 Supports rare diseases projects in France, across Northern Africa and the broader Middle East. IRDiRC sponsor.
The World Academy of Sciences (TWAS – UNESCO) Italy http://twas.org/opportunities Supports research projects (including rare diseases) in the developing world. Regional offices in Egypt, Brazil, China, Kenya and India.

Table 1: A Selection of Current European, US and International Grant Funding for Rare Diseases

Dr Ritchie Head is Director of Ceratium Limited.

Christina Olsen, European grants consultant and project manager for Ceratium Limited (www.ceratium.eu).

Dr Marc Van de Craen, co-founder of the Biotechsubsidy group (www.biotechsubsidy.com).

Dr Nick Rhodes, Reader in Tissue Engineering & Regenerative Medicine at the University of Liverpool (www.liverpool.ac.uk).

References

1 The Global Genes Project, 'The Global Genes Project' (2014). (Accessed August 2015). https://globalgenes.org/rare-diseases-facts-statistics/

2 Dunkle M. (2014). A 30-year retrospective: National Organization for Rare Disorders, the Orphan Drug Act, and the role of rare disease patient advocacy groups. Orphan Drugs: Research and Reviews Volume 2014:4 Pages 19—27.

3 Search orphan drug designations and approvals. FDA. (Ac-

cessed July 2015). www.accessdata.fda.gov/scripts/opdlisting/oopd.

4 D. E. Fagnan, N. N. Yang, J. C. McKew, A. W. Lo, Financing translation: Analysis of the NCATS rare-diseases portfolio. Sci. Transl. Med. 7, 276ps3 (2015).

5 Stehr and Forkel. Funding resources for rare disease research. Biochimica et Biophysica Acta, 2013, 1832: 1910-1912.

6 Communicating EU research and innovation guidance for project participants (EC 2014). (Accessed July 2015). http://ec.europa.eu/research/participants/data/ref/h2020/other/gm/h2020-guide-comm_en.pdf.

7 European Patients' Academy on Therapeutic Innovation. 2013. EUPATI. (Accessed July 2015). http://www.patientsacademy.eu/index.php/en/

Chapter 12

Orphan Drug Legislation and Adaptive Licensing

Anthony Hall
Findacure

Introduction

The orphan drug legislation is covered in detail elsewhere and will not be repeated here.[1,2] One recent change since these publications is that the requirement for a Letter of Intent (at least 2 months before the planned orphan designation application submission date) has been dropped, making the procedure more streamlined and potentially faster. There is a wealth of online resources available to guide the interested reader through the legislation and procedures. For example, the European Medicines Agency (EMA) website[3] or the Food and Drug Administration (FDA) website.[4]

The orphan drug legislation has done a lot to stimulate the development of treatments for rare diseases but the time it takes to develop treatments remains an issue. Due to the urgency to make treatments available as soon as possible for progressive and fatal conditions, such as Duchenne muscular dystrophy, many patients are willing to accept greater risks and greater uncertainty about risks than patients affected by less serious conditions.[5]

A legal framework already exists for the authorisation of drugs under exceptional circumstances (where the patient population is too small to allow a normal drug development to take place) and conditional approval (where early registration is desirable and additional evidence is supplied later). Both these pathways to registration in Europe, together with their US counterparts where applicable, are discussed in detail in Rare Diseases: Opportunities for social entrepreneurs, Chapter 4.[1]

The concept of early approval is now being pushed further, with the current interest in 'Adaptive Licencing'. The objective of this approach is to try to stimulate the arrival of more new medicines for unmet medical need reaching the market and provide earlier access to those in need. Historically, drug development has had a somewhat binary nature to it; with a molecule being an experimental 'product in development' all the way up to the 'magic moment' at which it becomes ostensibly a fully vetted, safe and efficacious therapy (see Figure 1).

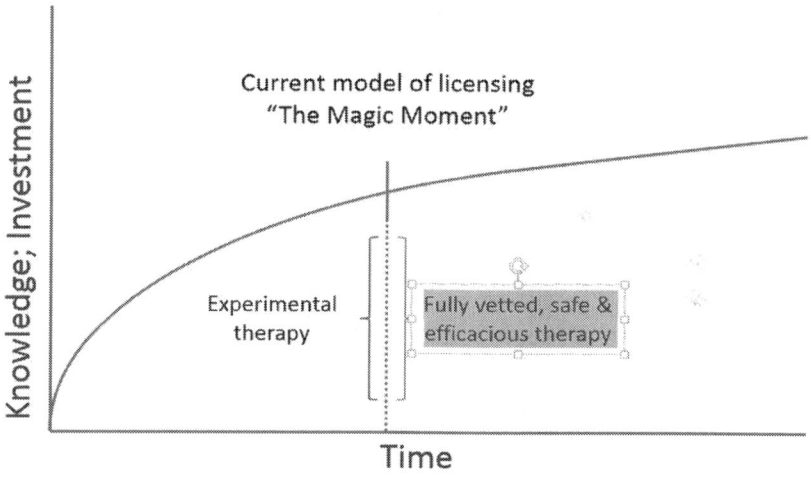

Figure 1. The binary nature of drug development. Adapted from Eichler, EMA. 2012.[6]

Clearly, the current licencing mechanisms do not reflect reality, since one is continually learning about the product during the development and one continues to learn after marketing authorisation, so in reality there is no 'magic moment'.

The European Medicine Agency (EMA) Roadmap to 2015 laid the foundations for adaptive licencing with its statement that, "…a key issue for regulators will be whether a more 'staggered' approval (or progressive licensing) concept should be envisaged for situations not covered by conditional marketing authorisations or marketing authorisations under exceptional circumstances…"[7]

The document also states, "It should be emphasised that progressive licensing should not lead to a reduced level of evidence for first-time marketing authorisation."

Definition of Adaptive Licencing

Adaptive licensing may be defined as a prospectively planned, adaptive approach to bringing drugs to market.[8] The prospective planning is an essential component; it is not intended that drug developers should come with a development programme that failed to produce convincing results and request an early authorisation whilst further data is collected.[9]

In its current form, Adaptive Licensing is not aimed at creating new regulatory tools or introducing new laws. Rather, the intention is to raise awareness of, and make better use of, existing tools within the current regulatory framework, such as (multi-stakeholder) Scientific Advice, Conditional Marketing Authorisation, Marketing Authorisation under Exceptional Circumstances, registries and pharmacovigilance tools (Risk Evaluation and Mitigation Strategies, Periodic Safety Update Reports, renewal of marketing authorisations). This 'conservative' approach, using existing tools, may eventually give way to a more transformative approach (See Eichler, 2012).[8]

The European Medicines Agency envisions two different scenarios for Adaptive Licencing, as illustrated in Figures 2 and 3.[10]

1. Approval is granted in a well-defined, high medical need subgroup, and subsequently widened to a larger patient population.

2. Conditional approval is prospectively planned, eg. on the basis of surrogate endpoints, and uncertainty is planned to be reduced through obligations to collect data post-approval.

Widening of the indication Scenario
(Final target indication in blue and red)

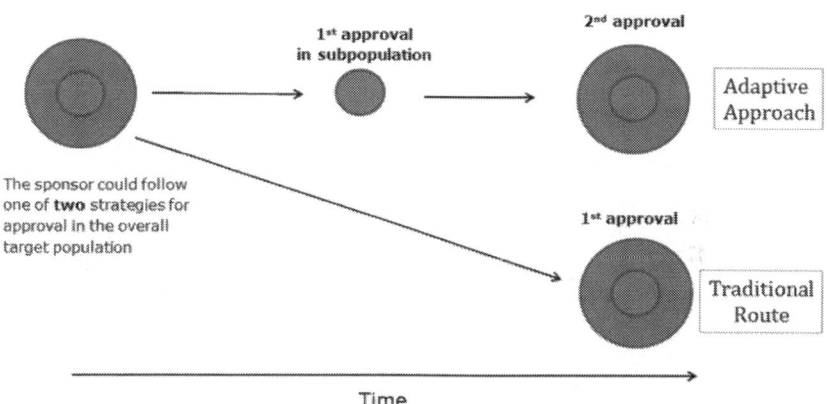

Figure 2. Different scenarios for Adaptive Licencing: Starting with a sub-population and widening to a larger population. (Reproduced from EMA 2014).[10]

This approach would fit with the threshold approach outlined by Eichler.[8] It is ideal for rare diseases, where the initial conditional marketing authorisation would be based on a small study with larger alpha (Type I error). Further randomised controlled trials (RCTs) would likely be impossible and patients would need to be informed of the increased uncertainty associated with early approval. Following the authorisation, knowledge expansion would rely on uncontrolled studies, as shown in the schematic below (Figure 4).

European Medicines Agency (EMA) pilot project

On March 19 2014, the EMA launched the Adaptive Licensing Pilot Project (the name has since been changed to Adaptive Pathways, as explained below).[9] The key features of this pilot

Prospectively planned Reduction of uncertainty Scenario

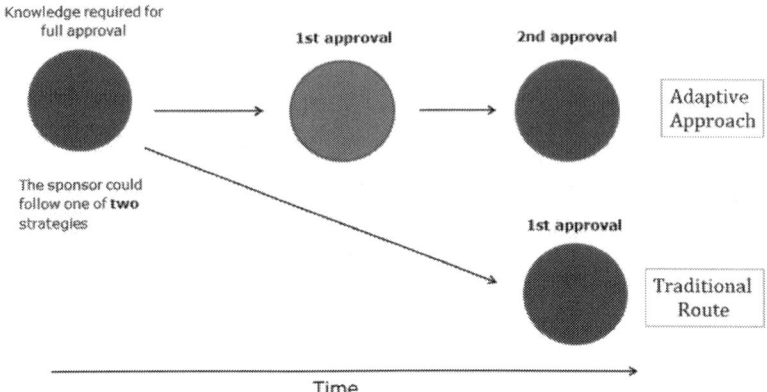

The AP discussions are conducted in a safe harbour environment and all submissions are strictly

Figure 3. Different scenarios for Adaptive Licencing: Conditional approval with a reduction in uncertainty over time. (Reproduced from EMA 2014).[10]

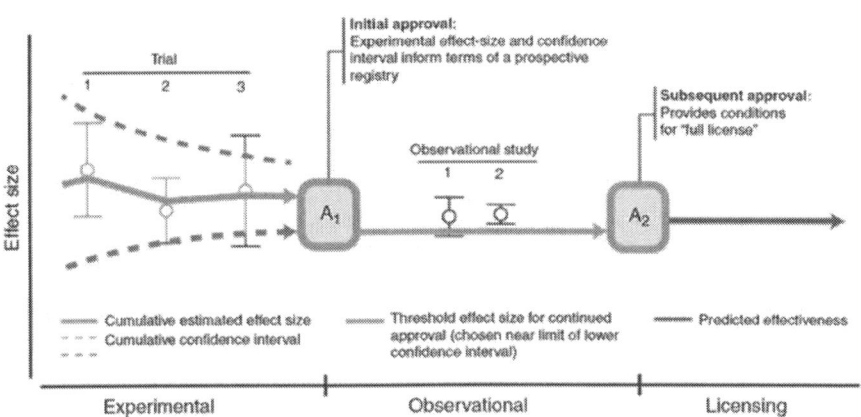

Figure 4. The threshold approach to evidence generation when randomised controlled trials (RCTs) are not practically or ethically feasible after an initial licence. Reproduced from Eichler et al. 2012.[8] and with permission from Wiley. © 2012 American Society for Clinical Pharmacology and Therapeutics.

project were for drug developers to undertake an iterative development plan, engage Health Technology Assessment bodies (HTAs) and other downstream stakeholders early on. There should be clear proposals for the monitoring, collection and use of real-world data, post-authorisation, as a complement to RCT data, to inform updates to the regulatory label and to the positions of other stakeholders.

Toward the end of 2014, the EMA published a report of the initial experience with the pilot project; 34 applications had been received, of which 10 fulfilled the criteria to enter the project and were selected to go into a Stage I discussion and of these, six were selected to go to a Stage II meeting.[10]

The EMA also changed the name of the project to Adaptive Pathways. This was to better reflect the objectives to "foster and facilitate the pathway of product development to potentially achieve earlier access to medicines through an early dialogue involving all stakeholders" (regulators, sponsors, HTA bodies, groups responsible for guidelines, patient organisations), with discussions in a 'safe harbour' environment rather than to create a new regulatory tool for licensing. The 'safe harbour' was created not only to assure applicants that the discussion would be confidential, but also would not be legally binding if the applicant decided to revert to traditional regulatory pathways. And the approach was changed in name from Adaptive Licensing to Adaptive Pathways to illustrate that the process required all stakeholders to be engaged in early dialogue, and in particular the payers. While the current regulatory process can be considered too long and too expensive, one of the main challenges in today's healthcare is the ability to pay for the new medicines, and make them available to patients once they have been granted a Marketing Authorisation. Pushing an approach such as Adaptive Licensing through, without considering how the reimbursement of the drug would work is considered by many to be counterproductive in the long term. An Adaptive Pathway aims to bring such issues to the development plan from the offset.

In the US, similar initiatives are also taking place. On 26 January 2015, the '21st Century Cures Act' discussion document was published.[11] The key features of this document are:

- Patient-Focused Drug Development
- Surrogate Endpoints
- Approval of Breakthrough Therapies
- Priority Review
- Accelerated Approval
- Expanded Access
- Modernizing Clinical Trials

Obstacles & Disadvantages of Adaptive Licensing

Whilst Adaptive Licensing may seem like an ideal solution for both patients and drug developers alike, bringing much needed new treatments to market faster is not without its difficulties. These are outlined by Eichler (2012) and summarised below.[8]

a. Gradual market entry may lead to lower return on investment. Even though development time may be shorter / cheaper, there is a potential for the gradual entry to reduce revenues and drug developers may prefer to stick with the traditional 'global launch' approach.

b. Difficulties with global launches. Use of an Adaptive Licensing pathway in Europe, for example, will not lead to an earlier launch in other territories, where it may still be necessary to go through traditional pathways. This will make it impossible to plan a global launch, since there could be considerable gaps between the launch dates in different regions of the world.

c. Risk of litigation. Companies may be concerned over the additional risk of litigation in case of unanticipated safety issues with a drug that has not yet been tested in a sufficient number of patients to give the usual degree of certainty regarding safety.

d. Need to collect data post-approval. This may also deter companies, since the logistics and costs of collecting this data may be very high. Good quality registries are often a post-approval commitment and these can be extremely expensive to run over a protracted period.

e. Concerns over reduced standards. Keeping in mind the fact that there are often calls for companies to delay market entry in order to collect more safety data before the public is exposed to the medicine, it could be seen as a lowering of standards in bringing medicines to market with less safety data.

f. Variable acceptability of increased uncertainty. Not everyone will have the same level of willingness to accept additional risk and uncertainty. This will vary in particular between diseases, but there may also be cultural aspects too.

g. Possible need for new legislation. Although the intention is to introduce Adaptive Licensing using existing legislation, as outlined above, for it to work successfully it is possible that new legislation may be required.

h. Questions over industry commitment. It is too early to know whether the industry will be open to the Adaptive Licensing approach.

i. Restricting prescriptions to the target population. If an early licence is granted for a restricted population (scenario (a) in Figure 2) there may be extensive pressure on treating physicians to prescribe also for a wider population where efficacy and/or safety has not yet been established. There may also be pressure on HTAs to reimburse when treatment is prescribed in this wider population and reluctance from HTAs to do so.

j. Ethics of RCTs after marketing authorisation. One of the key features of Adaptive Licencing is that additional data is collected post initial approval. However, it may be extremely difficult to collect informative data in such circumstances. In general, randomised, placebo controlled clinical trials are the gold standard for determining the efficacy and safety of a drug. Once a drug is on the market, however, it would be almost impossible to conduct a placebo controlled trial. This means that further data is likely to come from other types of trial, such as historically controlled trials, where it may be more difficult to determine the benefit : risk relationship.

k. Local reimbursement in EU. Drugs for rare diseases, or diseases where there is a high unmet medical need tend to be highly priced. In many countries, this already leads to problems with reimbursement and this could well be compounded if the drug has a conditional marketing authorisation or authorisation under exceptional circumstances, whereby it may be difficult to determine the cost-effectiveness of the drug.

Conclusions

The orphan drug legislation was introduced to stimulate the development of drugs where the population is too small to make such development commercially viable and it has been successful in doing so.[12] However, the majority of rare diseases are still without an effective treatment and additional approaches may be required. Recent interest in Adaptive Licencing, based on already existing legal frameworks, offers the possibility to introduce new treatments perhaps years earlier than would be available through traditional approval pathways. However, Adaptive Licencing is not without its challenges and it is still too early to tell whether this will be successful in bringing drugs to patients faster without increasing concerns about safety.

References

1 Hall AK. The practicalities of clinical development of drugs for rare diseases. In: Rare Diseases: Challenges and Opportunities for Social Entrepreneurs (Sireau N, ed.). Greenleaf Publishing, Sheffield, UK, 2013; pp.62-86.

2 Hall AK, Carlson MR. The current status of orphan drug development in Europe and the US. Intractible & Rare Diseases Research. 2014; 3(1): 1-7.

3 EMA website (orphan drugs section). (Accessed 6 September 2015). http://www.ema.europa.eu/ema/index.jsp?curl=pages/regulation/general/general_content_000029.jsp&mid=WC0b01ac05800240ce

4 FDA website (orphan designations section). (Accessed 6 September 2015). http://www.accessdata.fda.gov/scripts/opdlisting/oopd/index.cfm

5 Duchenne Muscular Dystrophy and Related Dystrophinopathies: Developing Drugs for Treatment Guidance for Industry (draft guidance). US Department of Health and Human Services Food and Drug Administration Center for Drug Evaluation and Research (CDER). 26170dft.doc. 05/22/15

6 Eichler H-G. Adaptive licensing: a useful approach for drug licensing in the EU? (Accessed 6 September 2015). http://www.ema.europa.eu/docs/en_GB/document_library/Presentation/2012/04/WC500124930.pdf

7 European Medicine Agency (EMA) Roadmap to 2015. (Accessed 6 September 2015). http://www.ema.europa.eu/docs/en_GB/document_library/Report/2011/01/WC500101373.pdf

8 Eichler H-G et al. Adaptive Licensing: Taking the Next Step in the Evolution of Drug Approval. Clinical Pharmacology & Therapeutics. VOLUME 91. NUMBER 3. March 2012. pp. 436-437. http://onlinelibrary.wiley.com/

doi/10.1038/clpt.2011.345/abstract;jsessionid=A5FCD-
7C0E97E3C88E78388475DD8E85C.f01t01

9 Pilot project on adaptive licensing. EMA/254350/2012.
EMA 19 March 2014.

10 Adaptive pathways to patients: report on the initial experience of the pilot project. EMA/758619/2014. 15 December
2014.

11 21st Century Cures Act. (Accessed 6 September 2015).
https://www.congress.gov/bill/114th-congress/house-bill/6/
text

12 European Parliament and Council of the European Union.
Regulation (EC) No 141/2000 of the European Parliament
and of the Council of 16 December 1999 on orphan medicinal products. Official Journal of the European Communities. 2000; 22.1.2000.

Chapter 13

Early Interaction with Regulators and Parallel Scientific Advice with Health Technology Assessment Organisations

Christian Hill
MAP BioPharma Ltd

Introduction and background

Market Access refers to the conditions set by countries to allow products onto their markets. Market Access for medicines is often described as confusing and full of risk for the innovative company that is trying to bring a new product to patients. However, this is probably more perception than reality. Once you understand the options and the processes, it is fairly straightforward to navigate and achieve market access.

In this section, we describe how companies can engage with Health Technology Assessment (HTA) organisations earlier than has usually been the case. We give some examples for individual countries and for the European Union (EU) as a whole. We relate this to the rapidly evolving regulatory process. This will help you to look at the process as a whole rather than as several elements in isolation.

Links to the regulatory process

First, here is a reminder of the regulatory process. Earlier in this chapter, we described how the European Medicines Agency (EMA) regulatory process for a new medicine can include a series of steps to enable early marketing authorisation. With the standard process of approval, it takes 210 days to get an opinion from a Committee for Medicinal Products for Human Use (CHMP). This is followed by approximately 67 days to get the full European Commission (EC) authorisation.

The early marketing authorisation can either be a shortened process or it may be given at an earlier date than normal. An example of a shortened process is getting a CHMP opinion in 150 days instead of the normal 210. An example of an early process is where there is a particular unmet clinical need and the EMA provide a marketing authorisation based on less clinical data than normal.

The types of approval can either be:

- Positive, either through the standard or accelerated process;
- Positive under exceptional circumstances, where comprehensive data cannot be provided and the risks and benefits are reviewed annually; or
- Conditional, where additional data is needed, but the immediate availability to public health outweighs the risk. This authorisation is valid for one year, on a renewable basis. Once the pending studies are provided, it can become a normal marketing authorisation.

Adaptive licensing was described earlier in this chapter. It brings HTA organisations and regulators together. It does not necessarily have an effect on the timelines in the current process, but it may bring the approval date forward.

The pros and cons of scientific advice for Health Technology Assessment and other routes to reimbursement

Regulators and HTA organisations aim to help companies to develop robust clinical trials through a range of activities. By providing advice, they also improve the chance of approval and reduce the burden on scarce resources. In particular, early advice by the HTA organisation should allow companies to ensure that their clinical trials program includes everything they require to get positive recommendations after regulatory approval. This will include consideration for possible early access programs, which may become possible or change in scope based on the early advice.

The benefits of a company engaging in getting early advice should include the following:

- Reducing the risk in the drug development programs of an innovative company. Particularly for those programs at earlier stages (Phase I or II);
- Improving efficiency in the use of scarce resources. These can be both financial and in manpower, especially for small and medium-sized enterprises (SMEs);
- Better two-way communication, to share expertise and validate current research, processes and methods;
- More transparent regulatory and repayment processes.

Risks for companies and authorities:

- Change. This is often described as the only constant, but this requires an evolution of skills, training and good communication. Also, it needs additional safeguards to make sure that company confidential information remains just that, confidential.
- Company culture and prior experience can be a major barrier to greater transparency, sharing of information and corporate strategy. This may initially increase the resources needed, if companies are to properly assess the opportunities and risks.
- The costs required to follow the scientific advice procedures can be substantial. Some companies may struggle to complete the actions expected by the regulators and the HTA organisation to a sufficient level.
- Different HTA organisations often ask for different ap-

proaches. For example, this may be in the choice of factors compared; their reliance on models of long-term quality of life versus quantified clinical benefits in the short term; their approach to surrogate markers for clinical benefit. It would be helpful to have advice if it could be interpreted and applied uniformly across the continent. However this is unlikely to be the case and some advice may be conflicting across member states.

The scientific advice available to companies

There are currently three possible ways to obtain scientific or HTA advice in Europe. These are:

- At the national level: for example with the National Institute for Health and Care Excellence (NICE) in the UK;
- On the EU level: for example, parallel scientific advice from the EMA and EU HTA bodies on regulatory, scientific and HTA issues;
- Involving multiple HTA organisations, such as through cooperative advice from EU national HTA bodies and projects sponsored by the EC.

EU level procedures

In 2005, the EC recognised the need to establish a sustainable European network of HTA bodies. It oversaw the setting up of the EUnetHTA (EU network of HTA) Project, a network of HTA organisations. The objective was to work together in order to develop reliable, timely, transparent and transferable scientific information for assessing health technology across Europe.

The EC also set up the HTA Network, a voluntary initiative that brings together the competent authorities responsible for assessing health technology. "All Member States have appointed a representative and the network held its first meeting at the end of 2013 to host a strategic discussion on European collaboration when it comes to health technology assessment. The HTA Network will be supported by a scientific and technical cooperation mechanism, a function which will be fulfilled by Joint Action EUnetHTA until the end of 2015," explained Flora Giorgio, Scientific Officer at Commission.[1]

In 2010, the EMA introduced a pilot project involving the participation of HTA organisations in Europe. This was based on the provision of Parallel Scientific Advice (see Figure 1 for timelines). It is aimed at developers who can receive 'parallel' feedback at the same time, from both regulators and HTA organisations, on their clinical development plans for new medicines. It is possible to apply for CHMP scientific advice/protocol assistance and advice from the HTA bodies at the same time. This is welcomed by the EMA, who advise interested companies to contact the scientific advice secretariat directly to arrange a discussion using the General Scientific Advice Inbox: ScientificAdvice@ema.europa.eu.[2]

Parallel Scientific Advice topics and criteria are:[3]

- Clinical trial design: Duration; Comparator (placebo or active) – (EMA vs HTA bodies); Primary and secondary endpoints.
- Patient population: Pathology; Pre-existing therapies; Number of patients needed to evaluate efficacy and safety (orphan disease).
- Doses: Acceptability of doses to be tested in the clinical program.
- Orphan designation: Significant benefit (question to Committee for Orphan Medicinal Products; COMP); Scope of the orphan designation (question to COMP); Benefits of orphan status on requirements (EMA vs HTA bodies).
- Target therapeutic indication: Indication that best reflects the clinical trial program.
- Patient reported outcomes: What is acceptable to be included in the product label (question to EMA); Which instruments can be used to measure the benefit to pa-

tients (question to HTA bodies).
- Statistical considerations: Request for advice on planned statistical analyses (eg. subgroups).

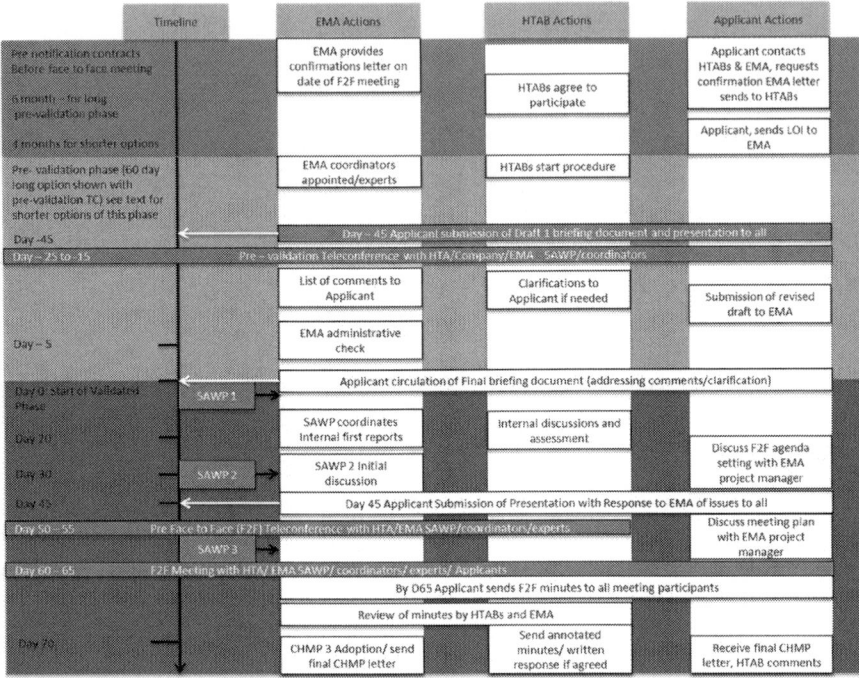

EMA – European Medicines Agency
SAWP – Scientific Advice Working Party
CHMP – Committee for Medicinal Products for Human Use
HTAB – Health Technology Assessment Bodies
HTA – Health Technology Assessment

Figure 1: Overview of parallel scientific advice and actions by each party.[4]

In addition to this initiative, HTA organisations have completed several early dialogue procedures. These included multiple HTA organisations, in the framework of the EUnetHTA Joint Actions (EUnetHTA JA) 1 and 2. The EMA was invited to participate as an observer in the early dialogue procedures of EUnetHTA JA2.

The final EU level option was introduced from September 2013. Fourteen HTA organisations began the 'Shaping European Early Dialogues' for health technologies project (SEED), under the coordination of the French National Authority for Health (Haute Autorité de Santé; HAS). The EU Commission financed the start of 10 additional early dialogues between multiple HTA organisations, to explore possible scenarios for having other early dialogues in the future.

National Level Procedures

UK – NICE

NICE was set up in 1999. It provides national guidance and advice to improve health and social care. This includes evidence-based guidance and advice, quality standards and performance metrics, and information services. NICE has around 600 employees and of these, two technical and two administrative staff work full time on scientific advice. There are also two external experts per project. NICE provides HTA advice on around 20 products per year. It is looking to expand this, with a particular focus on attracting SMEs to take up their services.

Typically, the scientific advice process takes 21-23 weeks. It starts with a briefing book, with questions, being submitted to NICE and finishes with the final report (see Figure 2). There is a 3-hour face-to-face meeting with NICE about 11 weeks after the submission of the briefing book. The meeting itself is relatively informal and interactive. The scientific advice given is not legally binding for any future appraisal. Fees for the advice depend on the size of the project–£38,000 for a medium project and £50,000 for a large project. NICE have recently introduced a scaled down version for SMEs. In this new process there is no face-to-face meeting but there is a teleconference with NICE to discuss the briefing book and an advice letter is produced. This process takes around 13 weeks to complete and the fees are £15,000.

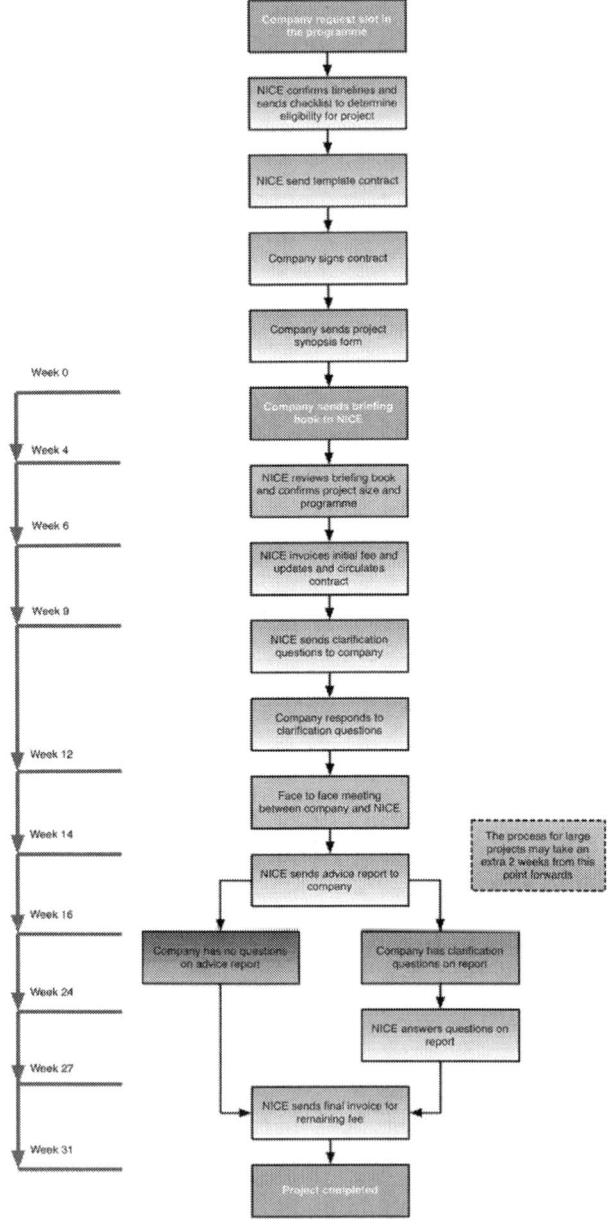

Figure 2. NICE Scientific Advice Process and Timelines

Germany – G-BA

Pharmaceutical companies can request consultation by the Federal Joint Committee (Gemeinsamer Bundesausschuss; G-BA) in accordance with the German Social Code, Book Five (SGB V, section 35a). The consultation can include advice on the documents needed for dossier submission, procedural steps, appropriate comparator, endpoints, study population and subgroups. A consultation before the start of phase 3 studies must involve the Federal Institute for Drugs and Medical Devices or the Paul Ehrlich Institute. The pharmaceutical company must pay the costs of the consultation, which can range from 2,000 – 10,000 Euros depending on the advice being sought.

An overview of the process is provided in Figure 3. Typically the process takes around 8 weeks up to the advice meeting. The meeting itself is formal in nature and led by the G-BA. During the meeting no presentation by the manufacturer is allowed. During the meeting the G-BA will provide its advice including an explanation and discussion of key themes in response to the manufacturer's questions. Following the meeting an advice report is provided within 14 days. Like NICE Scientific Advice, it should be noted that any scientific advice given is not legally binding for any future appraisal.

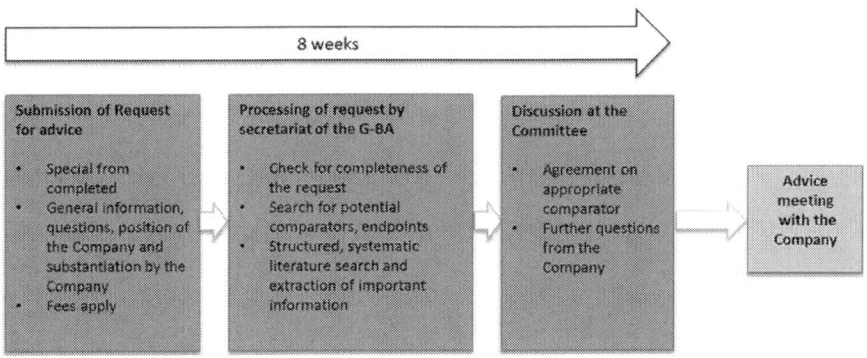

Adapted from G-BA advice presentation 2014

Figure 3. G-BA process for provision of advice for a health technology assessment

France – HAS

The French National Authority for Health (HAS) was created in August 2004 to improve the quality of patient care. Its remit covers:

- The assessment of drugs, medical devices, and procedures;
- Publication of guidelines to accreditation of healthcare organisations and certification of doctors;
- Training in quality issues and information provision.

HAS has more than 400 employees, with 100-110 involved in HTA activities. HTA advice takes up around 20 person days per project plus coordination, and provides advice on about 10 projects per year. Cost-effectiveness studies are now part of the market access requirements for all drugs where an 'improvement of actual medical benefit' (l'amélioration du service médical rendu; ASMR) rating of I, II or III is claimed and the drug has a potentially significant budget impact. This may mean that HTA advice on comparator and health economic evidence requirements will become more important.

Italy – AIFA

The Italian Medicines Agency (Agenzia Italiano del Farmaco; AIFA) is the Italian national authority responsible for both drug regulation and pricing-reimbursement. It has around 380 employees. Of these, 11 people (administrative, legal, statisticians, pharmacists, clinical and health economics specialists) spend 20% of their time on HTA advice. AIFA provides HTA advice on 1-4 products per year.

Sweden – MPA/TLV

Joint scientific advice meetings between the Dental and Pharmaceutical Benefits Agency (Tandvårds- och läkemedelsförmånsverket; TLV) and the Medical Products Agency (MPA) is available in Sweden. The aim of providing joint scientific advice is to fulfil the Government's instructions to the agencies to contribute to a rational and cost-effective use of pharmaceutical products, as well as meeting inquiries from the pharmaceutical industry. The application form at the MPA website has a section where participation of the TLV can be requested. It should clearly state which questions are directed to which authority ie. MPA or TLV. There is a face-to-face meeting, which typically lasts 90 minutes. The fee per scientific advice meeting is 45,000 Skr. The additional scientific advice provided by the TLV is free of charge. The advice given is not binding either for the MPA, the TLV or the company.

Netherlands – ZIN

The Netherlands National Health Care Institute (Zorginstituut Nederland; ZIN) manages the basic Dutch healthcare package. It is also responsible for encouraging improvements in healthcare quality and supporting education and training for healthcare professionals. It has around 450 employees, of whom 140 are involved in HTA and health care quality ($\approx 50\%$ of full time employment on HTA). Of these, six people spend two per cent of their time on HTA advice. ZIN provides early advice on 6 to 10 products per year through EUnetHTA.

The Future

Thus EMA-HTA parallel scientific advice as undertaken in the pilot is set to continue and evolve. Scientific advice/early dialogue involving regulators and HTAs is now identified and in progress as an area of collaboration under the EMA-EUnetHTA three-year work plan 2013–2015.

Scientific advice on the national level has gained significant momentum over recent years and this is set to not only continue but to expand. Indeed several organisations, including NICE in the UK, are actively reaching out to companies through workshops to increase uptake of their services.

Further updates on how the process has worked and what can be learned are scheduled to become available through 2015-16.

Christian Hill, Managing Director, MAP BioPharma Limited, Cambridge, UK. www.mapbiopharma.com

References

1 European Medicines Agency. EMA-HTA workshop: Bringing together stakeholders for early dialogue in medicines development – Report from the public workshop hosted by the European Medicines Agency (EMA) in London on 26 November 2013. 2014. Available at: http://www.ema. europa.eu/docs/en_GB/document_library/Report/2014/05/ WC500166228.pdf. Accessed 28 October 2015.

2 European Medicines Agency. European Medicines Agency Guidance for applicants seeking scientific advice and protocol assistance. 2014. Available at: http://www.ema.europa. eu/docs/en_GB/document_library/Regulatory_and_procedural_guideline/2009/10/WC500004089.pdf. Accessed 28 October 2015.

3 Rigourd, S. Experience of the Parallel European Medicines Agency (EMA)/ Health Technology Assessment (HTA) Scientific Advice from an Orphan Disease Point of View. Presented at the 7th European Conference on Rare Diseases & Orphan Products (ECRD 2014 Berlin). Available at: http:// www.rare-diseases.eu/wp-content/uploads/2014/05/0403_ Samuel_RIGOURD.pdf. Accessed 28 October 2015.

4 European Medicines Agency. Best Practice guidance for Pilot EMA HTA Parallel Scientific Advice procedures (for consultation). 2014. Available at: http://www.ema.europa. eu/docs/en_GB/document_library/Regulatory_and_procedural_guideline/2014/05/WC500166226.pdf. Accessed 28 October 2015.

Chapter 14

How to navigate the regulatory process: The US regulatory landscape

Marilyn R. Carlson, DMD, MD, RAC
Agility Clinical, Inc.

Introduction

According to the United States (US) Food and Drug Administration (FDA), "Most rare diseases are serious or life-threatening disorders with unmet medical needs. Speeding the development and availability of therapeutics for these serious diseases
is important, as they are often the first available treatment or
have significant advantages over existing treatments. FDA has
developed distinct and successful approaches to making such
therapies available as rapidly as possible."

Expedited Drug Development for Serious Conditions

FDA has created several programs intended to facilitate and
expedite development and review of drugs to meet unmet needs
for serious and life-threatening conditions. Priority Review, Accelerated Approval, Fast Track, and Breakthrough Therapy are
examples of such approaches for drugs.

Accelerated Approval

If a drug being developed to treat a serious or life-threatening
illness has the potential to provide a meaningful therapeutic

benefit over current treatments, the drug may be eligible for accelerated approval. Sponsors developing these types of drugs are encouraged to work with the appropriate FDA review division to determine eligibility. Use of the accelerated pathway allows sponsors to seek approval on the basis of adequate and well-controlled clinical trials with a clinical endpoint other than irreversible morbidity or mortality, ie. a surrogate endpoint. Drugs that receive Accelerated Approval may be required to conduct additional studies post-approval to verify clinical benefit or the effect on irreversible morbidity or mortality.

Priority Review

An application for drug approval may be eligible to receive Priority Review if it is a major treatment advance or it provides a treatment when no adequate therapy exists. Priority Review is an opportunity to shorten the New Drug Application (NDA) or Biologics License Application (BLA) review from the standard 10 months to six months.

Fast Track

Preclinical or clinical data that indicate a drug will treat a serious disease and fill an unmet medical need may be eligible to receive Fast Track designation. Fast Track designation provides more frequent interactions with FDA during drug development and may allow sponsors to submit completed sections of the NDA or BLA for review, rather than waiting until every section is complete ('rolling review').

Breakthrough Therapy

According to FDA, Breakthrough Therapy designation may be requested for a drug intended, alone or in combination, to treat a serious or life-threatening disease. The designation request requires the sponsor to provide preliminary clinical evidence that the drug may offer "substantial improvement over existing therapies". Once granted Breakthrough Therapy designation, a drug is eligible for all provisions of Fast Track designation, eg. FDA guidance on efficient drug development program, and organizational commitment involving senior managers.

The designation of Breakthrough Therapy for drugs that have preliminary clinical evidence of the potential for substantial improvement over available therapies for serious and/or life-threatening diseases, was signed into law in 2012 in the Food and Drug Administration Safety and Innovation Act (FDASIA). Detailed information about Breakthrough Therapy, as well as the other expedited programs, is described in a guidance document issued by FDA in 2013.[1]

See Table 1 for a summary of the unique features of each of the programs.

Features	Accelerated Approval Pathway	Priority Review Designation	Fast Track Designation	Breakthrough Therapy Designation
Requirement	Not specified.	Not specified.	Basis for the intention to treat a serious condition; potential to address an unmet need; advantages over available therapy	Preliminary clinical evidence of potential for substantial improvement over available therapies
Submission Timing	Discuss with FDA review division	Submit with original application for approval or with efficacy supplement	Submit with IND or no later than the pre-BLA or pre-NDA meeting	Submit no later than end-of-Phase 2 meeting with FDA
Time to FDA Response	Not specified	Within 60 calendar days	Within 60 calendar days	Within 60 calendar days
Incentives	Use surrogate or intermediate clinical endpoint in clinical trial(s)	6-month review versus 10-month standard review	Frequent FDA communications. May allow rolling review and/or priority review	FDA guidance on efficient drug development in addition to Fast Track incentives
Regulation	21CFR§314, subpart H; 21CFR§601, subpart E; FD&C Act, §506(c) as amended by FDASIA	PDUFA 1992	FDAMA 1997 as amended by FDASIA	FD&C Act, §506(a) as added by FDASIA

Table 1. FDA Programs for Expedited Development and Review
Food Drug and Cosmetic (FD&C) Act
FDA Modernization Act (FDAMA) of 1997
Prescription Drug User Fee Act (PDUFA) 1992

Although these regulatory options are not specifically intended for orphan drugs, the designations may also apply to drugs in development for rare diseases.

Orphan Drug Legislation

In 1983, US FDA created a pathway for drug approval for therapeutic agents for orphan indications. The unique challenges of clinical development of drugs for orphan indications was recognized in the Orphan Drug Act (ODA). The ODA has been successful in bringing hundreds of new drugs to market for neglected diseases.

Based on the number of FDA programs available, it is of interest to note how the orphan drug designations and expedited approval pathways have influenced specific aspects of the clinical development process and the time to approval.

Downing et al (2014)[2] investigated the weight of the clinical trial evidence supporting FDA approval of novel therapeutic agents between 2005 and 2012. Their analyses identified 188 approvals of novel therapeutic agents (81.9% pharmacologics), including the weight of the clinical trial evidence for products with orphan drug designation (16.5%) and those approved by an accelerated pathway (11.7%). A total of 488 pivotal trials were conducted for 206 indications.

Compared to the design of clinical trials for non-orphan and non-accelerated approvals, fewer pivotal trials for orphan indications and accelerated approval were randomized, double-blind and/or placebo-controlled, and these differences were statistically significant ($p < 0.001$). As would be expected, more orphan drugs and drugs with accelerated approval relied on surrogate outcomes. (See Table 2).

For novel therapeutic agents approved by FDA between 2005 and 2012, the number of subjects exposed to the drug during pivotal efficacy trials was approximately one third for drugs with orphan designation and those with accelerated approval, compared to drug exposure in standard drug development programs. The differences were statistically significant ($p < 0.001$).

	Randomized*	Doubl—Blind*	Placebo—Controlled*	Surrogate Outcome*
All (N=448)	400 (89.3)	356(79.5)	247 (55.1)	219 (48.9)
Orphan Status				
Yes (n=56)	30 (53.6)	21 (37.5)	16 (28.6)	41 (73.2)
No (n=392)	370 (94.4)	335 (85.5)	231 (589)	178 (45.4)
p-value	<0.001	<0.001	<0.001	
Accelerated Approval				
Yes (n=40)	18 (45.0)	12 (30.0)	12 (30.0)	38 (95.0)
No (n=408)	382 (93.6)	344 (84.3)	235 (57.6)	181 (44.4)
p-value	<0.001	<0.001	<0.001	

*N (%) [95% Confidence Interval]

Table 2. Design of Pivotal Efficacy Studies Providing Basis of FDA Approval for Novel Therapeutic Agents, 2005-2012. Adapted from Downing et al (2014).

The duration of the trials, and the completion rates, were similar for all pivotal trials analysed for novel therapeutic agents during the years 2005 to 2012 (See Table 3).

	Randomized*	Doubl—Blind*	Placebo—Controlled*	Surrogate Outcome*
All (N=448)	400 (89.3)	356(79.5)	247 (55.1)	219 (48.9)
Orphan Status				
Yes (n=56)	30 (53.6)	21 (37.5)	16 (28.6)	41 (73.2)
No (n=392)	370 (94.4)	335 (85.5)	231 (589)	178 (45.4)
p-value	<0.001	<0.001	<0.001	
Accelerated Approval				
Yes (n=40)	18 (45.0)	12 (30.0)	12 (30.0)	38 (95.0)
No (n=408)	382 (93.6)	344 (84.3)	235 (57.6)	181 (44.4)
p-value	<0.001	<0.001	<0.001	

**Median (interquartile range [IQR])

Table 3. Exposure to Novel Therapeutic Agents Approved by FDA between 2005 and 2012 during Pivotal Efficacy Trials. Adapted from Downing et al (2014).

In a comparison of the regulatory review times for 510 novel therapeutic agent applications by FDA, European Medicines Agency (EMA) and Health Canada (HC), Downing el al (2014) reported that FDA reviewed and approved applications more quickly on average than EMA and HC. The median length of time to approval was 303 days (185-372) for FDA, 366 days

(310-445) for EMA and 352 days (255-420) for HC. The difference was statistically significant (p <0.001). The median total review time was also shorter at FDA (p=0.002).

Pediatric Legislation

FDA has enacted legislation and created programs to mandate and to encourage the study of pediatric populations during the drug development process. These include; Best Pharmaceuticals for Children Act (BPCA) in 2002,[4] Pediatric Research Equity Act (PREA) in 2003,[5] and pediatric priority review vouchers in 2012.[6] In 2012, both BPCA and PREA were permanently reauthorized under the Food & Drug Administration Safety and Innovation Act (FDASIA).[7]

In 2002, the BPCA became law. BPCA provides incentives for sponsors to conduct FDA-requested pediatric studies by granting an additional six months to any existing marketing exclusivity.

In 2003, the PREA gave FDA the authority to require sponsors to submit an assessment of the safety and effectiveness of a drug for the claimed indications in all relevant pediatric subpopulations as part of certain NDAs, BLAs and supplement applications. In certain cases, PREA allows for deferrals and waivers. Additionally, PREA exempts orphan designated products.

Prior to the implementation of these laws, over 80% of drugs contained no pediatric information. Since implementation of these laws, more pediatric trials have been conducted than in the 50 years preceding and 500 labeling changes have been made to incorporate pediatric-specific information, which provides doctors with important information about correct dosage, safety and effectiveness in children.[3]

Under FDASIA for the first time, PREA includes a provision that requires manufacturers of drugs subject to PREA to submit a Pediatric Study Plan (PSP).[8] The intent of the PSP is to identify needed pediatric studies early in drug development and begin planning for these studies.

A sponsor who is planning to submit a marketing application for a drug or biological product that includes a new active ingredient, a new indication, a new dosage form, a new dosing regimen, or new route of administration (ie. that triggers PREA) is required to submit an initial PSP (iPSP) (unless the indication is already in pediatrics or the indication has been designated as exempt from this requirement, ie. orphan designated products) no later than 60 days after the End-of-Phase 2 meeting with FDA.[9]

In the iPSP, a full or partial waiver may be requested, but will not be formally granted or denied by FDA until the NDA or BLA is approved. If FDA grants a waiver for pediatric studies because there is evidence that the drug would be ineffective or unsafe in any pediatric age group, this information must be included in the product labelling.

Vouchers

The Rare Pediatric Disease Priority Review Voucher (PRV) program was also created under FDASIA which added Section 529 to the Federal Food, Drug, and Cosmetic (FD&C) Act. In November 2014, FDA issued a new guidance intended to assist developers of rare pediatric disease products to assess whether their product may be eligible for rare pediatric disease designation and a PRV.[10]

Sponsors may also request designation of their drug for a "rare pediatric disease" although this designation is not required in order to be eligible for a voucher. Product-specific questions should be directed to the FDA review division.

General questions related to the rare pediatric disease priority review voucher program and requests for pediatric disease priority review vouchers should be submitted to the FDA's Office of Orphan Products Development (OOPD) at orphan@fda.hhs.gov.

Regulatory Status

In 2014, more orphan drugs for rare diseases were approved by FDA than any previous year in the history of the program.

Among the hundreds of newly approved drugs in 2014, FDA considered 41 to be "novel" new drugs. Many were first-in-class and most used one or more of the expedited development and review pathways, including those that allowed more frequent communication with FDA during drug development.[11] For example:

- 78% (32/41) were approved after the first review cycle without FDA requests for more information that would have delayed approval or required a second review cycle;
- 61% (25/41) were designated for Priority Review after FDA determined the drug had the potential to provide a significant advance in medical care and set a target to review the application within six instead of 10 months;
- 41% (17/41) were designated as Fast Track for having the potential to meet unmet medical needs;
- 22% (9/41) had preliminary evidence demonstrating the drug may result in a substantial improvement on at least one clinically significant endpoint over available therapies and were designated as Breakthrough Therapy; and
- 20% (8/41) were approved under FDA's Accelerated Approval program which allows early review of a drug for a serious or life threatening illness that offers a benefit over existing therapies.

Of these 41 "novel" new therapies, 17 also had orphan drug designation and 63% (26/41) were first approved in the US.

Summary

Since the Orphan Drug Act became law in 1983, FDA has created expedited development and review pathways that benefit orphan drug development programs. An orphan drug in development may receive designation for one or more of these programs and shorten the development time, as well as the time to approval.

Some orphan diseases affect far fewer than 200,000 persons in the US. When developing new drugs for these diseases, there may be limited medical experience and a lack of information about the natural history of the disease. Acknowledging these unique challenges, FDA recently issued a draft guidance that provides the Agency's current thinking on how to create a successful drug development process for a rare disease.[12]

Marilyn R. Carlson, DMD, MD, RAC
Vice President, Medical, Regulatory & Scientific Affairs, Agility Clinical, Inc.

Product-specific questions should be directed to the FDA review division. General questions related to the rare pediatric disease priority review voucher program should be directed to OOPD at orphan@fda.hhs.gov or 301-796-8660.

References

1 Guidance for Industry: Expedited Programs for Serious Conditions – Drugs and Biologics. May 2014. http://www.fda.gov/downloads/drugs/guidancecomplianceregulatoryinformation/guidances/ucm358301.pdf

2 Downing NS, Aminawung JA, Shah ND, Harlan M, Krumholz HM, Ross JS. Clinical Trial Evidence Supporting FDA Approval of Novel Therapeutic Agents, 2005-2012. JAMA. 2014;311(4):368-377.

3 FDA Report: Complex Issues in Developing Drugs and Biological Products for Rare Diseases and Accelerating the Development of Therapies for Pediatric Rare Diseases Including Strategic Plan: Accelerating the Development of Therapies for Pediatric Rare Diseases, U.S. Department of Health and Human Services, Food and Drug Administration, 04 July 2014. http://www.fda.gov/downloads/Regula-

toryInformation/Legislation/FederalFoodDrugandCosmeti-cActFDCAct/SignificantAmendmentstotheFDCAct/FDASIA/UCM404104.pdf

4 Best Pharmaceuticals for Children Act (BPCA). https://www.federalregister.gov/articles/2012/10/24/2012-26214/best-pharmaceuticals-for-children-act-bpca-priori-ty-list-of-needs-in-pediatric-therapeutics

5 Pediatric Research Equity Act (PREA). http://www.fda.gov/downloads/Drugs/DevelopmentApprovalProcess/Develop-mentResources/UCM049870.pdf

6 Pediatric Priority Review Vouchers. http://www.fda.gov/Drugs/DevelopmentApprovalProcess/DevelopmentResourc-es/ucm375479.htm

7 Food & Drug Administration Safety and Innovation Act (FDASIA). http://www.fda.gov/RegulatoryInformation/Leg-islation/FederalFoodDrugandCosmeticActFDCAct/Signifi-cantAmendmentstotheFDCAct/FDASIA/default.htm

8 Guidance for Industry: Pediatric Study Plans: Content of and Process for Submitting Initial Pediatric Study Plans and Amended Pediatric Study Plans, Draft. July 2013. http://www.fda.gov/downloads/drugs/guidancecomplianceregula-toryinformation/guidances/ucm360507.pdf

9 Guidance for Industry: How to Comply with the Pediatric Research Equity Act, Draft. September 2005. http://www.fda.gov/downloads/drugs/guidancecomplianceregulatoryin-formation/guidances/ucm079756.pdf

10 Guidance for Industry: Rare Pediatric Disease Priority Review Vouchers, Guidance for Industry, Draft. November 2014. http://www.fda.gov/downloads/RegulatoryInforma-tion/Guidances/UCM423325.pdf

11 Novel New Drugs 2014 Summary. US Food and Drug Administration. January 2015. http://www.fda.gov/down-

loads/Drugs/DevelopmentApprovalProcess/DrugInnovation/
UCM430299.pdf

12 Guidance for Industry: Rare Diseases: Common Issues in
Drug Development, Draft August 2015. http://www.fda.gov/
downloads/Drugs/GuidanceComplianceRegulatoryInforma-
tion/Guidances/UCM458485.pdf

Chapter 15

How Are Patients Involved in the Regulatory Process at the European Level: EURORDIS Perspective

Maria Mavris, Virginie Hivert, François Houÿez and Yann Le Cam
European Organisation for Rare Diseases

Introduction

In the previous chapters, you have been introduced to the importance of interacting with the various stakeholders involved in the research and development of medicines. Patients' groups have successfully collaborated with academic researchers and the pharmaceutical industry to promote and participate in research into their disease and to support these processes either financially or otherwise.[1,2]

Another important stakeholder group in the process of medicine development is the regulators. In this chapter, we will describe the role of patients at the European level with the European Medicines Agency (EMA). Since its creation in 1995, the EMA has always encouraged interaction and dialogue with patients' associations in Europe; this collaboration has increased and strengthened over time. While medicine agencies at the Member State level have also started to integrate patients into decision-making procedures such as France, Netherlands, United Kingdom and Sweden[3], this will not be described here.

In this chapter, we will outline the various areas where patients are involved with EMA and focus particularly on scientific advice (called protocol assistance for orphan medicines) as well as the current and future involvement of patients at the time of marketing authorisation. The aim is to demonstrate the importance and the impact of patient involvement and to describe the processes regarding how patients are invited and how they can prepare for their participation.

The European Medicines Agency and Interactions with Patients

The European Medicines Agency (EMA), like all regulatory agencies for medicines, ensures that the medicines they authorise work and are acceptably safe. The same standards apply to evaluation of medicines at the Member State level as at the European level. However, once a marketing authorisation is obtained from the EMA, it is valid for every Member State of the European Union. The EMA is specifically responsible for the evaluation of medicines for rare diseases, HIV, cancer, neurodegenerative disorders, diabetes, auto-immune and viral diseases as well as for biotech products, gene therapy and monoclonal antibodies, for which the centralised procedure is mandatory.

In brief, the process for requesting regulatory approval for a medicine requires compilation of a dossier containing all the information, from the manufacture of the medicinal product to the clinical trials conducted in the concerned patient group and submitted for evaluation. At various stages along the way, patients are involved in the evaluation; both in scientific committees as well as in an *ad hoc* fashion. These latter contributions are elaborated further in this chapter.

The EMA publishes an annual report, entitled 'Interaction with patients' and consumers' organisations',[4] that details the various areas of work in the EMA where patients are involved. As part of its commitment to transparency of the regulatory process, the EMA has enabled and expanded the information shared with the public and the areas where patients are involved.[4,5] In addition to membership of the Management Board of the Agency, where two positions are held by patients' representatives, currently four scientific committees have patients' representatives as full equal voting members in accordance with their respective regulations (the Committee for Orphan Medicinal Products (COMP); the Paediatric Committee (PDCO); the Committee for Advanced Therapies (CAT) and the Pharmacovigilance and Risk Assessment Committee (PRAC)).[6,7,8,9] The roles and responsibilities of patients in these committees has been extensively described and will not be the focus of this chapter.

While patients are not currently involved in the Committee for Medicinal Products for Human Use (CHMP), an important working party of the CHMP was created in 2006. The Patients' and Consumers' Working Party (PCWP)[10] provides advice to the Agency and its scientific committees on areas including transparency and communication, safety of medicines and medicines evaluation, with particular focus on matters of direct and indirect interest to patients in relation to medicines. Patients' associations interested in joining the PCWP must fulfil certain criteria and all information can be found on the EMA website.[11]

Further to this type of long-term engagement – scientific committee mandates last for 3 years – patients' representatives are involved in *ad hoc* meetings such as at early stages of development in Scientific Advice (known as Protocol Assistance in the case of orphan medicines) and later in the process at the time of request for marketing authorisation in Scientific Advisory Groups (SAG). In Figure 1, we use the example of an orphan medicine to demonstrate the various times at which patients' representatives can play a role in the research and development and overlay this with regulatory processes.

The research and development processes are shown with the regulatory process, and documents destined for the public that are reviewed by patients are also indicated.

If the medicinal product is destined to treat a population of patients with a rare disease, then it might be sent to the Committee for Orphan Medicinal Products to receive an orphan

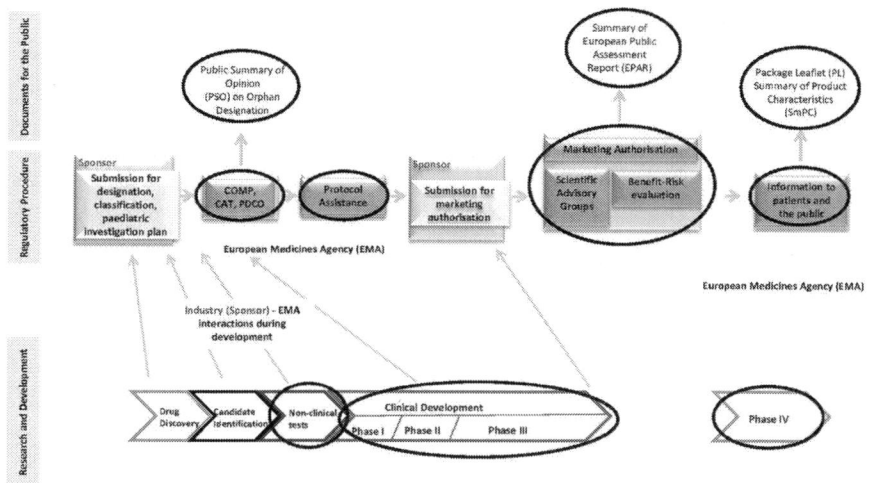

Figure 1: Schematic of research and development of a medicinal product and the associated regulatory processes. Circles indicate patient involvement.

designation. If it is an advanced therapy, it may be sent to the Committee for Advanced Therapies (CAT) to be classified according to the type of advanced therapy it is. Finally, a Paediatric Investigation Plan (PIP) must be submitted to the Paediatric Committee, to ensure that it is developed in the correct way for children, or for the sponsor to receive a waiver in the case that children are not concerned by this disease.

Scientific Advice

The process

A sponsor submits an application requesting orphan designation for their product to the Committee of Orphan Medicinal Products (COMP). Patients' representatives are involved in this committee and deliberate on whether the product meets the criteria[6]. Once a positive opinion is reached by the COMP, followed by adoption of a decision to grant orphan status by the European Commission, the sponsor may then seek Scientific Advice (Protocol Assistance).[12]

Scientific advice is voluntary and applicants ask questions to a working party of the Committee for Human use Medicinal Products (CHMP), which is the committee that provides an opinion on whether a medicinal product should receive marketing authorisation based on its quality, safety and efficacy and a positive benefit-risk balance. This dedicated group, called the Scientific Advice Working Party (SAWP) is comprised of approximately 30 experts from national authorities, universities and hospitals. Scientific advice can be obtained at any time in the medicines development process and on any area such as quality, non-clinical, clinical, statistics and significant benefit; the latter relates specifically to orphans.

The sponsor seeking scientific advice submits questions to the SAWP along with supportive documentation for their reasoning. In return, they expect a report with the opinions of the members of the SAWP dedicated to their dossier. In some cases, a report will be written while in other cases, a face-to-face meeting with the sponsors takes place.

Two important additional options are available for scientific advice: i) request joint scientific advice between the EMA and the US Food and Drug Administration (FDA) and ii) request parallel scientific advice between the EMA and the Health Technology Assessment bodies. Both options provide an opportunity for sponsors to establish the appropriate tests and studies that both parties require to determine a medicine's benefit-risk balance and value.[12]

The role of patients

Patients' representatives have been involved in scientific advice for orphan medicines for more than six years. Given the lack of expertise that exists with rare diseases and the fragmentation of knowledge, the input of the concerned patients or carers becomes invaluable for aspects concerning clinical trials such as inclusion and exclusion criteria for patients, endpoints and objectives of the study, the methodology and medicinal products used as comparators.

While not all procedures require the input of a patient representative, such as those with questions on non-clinical aspects, statistics or follow up confirmatory discussions, the objective is to include as many patients as possible to ensure the patient voice is heard for both the sponsor and the regulator.

What is the impact of patient input in scientific advice?

The majority of experience of patient input into scientific advice processes has been with rare disease patients participating in Protocol Assistance. Based on the positive outcome of these patient contributions, patients representing non-rare diseases have also been invited to participate in scientific advice.

Figure 2 shows the number of patients implicated to date and the number of dossiers received. In addition, the SAWP secretariat reports that in 50% of the cases where patients are involved, they influenced the advice provided by the SAWP to the sponsors (personal communication).

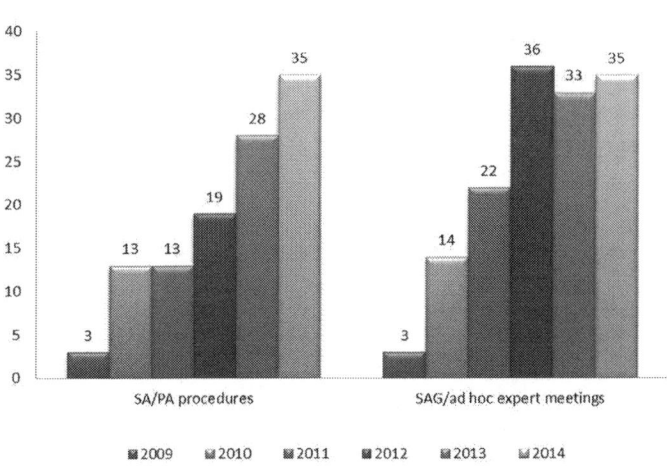

Figure 2: Patient involvement in Protocol Assistance procedures since 2008 and in scientific advice for 2013.

These types of interactions are very positive as they increase the trust between sponsors, regulators and patients; the processes are transparent and they are open to the concerned stakeholders. Extension of this type of patient involvement has been seen further down the regulatory process too, at the time of assessment of the dossier for marketing authorisation (see Figure 1).

Scientific Advisory Groups

The CHMP establishes a scientific advisory group (SAG) at the time of evaluation of a marketing authorisation application, to provide advice in connection with specific types of medicines or treatments. In most cases, the CHMP addresses these questions directly with the sponsor during an oral explanation. However, in some cases, an expert group known as the Scientific Advisory Group (SAG) may be consulted to provide advice.

As with the SAWP meetings, SAG meetings with the sponsor are relatively small, comprising around 10-15 people. Participants include the core SAG members, additional experts including patients, EMA staff and the sponsor and takes up approximately half a day. The meetings are informal and there is an opportunity for the patients' representatives to introduce themselves, to respond to questions regulators may have, and to ask questions for clarification.

The process

Currently, the CHMP chooses to convene a SAG meeting. However, the SAG can be consulted by other EMA scientific committees, the European Commission and by the SAWP. Similarly, the sponsor may also request a SAG to be convened when a dossier submitted for marketing authorisation is re-examined. A SAG is considered necessary when there is a major public health interest or potential controversy, substantial disagreement between the rapporteurs and CHMP members, complex technical issues, rare diseases with a need for expert input, questions about risk minimisation measures, design and feasibility or major post-authorisation safety issues.[13]

First, the questions put forward by the sponsor are explained. The company then presents their viewpoint, which is followed by a discussion with the sponsor. The SAG will then discuss internally, in the absence of the company and, after agreement, will prepare a written answer to the sponsor.

The role of patients

The SAG is composed of European experts, such as clinicians specialised in the field being discussed or patients' representatives with experience of the disease. The patients' input enhances and complements the discussions as they bring real life experience.

It is very important that patients' representatives understand that they are not expected to be scientific, medical or regulatory experts; their experience with the disease is the valuable input that other scientific experts do not have. According to the level of conflict of interest, the participation of patients can be restricted to some aspects of the discussion but not all (for example excluded from the overall conclusion and response to CHMP).

What is the impact of patient input in the SAGs?

In 2014, a total of 35 patients participated in 25 different SAG/expert meetings, providing their views on specific questions posed by the CHMP (Figure 2). The areas covered were: diabetes, HIV infection, cardiovascular, anxiety, multiple sclerosis, renal cell carcinoma, peripheral T-cell lymphoma, burns, axial spondyloarthritis, hepatitis B, Hodgkin lymphoma, short bowel syndrome, obesity, lipoprotein lipase deficiency, anti-infectives, haematopoietic stem cell transplantation therapy, cervical cancer vaccine, Leber's Hereditary Optic Neuropathy, schizophrenia/bipolar disorder, bone disorders, alcohol dependence, small pox vaccine and migraine.[4]

Oral presentations at CHMP meetings

The process

The CHMP assesses the dossiers it receives on a scientific basis to determine whether the medicines concerned meet the necessary quality, safety and efficacy requirements. This ensures, as much as possible, that medicines have a positive risk-benefit balance in favour of patients/users once they reach the marketplace.

The role of patients

The decision to include patients in an oral explanation is on a case-by-case basis. As with the SAWP and SAGs, the patients' representative will have experience of the disease, either as a patient or a carer. The patient representative can contribute to the discussion with the sponsor and with the CHMP after the oral explanation, can ask questions to the committee and the sponsor and in some cases, questions may be addressed directly to the patient. The patient representative does not have the right to vote during these meetings and, in addition, must leave the meeting room at the time the CHMP votes.

With respect to the contributions of the patient, the specific experience of living with the disease on a daily basis is valued. In addition to the aspects previously described for scientific advice, where patients' representatives can contribute to any part of the discussion, in this case, benefit risk has an additional importance. It is not surprising that the patient viewpoint on benefits and risks of a particular medicine may vary to that of a regulator or a healthcare professional. This is not because patients are less careful or less aware of the risks, but primarily because patients' representatives live with the disease either as the affected person themselves or as a family member. The perspective is different and provides an alternative opinion; this is particularly true for rare disease patients.

Patients' input into the assessment of benefit-risk

The experience of patients' input on benefit risk via Scientific Advice (Protocol Assistance) and the SAGs has been demonstrated to be very valuable. In this light, a one-year pilot phase has been launched to involve patients' values on benefit risk during the CHMP meetings. Initially, patients will be invited to contribute to product-specific oral explanations on products for the disease that concerns them. Examples that merit patient involvement include: a probable negative CHMP decision, or when the CHMP and the Pharmacovigilance and Risk Assessment Committee (PRAC) are likely to withdraw, suspend or revoke a marketing authorisation.[4]

Other procedural aspects potentially involving patients

Occasionally, patient organisations may directly address an EMA scientific committee on a specific issue such as withdrawal of a product from the market; the scientific committee will consider the matter and will decide whether further dialogue or interaction is necessary. In all cases, the scientific committee, together with the EMA secretariat, will acknowledge the request and will respond in writing to the patient organisation.

When a marketing authorisation applicant disagrees with the opinion of the CHMP, it can apply for a re-evaluation within 15 days after the initial opinion. Following the assessment of the grounds for appeal submitted by the applicant, the CHMP appoints two different rapporteur and co-rapporteur to re-assess the issues raised by the applicant. The CHMP can also ask advice from the Scientific Advisory Groups, and can involve patients.

How are patients invited to attend meetings at EMA?

The EMA receives the requests for scientific advice/scientific advisory groups and proceeds with the necessary processing and validation of the dossiers. Based on the type of questions submitted by the applicant sponsor, the requests are sent to the patients' organisations to identify an appropriate patient representative to participate in the procedure.

In the case of Scientific Advice, a first meeting of SAWP is held to discuss questions raised by the sponsor and to determine if a discussion meeting with the SAWP and the sponsor will take place, or if a response will be written.

The sponsor is informed of the decision and a response is written, or a discussion meeting is organised. Concurrently, the patients' representatives are nominated by the EMA or the contact patients' organisation, confidentiality and conflicts of interest are submitted, signed and assessed. Once all is in order, the confidential documents are sent to the patient representative who reviews and either, makes comments in written form, prepares to attend the discussion meeting at the EMA in London, or can join via conference call if unable to physically be present.

Throughout the process, patients' representatives are supported by the EMA staff as well as by the contact patient organisation. The EMA staff assists with procedural aspects such as completing and submitting the confidentiality and conflict of interest forms, as well as orienting them to the questions they should concentrate on. In addition, the contact patient organisation will support the patient representative by explaining logistical aspects, as well as help draw attention to the important questions. EMA organises all travel and accommodation where necessary.

For attendance to CHMP meetings, patients will be invited through the same channels, have to fill the same forms and go through the same process. However, in this case a mentor will also be appointed. The mentor will be a patient representative (from the PCWP), who has experience in EMA procedures and would provide support.

A video has been prepared by EMA for patients attending SA/SAGs that can also be used to support patients attending the EMA discussions in general.[14]

How can patients prepare to participate in meetings at EMA?

All meetings at EMA and reports are in English. It is therefore important that the nominated patient representative can speak and read English. At times, more than one representative has been nominated to provide support for each other and to review the documents together. However, in the case of scientific advice, only one patient representative can attend the meeting, whereas for SAGs and CHMP oral explanations, two may be invited to attend. It is important to remember at all times that the information is confidential and cannot be shared with anyone who has not signed the EMA confidentiality forms.

It is important for patients' representatives to feel supported and valued. They have experience with the disease being discussed; living with it themselves on a daily basis or caring for someone affected by the disease. They have knowledge of the impact on their lives and of their medical history, which medications and procedures they have tried and what are the real aspects that should be considered when examining the positive impact on the life of someone living with the disease. These are the valuable aspects that patients' representatives bring to the discussion.

Patients' representatives are encouraged to be prepared for the meeting by reading the documents provided, to ask questions to the EMA staff or to the patients' organisation that contacted them to be sure they understand the process. They should remember that they are there speaking on behalf of patients concerned by a specific disease and not as a medical or scientific expert (Figure 3).

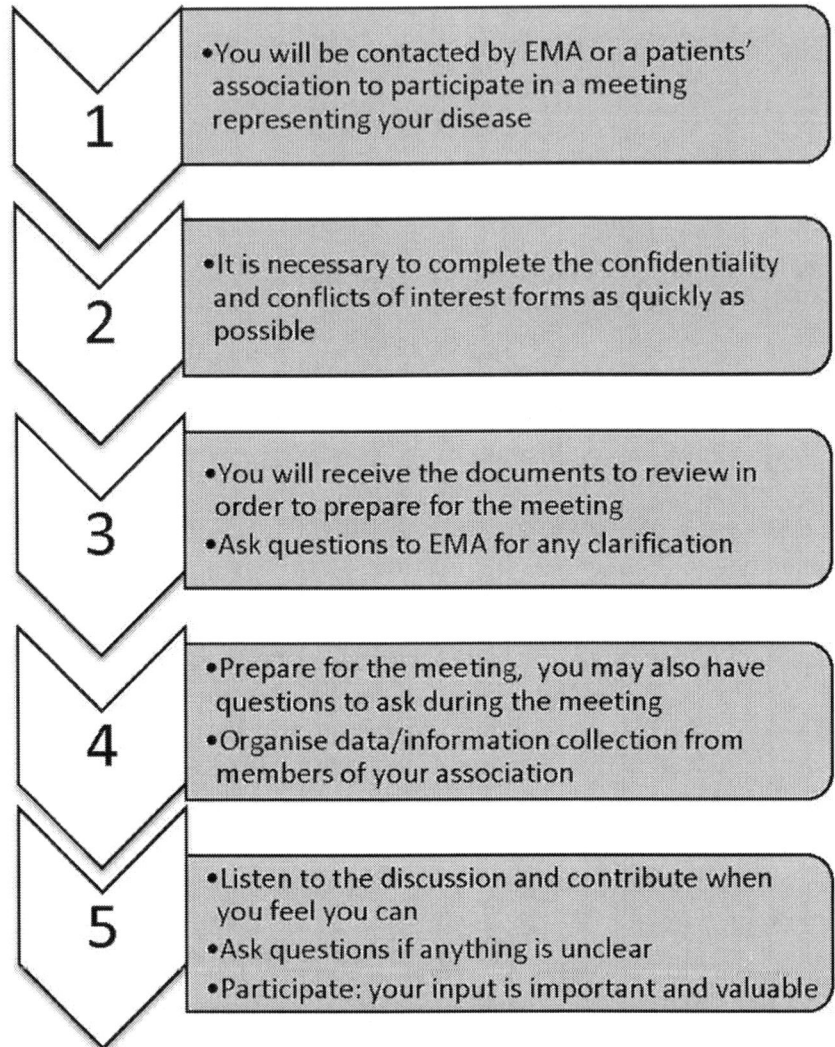

Figure 3: Advice for patients' preparation for attending meetings at EMA

It is understood that it can be intimidating to attend such a meeting and the EMA staff go to great lengths to prepare patients as much as possible and to make them feel at ease. Their input is very valuable and so the best advice is for patients to try to enjoy the process and to feel proud of the input that they are offering for other people living with the same disease and to the patient community in the EU.

Conclusions

The importance of including the patient voice in many aspects of medicine development has been recognised extensively by many of the stakeholders involved in this complex process. Early and continuous dialogue with the concerned patient group will encourage trust between sponsors and patients and regulators and patients, etc. Collaboration of this type can lead to protocols with more meaningful outcomes for patients, methodology that encourages more adherence by patients during the trials, as well as more efficient regulatory processes.

Underpinning this patient input is of course the invaluable personal experience of people living with a disease – either personally or as a family member or carer. However, there is also a need to educate patients' representatives in medicine development and regulatory processes and beyond, and initiatives such as the EURORDIS Summer School[15] and the European Patients Academy in Therapeutic Innovation[16] are taking on the task of achieving this objective.

Maria Mavris, Virginie Hivert, François Houÿez and Yann Le Cam
European Organisation for Rare Diseases, Plateforme Maladies Rares, 96 rue Didot, 75014 Paris, France.

References

1 Role of Patient Groups in Research and their Priorities for the Future. (Accessed 17 July 2015). http://www.eurordis.org/sites/default/files/publications/3_FBignami_RDD2010.pdf

2 EURORDIS Survey on "European Rare Disease Patient Groups in Research: current role and priorities for the future." (Accessed 17 July 2015). http://www.eurordis.org/content/survey-patient-groups-research

3 Draft agenda – EMA Human Scientific Committees' Working Parties with Patients' and Consumers' Organisations

(PCWP) and Healthcare Professionals' Organisations (HCPWP) joint meeting. (Accessed 17 July 2015). http://www.ema.europa.eu/docs/en_GB/document_library/Agenda/2014/05/WC500166310.pdf

4 Documents on key areas of the Agency's work with patients and consumers. (Accessed 17 July 2015). http://www.ema.europa.eu/ema/index.jsp?curl=pages/partners_and_networks/document_listing/document_listing_000235.jsp&mid=WC0b01ac05800aa3cb

5 The European Medicines Agency and Transparency: The Rare Disease Patients' perspective; Regulatory Rapporteur 11 (4): 11-15.

6 Regulation (EC) No 141/2000 of the European Parliament and of the Council of 16 December 1999 on orphan medicinal products. (Accessed 17 July 2015). http://eurlex.europa.eu/LexUriServ/LexUriServ.do?uri=CELEX-:32000R0141:EN:HTML

7 Regulation (EC) No 1901/2006 of the European Parliament and of the Council of 12 December 2006 on medicinal products for paediatric use and amending Regulation (EEC) No 1768/92, Directive 2001/20/EC, Directive 2001/83/EC and Regulation (EC) No 726/2004. (Accessed 17 July 2015). http://eurlex.europa.eu/LexUriServ/LexUriServ.do?uri=OJ:L:2006:378:0001:0019:en:PDF

8 Regulation (EC) No 1394/2007 of the European Parliament and of the Council of 13 November 2007 on advanced therapy medicinal products and amending Directive 2001/83/EC and Regulation (EC) No 726/2004. (Accessed 17 July 2015). http://ec.europa.eu/health/files/eudralex/vol-1/reg_2007_1394/reg_2007_1394_en.pdf

9 Regulation (EU) No 1235/2010 of the European Parliament and of the Council of 15 December 2010 amending, as regards pharmacovigilance of medicinal products for human use, Regulation (EC) No 726/2004 laying down Commu-

nity procedures for the authorisation and supervision of medicinal products for human and veterinary use and establishing a European Medicines Agency, and Regulation (EC) No 1394/2007 on advanced therapy medicinal products. (Accessed 17 July 2015). http://ec.europa.eu/health/files/eudralex/vol-1/reg_2010_1235/reg_2010_1235_en.pdf

10 Patients' and Consumers' Working Party (EMA website). (Accessed 17 July 2015). http://www.ema.europa.eu/ema/index.jsp?curl=pages/contacts/CHMP/people_listing_000017.jsp&mid=WC0b01ac0580028d32

11 The roles of patients as members of the EMA human scientific committees. (Accessed 17 July 2015). http://www.ema.europa.eu/docs/en_GB/document_library/Other/2011/12/WC500119614.pdf

12 Scientific Advice and Protocol Assistance (EMA website). (Accessed 17 July 2015). http://www.ema.europa.eu/ema/index.jsp?curl=pages/regulation/general/general_content_000049.jsp&mid=WC0b01ac05800229b9

13 Procedural Advice for CHMP on the need to convene a Scientific Advisory Group (SAG) or Ad Hoc Expert Meeting. (Accessed 17 July 2015). http://www.ema.europa.eu/docs/en_GB/document_library/Other/2011/07/WC500109577.pdf

14 Introductory video intended for patient representatives invited to participate in scientific advice (SA) or scientific advisory meeting (SAG) at the European Medicines Agency (EMA). 2015. (Accessed 17 July 2015). https://www.youtube.com/watch?v=pzrTwxLesEk

15 EURORDIS website – Training Resources. (Accessed 17 July 2015). www.eurordis.org/training-resources

16 European Patient Academy on Therapeutic innovation (EUPATI). (Accessed 17 July 2015). www.patientsacademy.eu

Chapter 16

Empowering Children to Become Involved in the Research Agenda

Elin Haf Davies PhD
Aparito

The European Union has long supported and promoted the importance of allowing children to "express their views freely" and be "taken into consideration on matters which concern them in accordance with their age and maturity".[1] The Council of Europe in their strategies 'Building Europe for and with children' (2009-2011) and the Rights of the Child (2012-2015), specify that "Children should be considered as active members of society, and not as mere passive subjects of decisions taken by adults. Taking their age and maturity into consideration, they should be consulted and given the opportunity to take part in social decision-making processes on all health care issues".[2,3]

The 'Committee of Experts on Child Friendly Health Care' also promoted the need to find ways to promote children's participation in decision-making regarding their own health care and in broader children's health care, and to examine approaches that can increase the coping potential of children, their families and caregivers, including the importance of bringing parents into the arena.

In recent years, extensive work has been carried out in the area of patient and public involvement (PPI) in the adult population. Numerous organisations, both general and disease-specific, now work to provide more information to patients with regards to participation in clinical trials and involvement in the design of clinical trials. It has also been reported that patient involvement in research boosts study success, with studies that included collaboration with patients in designing or running the trial being 1.63 times more likely to recruit to target than studies which only consulted patients. Studies that involved more partnerships were 4.12 times more likely to recruit to target.[4]

It has also been reported that listening to children/ youth opinions before making decisions helps to increase their adherence.[5] Doctors, ethics committees, industry and policy-makers now acknowledge that, in order to make paediatric clinical drug trials both acceptable and more relevant to patients and parents, early and meaningful engagement with children and their families is essential. With best practice now based on involving young people in setting the research agenda, project development, development of protocols and design of interventions.

An evaluation of communication and involvement of paediatric patients in research by the EU project **RESPECT**,[6] emphasised a need for enhanced patient involvement and empowerment, and the need for tailoring information to the child and parents.[5]

Of late, there is also increased attention to the importance of patient participation in trial design and outcomes selection, for children and young people too. In particular, the following groups have a specific focus on seeking the views of children and young people on all things research: the **Young Persons Advisory Group** of the Medicine Children Research Network (MCRN) and the ScotCRN in the UK; **KIDS** (Kids and Families Impacting Disease Through Science) in the USA; and **Young Advisors of CFRI** in Canada. More groups are sure to be established soon.

Embracing the value of engagement, the Paediatric Committee (PDCO) at the European Medicine Agency (EMA) also explored ways to facilitate the involvement of children and young people in the drug development process. It has been the EMA's long-standing policy to involve patients in their decision-making processes. In fact, it has been engaging with patients since its creation in 1995, and this interaction has increased considerably over the years, with patient representatives now being systematically involved across a wide range of EMA activities.

This includes being members of its scientific committees and management board; taking part in scientific advisory meetings; responding to consultations on specific medicines; reviewing the lay information on medicines prepared by the Agency; and regularly taking part in its conferences and workshops. The EMA currently works with over 35 patient/consumer organisations and has a dedicated patients and consumers' working party (PCWP) that acts as a permanent forum for dialogue on issues of interest to patients in relation to medicinal products. The interaction with patient groups has proved to be extremely beneficial; as they offer a real-life perspective to the scientific discussions on medicines, and provide valuable insights that the scientific experts do not necessarily have. There is a need and expectation for public bodies to listen to the views and experiences of patients, including young people, as they are the ones most affected by the regulatory decisions.

As part of this endeavour, the EMA, in conjunction with the European Network of Paediatric Research (**Enpr-EMA**) at the EMA,[7] conducted an online survey to identify the extent of children's and young people's current involvement in paediatric clinical research by all 39 registered members of Enpr-EMA. Although the numbers currently active in this field were identified to be rather low, the survey identified a high level of interest to promote greater child and family involvement. There was also a request for guidelines on establishing and maintaining young people's advisory groups and it identified the need for training/support or mentoring for this activity.

For its first direct engagement with young people, the EMA collaborated with the European Patients' Forum (EPF), and participated in a meeting in Brussels on 10 July 2013. Twenty-six young patients from several EU Countries gathered for a four-day seminar, as part of 'emPATHY'–"Europe meets young patients"–a project organised by EPF together with other nine patient organisations with financial support from the Youth in Action Programme of the European Commission. The overall objective of this seminar was to promote a more holistic approach to addressing young patients' needs at EU-level decision-making processes.[8]

As part of this meeting, the EMA were given the opportunity to participate in a two-hour workshop in order to specifically discuss PDCO activities and ambitions. It also gave an opportunity to get the group's thoughts about formulations and consenting to take part in clinical trials.

The EPF was founded in 2003 to ensure that the patients' community drives policies and programmes that affect patients' lives, to bring changes that empower them to be equal citizens in the EU. EPF currently represents 61 member organisations which are chronic disease-specific patient organisations working at European level, and national coalitions of patients' organisations. EPF reflects the voice of an estimated 150 million patients affected by various diseases throughout Europe.[9]

Involving young patients in a meaningful way through empowerment was identified as a long-term goal for EPF. EPF's first youth initiative dates back to 2008, when the Young Patient Perspective Project was implemented. In an attempt to enable patient organisations recognition and representation of the needs of young patients, the 2010 Regional Advocacy Seminar was dedicated to sharing good practice of young patients' participation in patient groups. Following the outcomes of the 2010 Regional Advocacy Seminar a EPF Youth Strategy was developed and adopted by our 2011 Annual General Meeting. On that occasion, the EPF Youth Group was established and the first Youth Assembly was held in Brussels, on 19-21 August 2012.

These initiatives are now increasing in numbers and in momentum, and are a sure signal that the benefits of early dialogue and engagement with children and young people will benefit paediatric research. The following case studies illustrate some great examples of work already done.

Case study 1

Gaucher Association UK: Empowering Young Patients to Shape the Future

Type III Gaucher disease (GD) is a rare metabolic disease. In the UK there are fewer than 25 patients.

In 2006 one of the nurses from Great Ormond Street Hospital (GOSH) and the UK Gaucher Association joined forces and started a group called the 'Aunty Days'. The purpose of this group initially was to bring together a group of young girls with Type III GD aged 11 – 16 years, to support each other while taking part in a clinical trial, to enjoy each other's company while doing fun things and to have the opportunity to talk about life, school and living with a chronic neuronopathic condition.

Turning the clock forward eight years and the girls group has gone from strength to strength. Through the continued support of the Clinical Nurses at GOSH and the Gauchers Association, the girls have: organised, chaired and presented a Type III family conference in November 2013; written and published a book on transitioning from paediatric to adult care; and set up a project to buddy younger type III patients. Two of them now sit on the Board of the Gauchers Association and three of them are involved in projects where they are speaking at UK and International meetings, about the challenges of growing up with a chronic condition, and demonstrating how they have been able to empower themselves to shape their future, and support others to do the same.

In December 2012 the Clinical Nurses at GOSH received an award from the Gauchers Association for their work supporting young Type III girls through the 'Aunty' project. This award is given every two years in recognition of an individual or individuals making a significant contribution to Gaucher patients and their families.

In September 2012 the Gauchers Association received a Global Patient Leadership (PALs) award from Genzyme to take forward this project, entitled 'empowering Young Type III GD Patients to Shape the Future'. This grant ensures that young people remain at the forefront of setting the research agenda.

Case study 2

Nuffield Council's film resources: young people's perspectives on clinical ethics reviews

In March 2014, the Nuffield Council on Bioethics launched two films as part of its project *Children and clinical research: ethical issues*[10]. The films were produced in collaboration with researchers from the University of Sussex, the University of Nottingham, and the Institute of Education, and focused on young people's perception of the ethical review process.

Students from a junior school, a secondary school, and a sixth form college in Brighton were shown a film featuring a 'mock' adult Research Ethics Committee (REC). The REC debated ethical issues associated with a fictional research protocol that proposed a different way of treating childhood asthma; through the use of 'personalised' medicine.[11] The same research protocol was then presented to the students, and their reactions were filmed both before and after they were shown the deliberations of the adult REC.

A report, summarising the main findings of the school workshops,[12] emphasised the importance of approaching clinical research from a 'child-centred' perspective. For example, overly-technical information sheets were found to be boring and inaccessible, limiting rather than enhancing understanding. Concerns were also expressed about participants being put at (unnecessary) risk.

Participants in the workshops highlighted that young people's contributions to clinical research should be valued (although not necessarily in financial terms) and identified the importance of building meaningful relationships with the research team, and of creating a three-way exchange of information between young people, their parents/guardians, and the research team. Sixth formers, as well as the younger participants, also indicated that they would include their parents in making decisions about taking part in clinical research.

The findings of the films and workshops will form part of the evidence considered by the Nuffield Council when forming recommendations for its forthcoming project report.

Case study 3

The NIHR Clinical Research Network (CRN): Working alongside industry to involve young people in formulation development

Children have been at the forefront of patient and public involvement in research for some time. In 2006, the NIHR Clinical Research Network started its first Young Persons' Advisory Group (YPAG), based at the network's coordinating centre in Liverpool. Since then, four more groups have been established in London, Nottingham, Birmingham and Bristol. The initial remit of these groups was to engage young people with research and to work in partnership with, and offer support to, researchers. The group provides a forum for young people to learn about, and comment on, various aspects of the research cycle, from the identification of research questions to the dissemination of research findings.

The NIHR is increasingly trying to promote involvement with patients and the public at the earliest stage possible in protocol development, to ensure the outcomes and acceptability of the study suit the needs of patients and families. Several examples of this can be found in a recently published summary evaluation report.[13] However, one particular study has been identified as the 'gold standard' for the inclusion and involvement of young people in the development of a new formulation of metformin, for the treatment of polycystic ovary syndrome (PCOS) in young people. Metfizz is a clinical development program for an effervescent Metformin soluble, for the treatment of PCOS in adolescent girls. Metfizz receives funding from the Seventh Framework Programme of the European Union and is co-ordinated by EffRx Pharmaceuticals SA, a speciality pharmaceutical company.

This is the first time that a pharmaceutical company formed a partnership with the NIHR CRN: involving paediatric patients from the initial design stage right the way through to completion of the study. The overall expectation is that young people will be involved throughout, inputting on a range of aspects over time, including the presentation and packaging of medicines, the study protocols, the outcomes to be measured in the study, as well as patient information leaflets.

To date, two groups of young people have been consulted: (i) 20 members of the NIHR Liverpool Young Person's Advisory Group (YPAG), aged eight to 18, and (ii) a group of nine young women currently being treated for PCOS, aged 13 to 18. The YPAG members initially worked together as a group to shortlist possible flavours for the medicine, such as banana, strawberry and orange, and to develop a discussion guide which could be used for consultation and involvement with the PCOS group. The PCOS group was then interviewed individually via one-to-one, in-depth interviews, to explore their views on the medicine (flavour, packaging and colour). This group was also given a 'sniff test' of the shortlisted flavours to choose from. The majority of young people consulted recommended that the medicine should be orange flavoured. The research team therefore opted for this flavour, with the expectation that using a flavour that appeals to young people, will help support compliance with taking the medicine during the trial, and beyond.

The study is yet to start, but young people's on-going opinions about the new medication will be captured through weekly diaries, that young people in the trial will be asked to complete.

Young people also reported their views about what the packaging should be like, and many of their suggestions were taken on board. The research team felt that considering young people's views on the presentation and packaging of the medicine, will help to support effective participant engagement in the study, and thereby support its overall success.

Young people in the PCOS group have also designed patient information sheets and, more importantly, highlighted important outcomes that are relevant to them.

Robyn, a member of the PCOS group, highlights the importance of this collaboration: *"To be able to work alongside industry professionals and be taken seriously is really motivating. Having lived with this condition for several years it is great to see that industry is open to involving young people in their research to develop a more patient friendly end product"*.

- Key learning points: The NIHR CRN: Children, Patient Involvement Manager was grateful for the support of the staff in the NIHR Alder Hey Clinical Research Facility (CRF) and the clinical staff, as they were able to provide a physical space for the young people's consultations to take place and offer logistical and practical support.
- Setting up a specialist group for young women with PCOS proved time consuming and challenging and this needs to be borne in mind for any future projects of a similar nature. In this case, this process required the manager to liaise with a key contact, who was already working with young people with PCOS, who then contacted all the possible young people asking if they would like to take part. The young people then had to be interviewed and fully briefed before they could be asked for consent to participate in the study. The process of setting up the group took several months.

- Setting dates for meetings with the PCOS group was also challenging because of the distance that the young people would need to travel and their availability.
- The young people appreciated that their views were being taken into account and were pleased that their choices of flavour and packaging were selected. This highlights the importance of ensuring that young people's input is genuinely taken on board, and the benefit of feeding back to participants.

For further information of this project or young people's activities within the NIHR CRN: Children, please contact Jenny Preston (patient and public involvement manager) on Jennifer. preston@liverpool.ac.uk

How to get children involved

Patient groups

Patient groups are best placed to create a Young People's Advisory Group themselves. By taking the example of the Gaucher Association UK, groups can be formed by recruiting for young people from contacts already known in the organisation, via the managing physicians or even via social media / on the web. By creating a disease-specific young people's advisory group as part of an existing patient organisation, the young people can be supported by people that completely understand their needs, and can ensure that their rights are protected at all times.

Clinicians / Researchers

Depending on the issues to be discussed, a clinician / researcher may choose to contact either a generic Young People's Advisory Group that already exists, such as at the NIHR Clinical Research Network or a specific disease group. The review of language and terminology in assent forms etc. can probably be best done by a generic group, whereas specific questions related to assessment and study design, are probably best asked to the actual patients that are to be recruited. Clinicians and researchers can also be instrumental in supporting patient groups create a Young People's Group – particularly when qualified health care professionals can offer support during the events.

There is a clear distinction between involving patients and young people as a means to obtaining specific input and guidance on issues relating to them *vs* conducting research on their views. The opinion of an ethics committee should always be sought if there is uncertainty whether the work done is classified as research or not.

Pharmaceutical companies

Companies should always seek the input of children and young people through established groups, either disease-specific or generic. Issues to be discussed, and the questions to be asked, should always be checked with those established groups and/or clinicians and researchers first.

Again, if there is uncertainty whether the work done is classified as research or not, the opinion of an ethics committee should always be sought.

Elin Haf Davies
Email : elin@elinhafdavies.co.uk
Tel : +447884495357

References

1 Charter of Fundamental Rights European Union, Art. 24 (1) December 2012. (Accessed 21 July 2015). http://eur-lex. europa.eu/legalcontent/EN/TXT/?uri=CELEX:12012P/TXT

2 The Council of Europe Programme in 'Building a Europe for and with children – 2009-2011 strategy'. (Accessed 21 July 2015). http://srsg.violenceagainstchildren.org/sites/default/files/documents/docs/COE_2009-2011_StrategyProgramme_

EN.pdf

3 Council of Europe Strategy for the Rights of the Child (2012-2015). (Accessed 21 July 2015). http://www.coe.int/t/DGHL/STANDARDSETTING/CDcj/StrategyCME.pdf

4 Ennis, L. et al. 2013. Impact of patient involvement in mental health research: longitudinal study. British Journal of Psychiatry. 203(5):318-6.

5 McDonagh, JE, Bateman, B. 2012. 'Nothing about us without us': considerations for research involving young people. Arch Dis Chil Educ Ed. 97: 55-60

6 Chaplin, JE. 2012. RESPECT patient needs. Relating expectation and needs to the participation and empowerment of children in clinical trials.

7 European Medicine Agency Networks – European Network of Paediatric Research (Enpr-EMA). (Accessed 21 July 2015). http://www.ema.europa.eu/ema/index.jsp?curl=pages/partners_and_networks/general/general_content_000303.jsp&mid=WC0b01ac05801df74a

8 European Patients Forum EMPATHY announcement. (Accessed 21 July 2015). http://www.eu-patient.eu/whatwedo/Projects/EPF-led-EU-Projects/EMPATHY/

9 European Patients Forum. (Accessed 21 July 2015). www.eu-patient.eu

10 Nuffield Council on Bioethics. 2014. Films: young people's perspectives on clinical research ethics reviews. (Accessed 21 July 2015). http://nuffieldbioethics.org/children-and-research/children-and-research-films-young-peoples-perspectives-clinical-ethics-reviews.

11 The protocol was developed in association with Professor Somnath Mukopadhyay, whose own research focuses on the possibilities of personalising medication for children and young people who have severe asthma.

12 Spencer G, Boddy J and Reed R. 2014. Children and young people perspectives on ethics review of clinical research with children. (Accessed 21 July 2015). http://nuffieldbioethics. org/sites/default/files/files/Report_young_peoples_perspectives_on_ethics_review.pdf.

13 Resources. National Institute for Health Research. Clinical Research Network Children. NHS. (Accessed 21 July 2015). http://www.crn.nihr.ac.uk/children/resources.

Chapter 17

Natural History Studies

Marc K. Walton, MD, PhDJanssen Research and Development

Anne R. Pariser, MDFood and Drug Administration

> *"The whole art of medicine is observation"*
> — Sir William Osler (1849-1919).

The natural history (NH) of a disease is a description of the disease, in the absence of intervention, beginning either from the time of disease onset (often symptom onset leading to initial diagnosis) or prior to disease onset for those persons at risk of developing a disease (eg. due to exposure to a causal agent). A complete natural history description continues uninterrupted throughout the course of disease until recovery or death.[1] NH studies provide the opportunity to identify demographic, genetic, environmental, and other variables that correlate with the disease and its outcomes in the absence of disease modifying treatment.[2]

The careful description of a disease is a fundamental practice of medicine,[3,4,5] and NH studies have an essential role in describing the etiology, clinical manifestations and rate of progression of diseases.[6] Importantly, NH studies can provide an organizing framework around which first steps toward initiating research into individual disorders are often taken.[7,8,9] The information derived from NH studies provides foundational and translational research support, which can be applied toward several major purposes, including the establishment of clinical research and therapeutics development, epidemiology, data standards programs, research and communication networks, and toward public health programs, such as improvement in patient care practices and healthcare delivery.[10,11,12]

Value of Natural History Studies for Rare Diseases

Description of disease NH is especially important for rare diseases. Rare diseases are a highly diverse collection of disorders, which often have substantial phenotypic heterogeneity within the individual disorders, and most of which are incompletely understood.[13,14] Rare diseases are defined in the United States (US) as conditions affecting less than 200,000 individuals in the United States,[15] and in Europe as a condition with a prevalence not more than 5 in 10,000.[16] There are estimated to be approximately 7000 rare diseases. Consequently, while individual rare diseases affect small numbers of patients, collectively they affect a significant portion of the population (ie. approximately 25-30 million people in the US). Most rare diseases are serious or life-threatening disorders with unmet medical needs, and in addition to the pain and suffering they inflict upon individual patients and their families, they represent a large public health concern for which the need for research support and NH study development has been identified internationally.[17,18,19,20,21]

There are several important applications for the information derived from NH studies, including (see Table 1):

- General disease tracking, providing epidemiologic estimates, patient identification and demographic data, and for communication purposes;
- Patient care, such as understanding the current standard of care practices and identification of treatment centers;

- Research prioritization and needs evaluation; and
- Therapeutics development and clinical trials support.

Table 1 Value of a Natural History Study

Communication, patient identification and demographic data collections
Inform patient care, develop standards of care and best practices, support development of treatment centers

Foundational and translational science development to:
 	
  • Describe full range of disease and important phenotypes, genotypes, and subpopulations within a disease (or group of related disorders)
  • Identify knowledge gaps, research priorities

Therapeutics development and clinical trials support
 	
  • Inform design and conduct of clinical trials
  • Develop and pilot clinical assessment tools, measures and outcomes for use in interventional trials
  • Identify and develop predictive, prognostic and response biomarkers for use in interventional trials
  • Refine disease definition and diagnostic criteria
  • Identify appropriate controls. Rarely, may serve as an historical control

General Disease Tracking

A frequent early step in beginning a NH study is an assessment and collection of information on patients known or thought to have the disease or condition. General information collected will include demographic and contact information, sometimes referred to as a communication registry (a communication registry can stand on its own or as part of a NH study). Vital functions of general disease tracking information include formation and strengthening of disease communities and the provision of a vehicle through which patients, their families and other stakeholders receive information relevant to the disease (eg. disease information and support, upcoming or ongoing research). Importantly, it can have a powerful effect upon the research and drug development communities, influencing decisions regarding planning for and initiating research activities. For example, availability of some prevalence information regarding a rare disease, the geographic location of patients and basic demographic information (such as age) may inform drug developers about a potential patient pool for a clinical trial. Having a well-organized and defined patient community with an accessible communication network can heavily impact decisions regarding the feasibility of conducting a clinical development program for a specific rare disease. The importance of establishing these networks cannot be overstated.

Patient Care and Research Prioritization

In a NH study, an orderly collection of the full range of care patients are receiving enables assessment of the scope of treatment practices for rare diseases. NH study clinics can also serve as a medical home for patients with a rare disease, particularly in situations where a condition has few experienced health providers or treatment centers. An assessment of care provided across treatment centers can better describe the range of existing patient care practices and assist with the development of best practices that may not otherwise be feasible for many rare diseases.[22,23] Similarly, documentation of clinical care and the often multi-disciplinary needs of patients with rare diseases (eg. developmental, nutritional, physical and occupational), is an effective way of recognizing gaps in patient care needs that can help identify and prioritize additional areas of research for a specific disease.

Therapeutics Development and Clinical Trials Support

One of the most important uses of NH study information is to inform drug development (Note: Drug and biological products will be collectively referred to as "drugs" unless otherwise specified). NH studies can establish a scientific foundation upon which rational drug development programs can be designed and conducted, and can help to make these programs more efficient. Of the approximately 7,000 different rare diseases, only a few hundred have drugs approved for their treatment.[24] Thus, most rare disease drug development programs are novel, are first-in-disease, and there is no existing model for clinical therapeutics research upon which to base a drug development program. Given the small number of patients with an individual disease, the opportunity for study of a candidate drug in clinical trials will be limited, and 'getting it right the first time' will be important. As a result, more (and more careful) planning is usually needed to develop therapeutic agents for rare disorders than for common diseases.

An important and essential role for NH studies in these situations is to provide comprehensive knowledge about the disease upon which clinical trials can be built, including:

- Full understanding of the entire spectrum of the disease, including the overall population and important subpopulations with the disease or condition. Many rare diseases have substantial phenotypic and genotypic variability within the disorder and, in order to fully appreciate the entire spectrum of the disease, the full range of disease manifestations, their time course, and variability of these manifestations between patients should be described.
- Disease definition and diagnostic criteria for the disease overall and important subpopulations within the disease. Diagnostic criteria could include a description of important medical events with the disease (eg. disease-defining criteria), and the use of objective testing, such as laboratory or genetic testing.
- Clinical assessments, such as patient reported outcomes, clinical events (eg. survival, clinical progression), assessment tools and measurement scales that may be used as endpoints in clinical trials. When no clearly appropriate clinical assessment tools are known, NH studies provide an opportunity to identify and pilot new assessments, or modified versions of existing assessments, in advance of a therapeutic clinical trial.
- Biomarkers, including the development of new or optimized biomarkers that may provide proof-of-concept information for the disease, patient identification

or drug selection, and for the evaluation of candidate drugs, may help guide dose selection and provide supportive information for efficacy and safety evaluations.

Knowledge of these elements is of most value when available prior to initiating clinical trials of a candidate drug, and will contribute to the efficiency of clinical evaluation in a therapeutic trial ('clinical trial readiness'). For example, for a drug to receive traditional approval in the US, substantial evidence of clinical benefit needs to be demonstrated, usually through the conduct of at least one adequate and well-controlled (A&WC) clinical study.[25] An A&WC study is one that has been designed and conducted in adherence to generally accepted principles of scientific research, including (but not limited to) identifying and selecting an appropriate patient population and using reliable outcome measures.[26] The design and conduct of A&WC studies necessitate a scientific foundation that includes knowledge of the disease's natural history, as well as an understanding of the candidate drug and its expected effect upon the disease.[27]

An additional important consideration for an A&WC study is the selection of a valid comparator or control group. Although consideration of NH studies as an historical control for an A&WC study is often raised, validity of NH knowledge as clinical trial control is uncommon.[28] Use of historical controls in A&WC studies is generally infeasible unless special circumstances apply. This includes a disease with a rapid, stereotypical clinical course with a well-defined clinical outcome that can be readily and objectively measured (eg. mortality) and for which the effects of the drug are self-evident (ie. effect is rapid following treatment and, usually, of sufficient magnitude such that it can be readily ascertained). Instead, use of NH study knowledge is a valuable contributor to the overall progress of a drug development program by providing the medical and scientific support upon which rational and scientifically sound clinical development programs can be built.

Study Design Considerations

Data Quality and Consistency

Conducting a single common NH study is more productive and can describe the disease better than conducting several smaller separate or single center studies. This requires coordination and advance planning to ensure that the data collected are of good quality across all study locations and are interpretable. The integrity of the data collected in a NH study is important, since the information will be used to inform the important purposes discussed earlier. Unreliable information has the potential to send these other initiatives (eg. clinical trials, patient care, analytics) in the wrong direction, resulting in delays, inefficiencies and increased costs; it can cause harm or, may undermine the overall findings.

NH studies do not evaluate an investigational intervention (eg. a drug), and thus, will not need to be conducted to a Good Clinical Practice standard used for clinical trials performed for drug regulation purposes.[29] We recommend, however, that all NH studies include processes and procedures that result in good quality data and capture. Important areas deserving of careful attention include:

- Use of a prospectively designed NH study protocol that documents procedures to be followed, time intervals for collections, and inclusion criteria (or at a minimum, working definitions) for patients to be included in the study (see Natural History Study Protocols, Related Documents and Processes section later in this chapter).
- Standardized data dictionaries, terminology/nomenclature, or common data elements to be used or enforced for data collections (eg. drop-down menus or restricted fields for some data fields).
- An information technology (IT) infrastructure that is suited to the study, considering the people conducting the study and providing data, and the evolution of the

study protocol over time. Plans for the long-term sustainability and growth of the IT systems are important. IT systems that can support remote data collections and access capabilities to facilitate inclusion of a broad patient population and to reduce patient burden (and hence, to minimize 'burn-out', drop outs and missing data) can be particularly valuable. Appropriate data security protections (both for access and alteration of the data) are also an extremely important consideration for the development and maintenance of the IT infrastructure. As part of the research plan, NH study designers are encouraged to consult knowledgeable IT expertise or existing structures[30] in order to build and sustain usable platforms to house and maintain these databases.

- Should biobanking, specimen or imaging collections, and incorporation of laboratory testing be included in the NH study, additional logistical and practical considerations for their capture and storage will need to be considered.

Patient Protections and Oversight

All research studies, including NH studies require some independent oversight to ensure protection of the rights, autonomy and safety of patients.

- The most significant risk to patients of participation in an NH study is the inappropriate dissemination of confidential information. Study procedures and data storage plans should provide protection against this.
- Informed consent documents should be used for all NH studies, which appropriately outline the procedures to be followed, information to be collected, and foreseeable risks.[31,32]
- In most cases, a NH study will require the use of an Institution Review Board (IRB) to provide study over-

sight. Given the broad geographic area to be covered for most NH studies, and anticipation of small numbers of patients from different locations or treatment centers, use of a Central IRB should be considered whenever feasible.[31,33,34,35]

- A steering committee that includes representatives and leadership from the patient and advocacy communities, in addition to scientific membership, is important.[31,36] The steering committee should oversee decisions for data access and use, and research prioritizations for and from the NH study. Additionally, because NH studies should evolve as they progress and the knowledge gained from them is evaluated, a steering committee with appropriate expertise and representation is needed to decide upon changes to the overall research plan. Since patients are expected to be most affected by any of these considerations, sufficient patient representation throughout the entire duration of an NH study, beginning with planning, is necessary. The steering committee will need to ensure that the study's demands on patients are realistic; this requires careful attention to the feedback from patients.

Categories of Natural History Study Designs

There are several different types of design characteristics for natural history studies (see Table 2). One of the most important characteristics categorizes studies based upon time-related features. This includes both a) the timing of when the study data are collected according to a study plan in relation to when the patients are evaluated, and b) the duration of observation for each patient. The patients may:

- have been evaluated during the course of non-study medical care visits to their individual health care practitioner prior to the study plan being created (called *retrospective* collection of study data);[37] or

- may be evaluated only after a study plan is completed, with the evaluations occurring as directed by the study plan (called *prospective* data collection).[38,39]

When the study data are retrospectively collected from medical care records, the term *'chart review'* is usually applied to the study design.[37]

A separate feature to categorize studies (applicable to either retrospective or prospective studies) distinguishes between studies where:

- evaluation data on a patient are obtained at only one point in time (called a *cross-sectional* study);[38] or
- evaluation data are obtained at multiple times over a period of months or years (called a *longitudinal* study).[39]

Table 2. Natural History Study Designs

Design	Description
Retrospective	Compilation of data already collected for another purpose
Literature review	Search and compile medical literature, usually case reports or case series
Chart Review	NH study data are collected from individual patient medical record
Prospective	Evaluations and data collections occur as directed by the study plan
Cross-sectional	Obtain evaluation data on a patient at one point in time only (eg. survey)
Longitudinal	Obtain evaluation data at multiple time points over an open-ended or specified period

There is value to each approach to a NH study, and each approach has different strengths and weaknesses. One design type usually cannot substitute for another. It is not uncommon that the best approach to understanding the NH of a disease is to use several design types in sequence, each step informing how to best design the next step in the progression of knowledge building. Most commonly, the first step to building a comprehensive understanding of the NH of a disease, is not to begin with a study of one of these types, but instead to begin with an intensive review of the extant published information (eg. medical literature) about patients with the disease. Compiling information from previously published reports and studies will restrict the type of information gathered, which is often inconsistent between different published reports. Nonetheless, the perspective obtained from this pooling of information can be a guide to designing the first planned NH study.

Retrospective Studies

Retrospective or chart-review studies have the advantage of often being the design that offers the fastest completion of the data collection because the evaluation of patients has already occurred by the time the study plan is written. This benefit is particularly pronounced for retrospective longitudinal studies. However, there are substantial limitations as to what can be expected from this approach. Because the medical care records usually include only the information the health care practitioner thought was useful to record for purposes of medical care of each individual patient, it is likely that information important to a comprehensive NH study was not recorded. In addition, each practitioner recorded information in a form that was useful to the practitioner's approach towards medical care for each patient. Together, these factors lead to chart record information often being incomplete, and with substantial variation in the level of detail recorded, especially between practitioners but also for each practitioner over time as they cared for different patients. Consequently, retrospective studies may be able to provide broad ranging information, but usually not with sufficient consistency or completeness to adequately define the NH of the disease for all of the uses to which NH knowledge can be applied.

Prospective Studies

Prospective studies plan in advance what information should be collected from each patient and precisely how the observations should be performed and recorded. This allows for including in the patient observations the types of information that will have great value in helping to guide therapy development (or other uses of the data), without restriction as to whether the information has immediate applicability to the medical care of the patient. The advantage is similar regarding consistency of timing of evaluations and of the form for recording the information. Therefore, if there is good adherence to the plan, the collected data are complete and in the form that is most useful for application in therapy development (or other purposes). The drawback, of course, is that the data cannot be collected until after the plan is created, and the amount of delay is related in part to the specifics of the plan.

Prospective cross-sectional studies will have less data-collection delay than longitudinal studies, because each patient must be evaluated only once and there is no study-required duration of time over which these evaluations should be spread. While generally not practical, there would be no disadvantage to evaluating all of the study patients on a single day, immediately after completion of the study plan. In general, however, for logistical reasons even single-visit (cross-sectional) studies will need a meaningful amount of time to recruit and evaluate all the planned patients.

Most diseases of interest are not short duration single event diseases. Most of the diseases for which NH knowledge will be valuable are long duration diseases (ie. chronic diseases) that are either continuously present (largely unremitting), progressive or recurrent (episodic). Cross-sectional studies can provide a description of the range of manifestations of the disease and of the severity of the manifestations. For therapies intended to provide largely immediate benefit when given to patients with an acute episode or flare of the disease, this may be sufficient NH knowledge. However, cross-sectional studies are generally unable to provide an understanding on the course of the disease within an individual patient. An understanding of the full spectrum of disease course across the range of patients is important to developing chronic therapies for most diseases.

Prospective longitudinal studies provide the most comprehensive and richest form of NH knowledge. The course of the disease can be understood as it occurs to the individual patients. This is important information for planning development of chronic therapies. The design of longitudinal studies can be guided by the information obtained in cross-sectional studies, influencing the choice of manifestations that are planned for examination in the study, and the methods to evaluate the manifestations. The goal for duration of patient observation that provides comprehensive information will be related in part to the time course of the disease. Diseases that are relatively slow to progress will usually require longer periods of patient follow-up than diseases that, albeit chronic, progress in shorter periods of time.

Although not a NH study itself, potentially valuable information that can guide design of prospective NH studies may come from patient focus groups. In focus groups, patients can describe how the disease affects them without being constrained to standardized data collection formats (see Data Elements for Collection section below). Such moderator-guided, but otherwise unrestricted discussion, among a small group of patients (or caregivers) can help inform what disease manifestations may be important to evaluate during a NH study.

Study-Site Organization Models for Natural History Studies

As with any clinical study, NH studies will need to have specific choices made for multiple aspects of how a study is implemented. Some of these issues are discussed here for prospective NH studies.

'Study site' refers to the location(s) where study personnel work and the observations of the patients occur during the course of the study. Study sites are enlisted to participate in the study prior to patients enrolling in the study for that site. For purposes of this discussion, study sites are usually located at medical centers or medical clinics, staffed by clinical professionals, and usually serve as centers of research and medical care for many patients and diseases. These clinics usually have prior experience of conducting a study according to a written protocol and providing high-quality data. Nonetheless, different sites can have different capabilities, depending on the type of clinical staff at the site, their general professional or specialized training, and the infrastructure available. These differences can influence decisions about whether any particular clinic is appropriate to be a study site for a particular NH study.

Models for the number of study sites that conduct the study can be loosely categorized as single-, pauci- or many-site models, or as a non-site study model. Each of these models has advantages and disadvantages. Which is adequate for any particular NH study will depend on the specifics of the disease, patient population, objectives of the study, and specific requirements for conduct of the study.

Single-site Studies

Single-site studies are those where a single clinical site, usually at an academic research medical center, is selected to conduct the study. All patients travel to the selected study site for evaluation and recording the information as planned in the study protocol. This can be a useful approach when some portions of the patient evaluation require specialized and expensive, or difficult to obtain, equipment that is not usually present in medical clinics. Or, when there is some specialized training that the clinical staff must have to perform the evaluation correctly and reliably. For most rare diseases, the number of patients that will be evaluated is not so large as to overwhelm the capacity of the staff at the single center to conduct the protocol. Even for evaluations that do not require specialized professional training but are susceptible to variation in results based on variation in how the examiner performs the evaluation, use of a single site and an unchanging study staff can decrease the variability in study data that is related to the examiner. Such variations are not informative about the patients who have the disease. This may be especially useful with rare diseases with very small numbers of patients where if there are many study sites, only one patient would be seen at each site and the evaluator-induced variation in study results may be large in comparison to the true disease-related range in the study results. A not inconsiderable disadvantage of the single-site model, however, is that all patients must travel to the selected site every time the protocol plans for an evaluation. This can require significant financial resources (either on the part of the study organizer or the study participants) for those patients who do not live near the selected site. The travel can also be physically difficult for some patients with some diseases. Alternatively, the burden of financial resources or physical difficulty may influence the study organizer to decrease the frequency of study visits in longitudinal studies below the level that would be most informative. This can result in the study data being more sparse than is optimal to gain the maximal advantages from a NH study.

Pauci-site Studies

Pauci-site studies are those where only a small number of study sites are selected to conduct the study, and all patients travel to one of these sites, usually the one that is closest to where the patient lives. 'Small number' of sites in this case does not imply any specific fixed range of number of sites, but rather that the number of sites is very few in relation to some study conduct aspects. One is that in comparison to the number of patients who will participate in the NH study; the number of sites is few enough so that a significant number of patients are seen at each clinical site. The overall influence on the data of evaluator variability for pauci-site study sites is greater than for single site studies. However, since there are still multiple patients at each site, the evaluator variability is less likely to confound interpretation of the study results than when there are only one or two patients per study site. This approach can be attractive when there is only a limited amount of uncommon specialized equipment or training necessary to conduct the study properly. An advantage of this model is that more patients will live closer to a study site than in a single-site study, thus reducing the burdens of difficulty of travel on the patients and of travel expenses. In general, however, there will not be so many sites so as to ensure that all patients will live conveniently close to a study site. Because there is more than one site, the study organizer will have an added oversight burden to monitor (ie. watch over in some manner) the performance of the study at the several sites, both to ensure the written protocol is followed and to periodically assure that any procedures that are subject to evaluator variability are being consistently performed. When there are only a few study sites, however, this should not be overly burdensome.

Many-site Studies

Many-site studies are those where there are multiple study sites scattered across the relevant geographic area. Because of the larger number of sites, the benefits and disadvantages of the pauci-site model are magnified. In this model, there is much more likelihood that any eligible patient will live reasonably close to a study site and it will not be as great a difficulty, or expense, for the patient to go to the site for study visits. This has the potential to increase the number of patients for whom participation is feasible, and who may choose to participate in the study. It also has the potential to allow for more frequent study evaluation time-point visits without the travel burden being so great for the patients, as to cause large amounts of missing data from missed visits, or for patients to drop out of the study entirely. If, however, the NH study depended upon some specialized equipment that is difficult or expensive to obtain or maintain, or uncommon specialized professional training, this model may not be feasible. In addition, there are many sites in comparison to the number of patients who participate in the study (and few patients per site) raising the concern about between-evaluator variation in how the evaluations are performed that might confound interpretation of the data. Consequently, the study organizer's role, to carefully monitor the conduct of the study at the study sites, becomes larger and more essential.

Non-site Studies

Non-site studies are those studies that do not use a prospectively identified and prepared study site where patients travel to and are evaluated, as planned in the study protocol. Instead, data collection occurs at the location of each individual patient. The most common concept for a non-site NH study is one where the patient, or the patient's family, provides all of the information collected in the study while at their own home. This may be done via paper questionnaires mailed to the patient and mailed back to a study operations center that enters the data into an electronic database. Increasingly, however, data collection via an internet web interface to direct electronic capture is being used. Patient self-evaluation for data collection will be limited to types of data that are appropriate for evaluation by non-clinically-trained people. There is a large amount of valuable NH information suitable for this means of data collection, such as reporting of the patient's activities or feelings during their daily routine, or asking about the relative importance to each person of different types of disease-related limitations.

Including self-report items in a NH study leads to concerns about the consistency of how individual patients understand the question asked. This can be further increased because many rare disease NH studies will be performed in multiple countries so as to have enough patients participate. Self-reports are made in response to some prompt; these prompts must be available in several languages, so that all enrolled patients can understand the questionnaire. The translation should lead to the same understanding of the question irrespective of the regional origin of the patient. Some questions, however, can require nuanced translation to ensure the meaning is the same in all languages.

In addition, there can be cultural differences in how the topic of the question is regarded. Multinational studies should prepare any needed translations in advance of initiating the study and confirm that language or cultural differences do not change the meaning, or otherwise lead to non-equivalent data being obtained in different geographic regions.

The non-site model does not automatically imply, however, that there are no clinical professionals involved in the patient evaluations or that no specialized equipment is used in the evaluations. There will always be some information about the patient's health status and functional abilities that is not suitable for self-report. Some of this additional information may be feasible to obtain within the non-site study model. For example, patients usually have a personal healthcare provider for their ongoing care near where they live. A protocol may plan study evaluations that, for accurate measurement, rely on the general healthcare professional training but not the specialized training of clinical investigators at academic medical centers. These evaluations might be performed by the patient's personal healthcare provider and given to the study organizer either by the healthcare provider directly, or via the patient.

Another option might be appropriate for some evaluations needed for the study. Some evaluations are not suitable for self-report because they require some limited amount of training, such as how to administer a specific functional ability performance test, or how to accurately judge what is observed when the patient does the activity. In these cases, NH study organizers can consider whether it is feasible to train a limited number of lay-person volunteers (eg. some members of a disease-specific patient advocacy organization) to correctly administer the evaluation and accurately record the result. These volunteers can be recruited, dispersed throughout the regions in which patients who join the study are located. If these study-trained persons travel to each patient's location at scheduled times to administer the evaluation and provide the measurement to the study organizers, the non-site model has the potential to include some moderately complex data collection procedures, without the burden on the patient to travel to a potentially distant study site.

Mixed Models

The considerations discussed here do not make any particular model the universal best model. The different models can be considered for each specific NH study, and the potential procedures or resources that may be available to address the study-model concerns in the particular case. In addition, NH studies should not be viewed as necessarily adopting any one of these models in a pure form to the exclusion of features of the other models. There are many different types of information that can be important to a good NH study, with a diversity of need for level of professional or other specialized training, specialized equipment, and frequency of collection. A study plan that employed a mixture of the different study-models to encompass the diversity of evaluations may be the most efficient approach to study design. A mixture of these approaches to study evaluations may be the most feasible for the largest number of patients, and thus, enable the maximal number of patients to participate. For example, the study organizers might plan for a small number of highly difficult or equipment dependent measurements to be infrequently evaluated during the study, at just the one or few sites capable of this, while less difficult measurements are made much more frequently using the many-site or non-site study model. The study organizers should plan the study carefully. They should take all the discussed factors into consideration and ensure that the study protocol is clear about what category of person performs each of the study evaluations, what new training (with certification and periodic re-certification if useful) will be needed for the study personnel, and how the quality of the evaluations and measurements will be assured.

Natural History Study Design and Design Evolution

Just as for any clinical study, the design features of a NH study should be determined based on the detailed specific objectives of the study (See Table 3). Consequently, the first step to designing a NH study is consideration of, and detailed statement of, the future uses of the data from the NH study and, as far as possible, the specific questions for which the NH study data should provide an answer. Clear identification of these questions is important because only by considering how each specific question can be addressed can the necessary data be determined. Therefore, people with experience in situations where those answers are relied upon (ie. experience in drug development) should be involved with creating the design for the NH study.

A common and important application of the knowledge derived from NH studies, is to provide answers to all of the questions directing choices that will be made in the process of designing a drug development program. The issues that arise during a drug development program related to study design are not all obvious and thus, people with broad experience in the clinical development of drugs can provide valuable advice on the study design and data collection. NH study design includes making choices about:

- the information to be collected;
- the evaluation to be used to collect each element of the information;
- the frequency for collection;
- the type of person (categorized from highly specialized clinical investigator through those with less intensive professional training, to patient self-report) to be used for each evaluation to assure that the data are of good quality; and
- other elements of study design.

Although the NH study design should be based on the best available information at the time it is designed, the design should not necessarily be viewed as unchanging. Instead, a longitudinal NH study is more usefully viewed as a study that evolves over the time it is being conducted. This might also apply to prospective cross-sectional studies, if substantial numbers of patients are enrolled over an extended amount of time. When NH studies are initiated for disorders for which there is very little information, many of the choices made regarding what information, how, and when to evaluate the patient, are not optimally formulated because of the lack of information. Thus, NH studies should plan (as appropriate) for periodic analysis of the accumulated data. These analyses should support a re-evaluation of the core NH study questions. In doing this, it might be determined that it is not useful to gather additional extensive information about a particular aspect of the patient's health and functioning that was an initially prominent interest, because the accumulated data are sufficient for the intended purpose. Alternatively, information on an aspect of the patient's health and functioning initially of uncertain usefulness, may be affirmed as having potential value for drug investigation studies. Consequently, a more intensive or refined evaluation of that aspect (eg. a more sensitive measurement tool, more frequent measurement) is warranted to increase the value of the NH study. This may lead to development of new evaluation tools for specific manifestations that have substantial potential to become a key focus for a drug's treatment benefit. In addition, new questions about an aspect of patient health and functioning might arise and evaluations to address that health aspect can be added.

Table 3. Key Principles for Natural History

View NH studies as precompetitive, with the goal of learning about the disease

- Consider the study's ultimate goal, such as the potential therapeutic development plan for the disease during the design phase
- Avoid using a study design that depends on a specific therapy or a narrow set of data collections

Involve the broad stakeholder community early and on a continuing basis

- Patient and advocacy group participation is critical to NH study success
- Plan for multi-center/site data collections, such as use of central IRBs
- Standardized data collections and data definition language will be needed

Studies

Data Elements for Collection

The rare diseases are diverse, with each disease having substantial variability in manifestations and progression. Thus, no single set of data elements can be expected to adequately describe all rare diseases, and data collection (both elements and methods) should be chosen to reflect the individual disease and the immediate aims of the study, as well as desired future applications of the data (eg. clinical trials, patient care). Prior to initiating a NH study, careful consideration of currently available disease knowledge should be explored, such as literature reviews and case records, and where applicable, disease experts, patient and caregiver interviews, and any existing data collections, such as registries (see Categories of Natural History Study Designs section).

Some common elements and approaches to consider when selecting a set of data elements for a specific disease or related group of diseases could include:

- Disease definitions and diagnostic criteria. This should include descriptions used for recognizing, defining and collecting important medical events, and any objective testing that could be used.
- Age at onset and diagnosis, including the specific problems that led to diagnosis.

- Description of the full range of disease manifestations, and should include an identification of important disease subtypes. This could include:
  - Clinical effects and outcomes of the disease. The nature and severity of how each involved body system is affected should be described. This assessment should be as inclusive as possible, and not be limited only to the most severe or prominent manifestations.
  - Assessments from the patient regarding which clinical manifestations are most important and relevant to them, and how their life is affected by the specific manifestations.
  - The time course evolution of the disease manifestations.
  - Genotypes, phenotypes and genotype-phenotype relationships important to the identification of disease subpopulations, and which may have predictive or prognostic implications.
  - Identification of potential clinical outcome measures, tools and instruments. These assessment tools may have utility in developing new clinical trial endpoints, which can undergo pilot testing in NH studies.
  - Identification of potential biomarkers.
  - Assessment of medical care and current practices across the disease, different treatment centers and health care providers. Standards of care are likely to change over time, and careful documentation can assist with establishing best practices. This can also help establish consistency in procedures across participating study sites during clinical trials.

The collection and long-term storage of biological samples (eg. tissue samples, blood, other body fluids) should be given consideration. The long-term storage of some biological samples can require substantial resources, and many organizations may find it difficult to develop the resources for this. However, if feasible, biobanking should be included. Storage of samples of multiple types from many patients for analysis at some future time, can lead to significant advances in understanding and potentially treating the disease. For example, when medical research identifies a potential key biomarker, disease-related gene, or therapeutic target, having an existing source of samples whose analysis can prove or disprove the relevance of the biomarker, gene, or putative target can support rapid advances.

An important perspective is that NH studies describe the disease, with the results being independent of any current or future investigational treatment agent. Thus, knowledge gained from these studies can be applied to multiple drug development programs. We recommend that an overall NH research plan first be developed, and the data elements be selected with this broader purpose in mind. NH studies should generally not be designed for a particular candidate drug or one narrow purpose. Patients and caregivers should also be involved in the planning and design of NH studies, and decisions regarding the information to be collected. This is particularly important to long-term NH studies, in order to minimize attrition and missing data, and to assess feasibility of the clinical plan.

Natural History Study Protocols, Related Documents and Processes

Consistency of data collection across different study locations (for any of the site-models other than single site) and over time (for all studies) is essential to obtaining interpretable data. Well written, comprehensive study protocols are the central means to optimizing this needed uniformity. Protocols should be well detailed with regards to nomenclature, identifying specific evaluations to perform, the logistics of data collection and recording of data in the central database, formats for recording measurements, etc.

Often there is value to a separate manual of procedures for the study that describes in substantial detail how to perform each evaluation. When some of these evaluations are not

familiar to study evaluators, a training program that all evaluators must complete can be very valuable to increasing the
quality of the data that is collected. When this is useful, planning for some form of certification of the intended evaluators
can help insure that the evaluations will be performed in the
proper manner. NH studies are often many years long, and periodic re-certification of the evaluators for the necessary study
skills can also contribute to maintaining the value of the study
data. Because there are many different levels of complexity to
evaluations that might be used in a study, and people with different levels of experience might be designated for performing
the different evaluations, the value of training, certification,
and periodic re-certification can apply to all evaluators in a
study, from established clinical investigators at medical centers
through to lay persons.

Plans should also be formulated for the periodic analysis of
the accumulated data. This may be mostly applicable to longitudinal studies. Periodically advancing the understanding of the
disease NH will enable thoughtful evolution of the NH study
protocol, as discussed above. Analysis plans for a NH study
are not subject to some of the issues that are important with
the drug testing studies intended to demonstrate efficacy. NH
studies are progressive learning and exploration studies, and
there is not the same overriding concern about false positive
findings (Type I errors) as with drug efficacy studies. Multiple
exploratory analyses of the data, including some further analyses suggested by the initial analyses are encouraged.

However, the 'learn, then confirm' concept is not entirely
absent from optimal use of NH studies. For example, one objective in a NH study might be to develop a new outcome measure
for use as a clinical trial endpoint. The outcome tool might be
refined several times during the course of the NH study to optimize the balance between reliability, sensitivity, and ease of use.
Once tool design has been adequately optimized via a learning
process to create the final version, further data collection in the
NH study can serve to confirm the hypothesis that the final version has good measurement properties.

Community-wide Collaborative Natural History Studies

The power of NH information to guide drug development derives from an integrated analysis of comprehensive data about as many patients with the disease as possible, and as widely available as possible to persons with an interest in developing a therapy. Consequently, fragmenting of the data from individual patients is counterproductive to maximizing the benefit of a NH study. By definition of the term 'rare disease', there cannot be multiple separate large databases for rare diseases because there are not sufficient patients to do so. Having all the available patient data in a single consistent database, collected under a common study protocol, will be important. All patients should have the same evaluations to measure health aspects performed in the same way and the measurements recorded in a standardized data format. Because of different prior experiences, different investigators and study organizers will often begin with different ideas of what is important to measure or how to measure those disease features. For the NH study to meet its goals, however, there should be collaborative efforts among the interested investigators from the outset to develop a single common protocol that is applied to all patients, with the data all being placed in a common database.

Similarly, the information obtained in a NH study will not have the desired impact if it is not accessible to persons and organizations who are working to develop new treatments. Many of the validly interested organizations will not have been participants in the creation and conduct of the NH study, and consequently access should not be limited to only investigators who participated in the conduct of the study. At the time of initial design, the NH study organizers should also plan how access to the observed information will be provided. Although it is uncommon to provide full copies of the primary data to anyone who requests the data, overly restrictive access policies can limit the usefulness of the study data. There are many different ways to provide access to the knowledge contained in the database, and NH study organizers should consider what level of access will be available to different types of requestors, and how that access will be provided.

Future Directions

Well-designed and planned NH studies should benefit researchers, regulators, drug developers, caregivers, and patients. The studies provide the essential foundational information that can initiate and sustain research into a rare disease, and provide the path through which the lives of patients with rare diseases can be improved. NH studies also emphasize the need for all stakeholders to make long-term commitments to work together to conduct these studies, and to harness the necessary resources to advance the acquisition of knowledge for a specific disease. Active engagement of the rare disease patient community benefits patients and helps move therapeutic development forward and may advance patient care.

The most successful NH studies are community endeavors involving all stakeholders. In many cases researchers design and carry out the studies, patient groups identify potential study participants, educate patients and families about the value of NH studies, sustain patient involvement, and assist with data collection and management. People with successful drug development experience, such as from the pharmaceutical industry, can provide drug development expertise and identify questions that NH studies need to answer. Regulatory agencies, such as FDA, can also provide advice on knowledge needs for rare disease drug development programs, and set clinical development standards. Public health agencies, such as NIH, can help ensure that NH studies are communal endeavors by leading, funding and coordinating NH studies.

The rare disease community recognizes that there are many hurdles to overcome, such as lack of funding, concerns with intellectual property, data sharing, and standardization of data collection, and has begun to address some of these issues. International efforts are also ongoing to develop common data elements, protocols and collaborative research networks, and to create tissue repositories for rare diseases.[40] However, more work needs to be done. The value of NH studies is increasingly being recognized by the rare disease community. NH studies engender ongoing and increasing collaborations among all rare disease stakeholders, and we hope that increasing interest in designing and conducting NH studies will continue to lead to benefits for patients with unmet medical needs.

Anne R. Pariser, MD
Office of Translational Sciences, Center for Drug Evaluation and Research, US Food and Drug Administration, Silver Spring, MD, USA.

Marc K. Walton, MD, PhD
Janssen Research and Development, Titusville, New Jersey, USA.

Disclaimer: The authors declare no conflict of interest relevant to the subject matter discussed in the manuscript. The opinions presented herein are those of the authors and do not represent the views or policies of the FDA.

References

1 Posada de la Paz M, Groft SC. Rare diseases epidemiology research. In : *Rare Diseases Epidemiology. Advances in experimental medicine and biology.* 1st ed. Springer Netherlands; 2010;686:1739.

2 National Cancer Institute. NCI dictionary of cancer terms. 2012. Available at: http://www.cancer.gov/dictionary?cdrid=538640 (Accessed 28 July 2015).

3 Last JM. The Iceberg: 'Completing the clinical picture' in general practice. Lancet. 1963;2:28-31. Reprinted Int J Epi-

demiol. 2013;42:1608-1613.

4 Last JM. Commentary: The iceberg revisted. Int J Epidemiol. 2013;42:1613-1615.

5 Belkin BM, Neelon FA. The art of observation: William Osler and the Method of Zadig. Ann Intern Med. 1992;116: 863-866.

6 Centers for Disease Control and Prevention. CDC's Vision for Public Health Surveillance in the 21st Century. MMWR. 2012;61(Suppl: July 27, 2012): 1-35.

7 Seminara J, Tuchman M, Krivitzky L, et al. Establishing a consortium for the study of rare diseases: The Urea Cycle Disorders Consortium. Mol Genet Metab. 2010;100:S97-S105.

8 Groft SC, de la Paz MP. Rare diseases – avoiding misperceptions and establishing realities: the need for reliable epidemiological data. Adv Exp Med Biol. 2010;686:3-14.

9 Krischer JP, Gopal-Srivastava R, Groft SC, Eckstein DJ. The Rare Diseases Clinical Research Network's organization and approach to observational research and health outcomes research. J Gen Intern Med 2014. 29(Suppl 3):S739-44.

10 Marshall BC, Nelson EC. Accelerating implementation of biomedical research advances: critical elements of a successful 10 years Cystic Fibrosis Foundation healthcare delivery improvement initiative. BMJ Qual Saf. 2014;23(Suppl 1):i95-i103.

11 Horton DK, Mehta P, Antao VC. Quantifying a nonnotifiable disease in the United States. The national amyotrophic lateral sclerosis registry model. JAMA. 2014;312:1097-1098.

12 Ross CA, Aylward EH, Wild EF, et al. Huntington disease: natural history, biomarkers and prospects for therapeutics. Nat Rev Neurol. 2014;10:204-216.

13 Braun MM, Farag-El-Massah S, Xu K, Coté TR. Emergence of orphan drugs in the United States: a quantitative assessment of the first 25 years. Nature Rev Drug Discov. 2010;9:519-522.

14 Griggs RC, Batshaw M, Dunkle M, Gopal-Srivastava R, Kaye E, Krischer J, Nguyen T, Paulus K, Merkel PA; for the Rare Diseases Clinical Research Network. Clinical research for rare disease: opportunities, challenges, and solutions. Mol Genet Metab. 2009;96(1):20-6.

15 Orphan Drug Act, Pub. L. 97-414. 96 Stat. 2049 (1983). Amended in 1984 by Pub. L. 98-551 to add a numeric prevalence threshold to the definition of rare diseases.

16 Regulation (EC) No 141/2000 of the European parliament and of the council of 16 December 1999 on orphan medicinal products. Official Journal of the European Communities. 22.1.2000. I. 18/1-5.

17 Institute of Medicine. Rare diseases and orphan products: Accelerating research and development. Washington, DC: : The National Academies Press; 2010. Available from: http://www.iom.edu/Reports/2010/Rare-Diseases-and-Orphan-Products-Accelerating-Research-and-Development. aspx. (Accessed 28 July 2015).

18 Eurordis position paper on research priorities for rare diseases. February 2008. Eurordis. http://www.eurordis. org/sites/default/files/publications/position-paper-EURORDIS-research-prioritiesFeb08.pdf . (Accessed 28 July 2015).

19 National Institutes of Health. Workshop on natural history studies of rare diseases: Meeting the needs of drug development and research. May 16-17, 2012. Workshop Summary. Available at: https://events-support.com/events/Natural_History_Studies. (Accessed 28 July 2015).

20 EURORDIS-NORD-CORD release a joint declaration of 10 key principles for rare disease patient registries.

2012. Eurordis. http://www.eurordis.org/content/euror-dis-nord-cord-release-joint-declaration-10-key-principles-ra-re-disease-patient-registries . (Accessed 28 July 2015).

21 Forrest CB, Bartek RJ, Rubinstein Y, Groft SC. The case for a global rare-diseases registry. Lancet. 2011;377:1057-1059.

22 Boyle MP, Sabadosa KA, Quinton HB, Marshall BC, Schechter MS. Key findings of the US Cystic Fibrosis Foundation's clinical practice benchmarking project. BMJ Qual Saf. 2014;23(Suppl 1):i15-i22.

23 McDonald CM, Henricson EK, Abresch RT, et al. The Cooperative International Neuromuscular Research Group Duchenne natural history study – a longitudinal investigation in the era of glucocorticoid therapy: Design of protocol and the methods used. Muscle Nerve. 2013;48:32-54.

24 US FDA. Office of Orphan Products Development. Search Orphan Drug Designations and Approvals. Available at: http://www.accessdata.fda.gov/scripts/opdlisting/oopd/. (Accessed 28 July 2015).

25 US Food and Drug Administration (FDA). Code of Federal Regulations (CFR) Title 21: Approval of an application and an abbreviated application. Pt. 314.105. US Government Printing Office. Washington, DC, USA 2014.

26 FDA. 21CFR: Adequate and well-controlled studies. Pt. 314.126. US Government Printing Office. Washington, DC, USA 2014.

27 Pariser AR, Yao LP. Rare diseases and orphan drugs. In: Pediatric Drug Development, Concepts and Applications. Second Edition. Eds. Mulberg AE, Murphy D, Dunne J, Mathis LL. John Wiley & Sons Ltd, West Sussex, UK. 2013.

28 US Department of Health and Human Services. FDA. Guidance for Industry. E 10 Choice of control group and related issues in clinical trials. 2001. Available at: http://www.fda.gov/downloads/Drugs/GuidanceComplianceReg-

ulatoryInformation/Guidances/UCM073139.pdf. (Accessed 28 July 2015).

29 FDA. Guidance for Industry. E6 Good clinical practice: Consolidated guidance. 1996. Available at: http://www.fda. gov/downloads/Drugs/GuidanceComplianceRegulatoryIn- formation/Guidances/UCM073122.pdf. (Accessed 28 July 2015).

30 Patient Registries. National Organization for Rare Disor- ders. NORD registry platform. 2014. https://rarediseases. org/for-patient-organizations/ways-partner/patient-registries . (Accessed 28 July 2015).

31 Dept. of Health and Human Services. CFR Title 45 and 46: Public welfare and protection of human subjects. 2009. Available at: http://www.hhs.gov/ohrp/humansubjects/guid- ance/45cfr46.html . (Accessed 28 July 2015).

32 Neff MJ. Institutional Review Board consideration of chart reviews, case reports, and observational studies. Respir Care 2008;53:1350-1353.

33 FDA. Guidance for industry -using a centralized IRB re- view process in multicenter clinical trials. 2006. Available at: http://www.fda.gov/downloads/RegulatoryInformation/ Guidances/ucm127013.pdf. (Accessed 28 July 2015).

34 Minikoff J. The paradoxical problem with multiple-IRB review. N Engl J Med. 2010;363:1591-1593.

35 Clinical Trials Transformation Initiative. Considerations to support communication between institutions and outside IRVS when responsibilities are being assigned for multi- center clinical trial protocols. 2013. Available at: http:// www.ctti-clinicaltrials.org/files/documents/CentralIRBCon- siderationsDocument.pdf. (Accessed 28 July 2015).

36 FDA. Guidance for clinical trial sponsors – establishment and operation of clinical trial data monitoring committees. 2006. Available at: http://www.fda.gov/downloads/Regula-

toryInformation/Guidances/ucm127073.pdf. (Accessed 28 July 2015).

37 Hess DR. Retrospective studies and chart reviews. Respir Care. 2004;49:1171-1174.

38 Coggan D, Rose G , Barker DJP. Case-control and cross sectional studies. In: Epidemiology for the uninitiated, Chapter 8. British Medical Journal Publishing. 1997. Available at: http://www.bmj.com/about-bmj/resources-readers/ publications/epidemiology-uninitiated. (Accessed 28 July 2015).

39 Coggan D, Rose G , Barker DJP. Longitudinal Studies. In: *Epidemiology for the uninitiated,* Chapter 7. British Medical Journal Publishing. 1997. Available at: http://www.bmj. com/about-bmj/resources-readers/publications/epidemiolo-gy-uninitiated. (Accessed 28 July 2015).

40 International Rare Diseases Research Consortium. Policies & Guidelines. April 2013. Available at: http://www.irdirc. org/?page_id=29. (Accessed 28 July 2015).

Chapter 18

Clinical Efficacy Measures and Surrogate Endpoints

Anthony Hall
Findacure

Introduction

The topic of clinical efficacy measures and surrogate endpoints is covered by the author in detail elsewhere and will not be repeated here.[1] In the previous book, the example of the clinical development of nitisinone for the treatment of alkaptonuria was used. Alkaptonuria is an inherited condition which, although present from birth, has a gradual effect on clinically measurable parameters, such as joint destruction by a process called ochronosis. The objective of treatment is to prevent these clinical manifestations but a clinical trial of sufficient duration to show the effect of a treatment in preventing these parameters would not be feasible. Therefore, the use of an easily detectable biochemical marker, homogentisic acid (HGA) was proposed as a surrogate endpoint. The particular challenge in this case was not the ability to measure the biochemical marker, but rather to validate it as a suitable surrogate for clinical outcome measures. Although the biochemistry is well characterised and the link between HGA and the clinical sequelae of the disease is well accepted, it is not known to what level HGA needs to be reduced in order to prevent the clinical sequelae, at what age treatment would need to begin, or what is the long-term safety of the drug in this patient population. Nevertheless, the European regulators (consulted through the Scientific Advice procedure) were understanding of the potential difficulties and helpful in determining a feasible development programme. The clinical programme is now underway, led by an FP7 sponsored consortium. The interested reader is referred to the above reference.

Since the publication of that first Rare Diseases book, the author has had the privilege to work on the development of new treatments for Duchenne muscular dystrophy (DMD), a devastating disease in desperate need of new treatments. The difficulties of developing drugs for the treatment of DMD provides an ideal example to highlight some of the issues regarding clinical efficacy measures and surrogate endpoints and a brief overview will be given here.

Clinical efficacy measures

At the time that the clinical programmes for the compounds currently in late clinical development for the treatment of DMD were being conceived, the natural history of DMD was much less well characterised than it is now. The clinical efficacy endpoint that emerged as being the best candidate to show efficacy of a disease modifying treatment in boys who are still able to walk was the six minute walk distance (6MWD) test. This test, which is a measure of both strength and endurance, had been used in the assessment of other conditions such as cardiac failure.[2,3] More recently it had been used in the assessment of efficacy for other neuromuscular conditions such as Pompe disease.[4] McDonald (2013), among others, has shown the natural history of the 6MWD in patients with DMD and it seemed reasonable to assume that a drug which improves muscle function would lead to improvements in 6MWD or at least delay the deterioration.[5]

However, as can be seen from Figure 1, not only is there a large variability in the 6MWD amongst boys, but also the distance walked tends to increase up to the age of about 7 years, as boys are growing, after which it inevitably decreases. In addition to inter-patient variability, there is also an intra-patient variability from day to day, which depends on many different factors such as the amount of encouragement the boy receives.

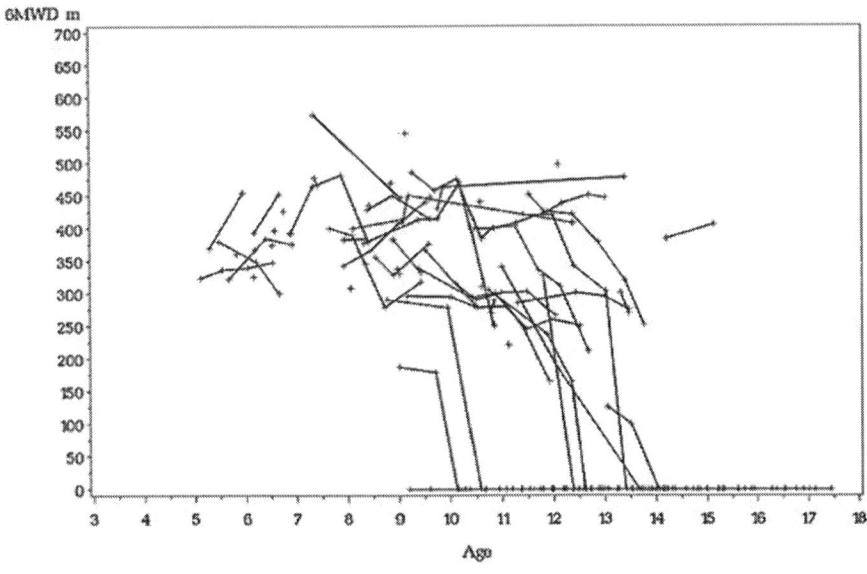

Figure 1. 6MWD by age of boy (From Goemans *et al*, 2013)[6]
Reproduced with permission from Elsevier

As might be surmised from the above natural history graph, the course of an individual patient will depend on (among other things) his age and baseline function. Indeed, it has been shown that, when patients are crudely divided according to these parameters, the course is quite different, as shown in Figure 2.[7]

It is clear that the natural variability in the 6MWD, with the unpredictability of the changes over time, makes it a difficult (intermediate) clinical endpoint to use in clinical trials. In addition, a wide range of other clinical measures are usually assessed during clinical trials in DMD, including the North

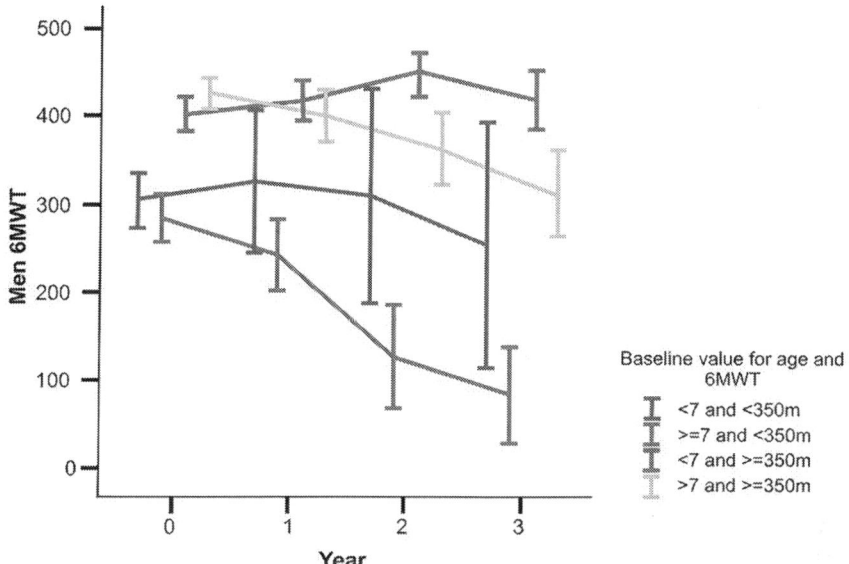

Figure 2. Course of the 6MWD in ambulatory boys with Duchenne muscular dystrophy over the course of 3 years, divided according to baseline age and 6MWD. (Reproduced from Pane *et al*, 2014).[7]
Copyright: © 2014 Pane et al. This is distributed under the terms of the Creative Commons Attribution License.

Star Ambulatory Assessment, 10-metre walk / run, rise from floor time, 4-stair climb and descent, measures of strength, pulmonary function tests, cardiac function and various patient reported outcome measures. It is a rapidly changing area, with new measures constantly under development, such as the computerised workspace evaluation, (which uses a computer-mounted camera to map out the area within which a patient can actively use their arms), the MyoTools (which, for example, measure grip pinch strength) and wearable technologies measuring overall movement during the course of the day.[8,9]

Surrogate endpoints and biomarkers

A surrogate endpoint may be defined as a biomarker intended to substitute for a clinical end-point. "Surrogate endpoints may be used as primary endpoints when appropriate (when the surrogate is reasonably likely or well known to predict clinical outcome)."[10]

In the DMD field, there is a great deal of interest in the possibility of using surrogate endpoints for accelerated approval of new therapies. Not only could these overcome the difficulties associated with the clinical measures, but they would also potentially be detectible sooner, thus shortening the amount of time required to perform (early phase) clinical trials. These include measurement of dystrophin, the protein that is lacking in DMD, in biopsies of muscle and magnetic resonance imaging (MRI) to assess the overall amount and composition of muscle. Until now, however, there is no clear surrogate that is universally accepted as being an alternative to clinical measures.

Regulatory Guidelines

In contrast to more common conditions, the vast majority of rare diseases do not have a guidance document from regulators to guide drug developers in the process of developing treatments. In 2013, the European Medicines Agency (EMA) published a guideline on the clinical investigation of medicinal products for the treatment of Duchenne and Becker muscular dystrophy.[11] In 2014, a consortium of stakeholders, including patients, parents and caregivers, clinicians, scientific experts and industry took the unprecedented step of producing an independent draft guidance and presenting it to the Food and Drug Administration (FDA) for consideration. After a public consultation process, a more concise draft was released by the FDA.[12] These are, however, the exception rather than the rule and the existence of these (draft) guidelines is in no small part due to the very proactive patient organisations that exist for DMD.

The FDA draft guidance document recognises the lack of a recommended or required set of clinical outcome measures for DMD and encourages sponsors to make proposals. The document outlines a number of clinical endpoints that may be used, including the 6MWD. It also goes on to discuss the potential use of biomarkers and intermediate clinical endpoints for accelerated approval. Although the guidance document is specific for dystrinopathies, it may also be helpful in gaining an insight into the regulatory thinking behind the outcome measures the regulators may expect to be studied and the approach to studying these, which can be translated to other rare diseases where no such guidance exists.

Benefit-risk considerations

The marketing authorisation for Glybera®, the first gene therapy to be registered, was initially rejected by the EMA on the basis that the sponsor had not demonstrated an acceptable benefit-risk relationship. The Committee for Medicinal Products for Human Use concluded that there was insufficient evidence of the benefits and safety of Glybera® to recommend approval at this stage. The studies provided had not shown a consistent long-lasting benefit of treatment, and there were, at the time, too few patients for whom sufficiently long-term data was available. There was also insufficient evidence at this stage of a reduction in the rate of pancreatitis.

In 2012, the EMA was asked to re-evaluate the application for Glybera® in a restricted group of patients and a positive opinion was adopted by the Committee for Advanced Therapies in June 2012, which was then endorsed by the CHMP. This underscores the difficulties when developing an advanced therapy with a very small patient population. The EMA Assessment Report noted:

"The Glybera® application also needs to be considered in the context of an extremely orphan indication with very limited patients together with a new emerging era of gene therapy medicinal products in clinical practice together with a limited but evolving scientific knowledge. Taking all this into account, and compared to other 'new concepts' in the past, (for example

monoclonal antibodies), it may be unrealistic to expect a similar level of evidence for the demonstration of quality, safety and efficacy and the overall benefit/risk as for 'classical' medicinal products."[13]

In its review of the MAA for ataluren, the first product registered for the treatment of (a subset of patients with) DMD, the EMA initially had difficulty assessing the benefit-risk. Indeed, following registration, the EMA took the unusual step of publishing a separate paper explaining the basis for approval.[14] This publication contains a number of important statements that highlight the agency's thinking on a flexible approach to licensing in rare diseases with high unmet medical need and some of these are quoted below to illustrate the ideas discussed in this piece.

"Although the efficacy data available lacked robustness, the beneficial effects of ataluren were considered plausible and clinically relevant for this rare disease with high unmet medical need." This demonstrates the fact that the agency is prepared to consider data, which may be less robust than in a traditional approval.

"Nevertheless, even the limited effect observed was perceived as meaningful by patient representatives. They considered that prolonged independent use of arms and hands permitting for example to feed and drink from a cup independently, are major achievements in an advanced stage of disease." Here we see the importance that the regulators place on the views of patient groups in rare diseases and the fact that non-standard endpoints may be acceptable in these circumstances.

"In order to enable early access by patients to medicines filling an unmet medical need for seriously debilitating or life-threatening diseases, the EMA may recommend the conditional approval of a new medicine with temporarily increased level of acceptable uncertainty over its benefits and risks." This emphasises the point that the benefit: risk assessment may be different in seriously debilitating or life-threatening diseases, as explained in the section on Adaptive Licensing. However,

as noted, *"Such conditional approval is subject to additional data being provided by the applicant company under an agreed timeframe, in order to reduce the uncertainty around the marketing authorisation decision to a generally acceptable level."*

In the case of surrogate endpoints, the *"FDA considers the totality of the available evidence when conducting a benefit-risk assessment. For example, if the effect size on a sensitive measure of muscle function is modest for a drug with substantial risks, evidence of the clinical impact of the effect provided by patient reported outcomes is likely to be an important basis of benefit-risk assessments"*.[12]

Conclusions

The above is a short overview of some of the considerations for clinical and surrogate outcome measures in clinical trials (and ultimately for the registration package) for drugs to treat rare diseases. The examples given are intended to illustrate the type of thinking that is needed in conceptualising a development programme in a complex rare disease with an often poorly documented natural history and no universally accepted outcome measures. Often the drug development and the learning are occurring in parallel. The important thing is that they are happening.

References

1 Hall AK. The practicalities of clinical development of drugs for rare diseases. In: Rare Diseases: Challenges and Opportunities for Social Entrepreneurs (Sireau N, ed.). Greenleaf Publishing, Sheffield, UK, 2013; pp.62-86.

2 McDonald CM *et al.* The 6-minute walk test and other endpoints in Duchenne muscular dystrophy: longitudinal natural history observations over 48 weeks from a multicenter study. Muscle Nerve 48: 343–356, 2013.

3 Enright PL. The Six-Minute Walk Test. Respir. Care 2003; 48(8):783–785.

4 van der Ploeg AT *et al.* A Randomized Study of Alglucosidase Alfa in Late-Onset Pompe's Disease. N Engl J Med 2010; 362:1396-406.

5 McDonald CM *et al.* The 6-minute walk test and other endpoints in Duchenne muscular dystrophy: longitudinal natural history observations over 48 weeks from a multicenter study. Muscle Nerve 48: 343–356, 2013.

6 Goemans N *et al.* Ambulatory capacity and disease progression as measured by the 6-minute-walk-distance in Duchenne muscular dystrophy subjects on daily corticosteroids. Neuromuscular Disorders 23 (2013) 618–623.

7 Pane M, Mazzone ES, Sivo S, Sormani MP, Messina S, *et al.* (2014) Long Term Natural History Data in Ambulant Boys with Duchenne Muscular Dystrophy: 36-Month Changes. PLoS ONE 9(10): e108205. doi:10.1371/journal.pone.0108205.

8 Han JJ *et al.* Validity, Reliability, and Sensitivity of a 3D Vision Sensor-based Upper Extremity Reachable Workspace Evaluation in Neuromuscular Diseases. Version 1. PLoS Curr. 2013 December 12; 5: ecurrents.md.f63ae7dde63caa-718fa0770217c5a0e6.

9 Seferian A M *et al.* Upper Limb Evaluation and One-Year Follow Up of Non-Ambulant Patients with Spinal Muscular Atrophy: An Observational Multicenter Trial. PLoS One. 2015; 10(4): e0121799.

10 ICH Harmonised Tripartite Guideline. General considerations for clinical trials E8. 17 July 1997.

11 Guideline on the clinical investigation of medicinal products for the treatment of Duchenne and Becker muscular dystrophy. Committee for Medicinal Products for Human Use (CHMP). 21 February 2013. EMA/

CHMP/236981/2011.

12 Duchenne Muscular Dystrophy and Related Dystrophinopathies: Developing Drugs for Treatment Guidance for
Industry (draft guidance). US. Department of Health and
Human Services Food and Drug Administration Center
for Drug Evaluation and Research (CDER). 26170dft.doc.
05/22/15.

13 EMA/882900/2011. Assessment Report Glybera (Alipo-
gene tiparvovec).

14 Haas M *et al*. European Medicines Agency review of ataluren for the treatment of ambulant patients aged 5 years
and older with Duchenne muscular dystrophy resulting
from a nonsense mutation in the dystrophin gene. Neuromuscular Disorders 25. (2015). 5–133.

Chapter 19

Statistical Considerations

Elizabeth Ludington
Agility Clinical Inc

Introduction

The statistical considerations related to developing and analyzing clinical trials in rare diseases can be more complex than those for more common diseases. In general, if a treatment or therapy has a small but clinically meaningful impact on the disease, a larger study will have a better chance of demonstrating that the observed treatment effect is more likely to be due to the intervention under study than to random chance. Unfortunately, in studies of rare diseases, it is often impractical or even impossible to recruit a large number of patients to participate in the study. Thus, it can be extremely challenging in small trials to demonstrate that an investigational treatment is beneficial to patients with the disease. Although there are statistical methods that can help in the analysis of the data, it is often more efficient to account for these complexities when designing the study.

Regulatory agencies have acknowledged the fact that aspects of drug development in common diseases may not be appropriate or feasible for rare diseases. Indeed, regulatory agencies may allow for a greater degree of flexibility to account for the unique challenges present in development of new treatments for rare diseases. For example, the FDA has four programs designed to help advance the development of certain drugs that would potentially fill an unmet medical need in serious conditions: fast track designation, breakthrough therapy designation, accelerated approval, and priority review designation (FDA, 2014). Importantly, a development program may be considered for more than one of the aforementioned programs. Similarly, in Europe, companies have been able to request accelerated assessment (European Parliament and Council of the European Union, 2004; CHMP, 2006), and in addition companies may obtain conditional marketing authorization or marketing authorization under exceptional circumstances (European Parliament and Council of the European Union, 2004, Commission of the European Communities, 2003; Commission of the European Communities, 2006). Both agencies have recently demonstrated examples of such flexibility with approvals and recommendations. For example, in August 2014 the FDA approved Cerdelga for the long-term treatment of adult patients with the Type 1 form of Gaucher disease based on a reduction in spleen volume. In April 2014 the EMA approved Cholic acid FGK for the treatment of inborn errors in primary bile acid synthesis for patients who lack specific liver enzymes, based on changes in bile acid levels and liver function. Both Cerdelga and Cholic acid FGK have orphan drug designation from the respective regulatory agencies.

Statistical Implications: Choice of Endpoints

From a statistical perspective, the probability of having a successful study if the treatment works is driven by three considerations: the size of the study, the effect of the treatment, and the variability of the data. For common diseases, it is often easy to increase the probability of success by simply increasing the sample size of the study. This is often not feasible in studies of rare diseases, and researchers must find other ways to increase the probability of success, such as choosing endpoints with less variability than others, or endpoints that are able to demonstrate a large effect compared to a control.

In designing clinical trials, it is very important to define endpoints that can show a treatment is effective, as regulators will not approve treatments that are not effective. From a clinical perspective, the most clinically relevant endpoint may be difficult to measure, take too long to measure, or be highly variable. For example, the most clinically relevant endpoint may be overall survival; however, it could take many years to conduct an adequate study that is designed to show improvement in survival rates.

It is also important to choose endpoints that are important from a patient's perspective. Companies that are developing new therapies can partner with patient groups to help identify endpoints that matter to both the patients and regulators. Choosing clinically relevant endpoints that are appropriate in small trials can be a challenging, complex process, and patient groups can help drive the research based on their detailed knowledge of patient population, heterogeneity, relevant predictive outcomes (eg. what doctors are measuring to determine disease progression), and the importance of those outcomes to disease and patients, including their quality of life.

Use of Surrogate Endpoints: Benefits

Because clinical endpoints (such as survival) can be difficult to study, it is often necessary to identify alternative endpoints, often referred to as biomarkers or surrogate endpoints. A surrogate endpoint can be defined as a biomarker intended to substitute for a clinical endpoint (CHMP, 2005). Surrogate endpoints may be used as primary endpoints when the surrogate is reasonably likely or well known to predict clinical outcome (ICH Expert Working Group, 1997). For example, tumor response may be appropriate surrogate endpoints in lieu of a clinical endpoint such as overall survival and can form the basis for regulatory approval, as can be seen by the FDA approval of

Sylvant for Castelman's disease (a rare disorder similar to lymphoma) in April, 2014.

From both statistical and clinical perspectives, the use of surrogate endpoints can be beneficial for many reasons:

- Speed – a trial may be able to demonstrate improvement in surrogate endpoints more quickly than clinical endpoints. For example, a reduction in blood levels of a particular biomarker could occur years before a clinical endpoint such as renal failure or death.
- Sample size – surrogate endpoints may have reduced variability compared to clinical endpoints, and the treatment may have a larger effect on the surrogate endpoint than clinical endpoints, resulting in a study that may require fewer subjects.
- Practical considerations – in certain situations where it may not be possible to directly observe a clinical endpoint, a surrogate endpoint may be considered (CHMP, 2005).

Use of Surrogate Endpoints: Challenges

There are, however, challenges that exist when using surrogate endpoints, as discussed in Fleming's article on the use of surrogate endpoints and the FDA's accelerated approval (Fleming, 2005). For example, the clinical relevance of the endpoint may not be well understood, and it may be difficult to demonstrate that the biological marker is predictive of clinical outcome. Because the exact relationship between the surrogate endpoint and clinical outcome may be unknown, it can be difficult to assess whether the potential risks outweigh a benefit that is indirectly measured. In addition, the relationship between the surrogate endpoint and clinical endpoints may vary across interventions, particularly for diseases that have multiple pathways. A surrogate endpoint may be associated with a pathway that influences the clinical output; however, since therapies could be effective through different pathways, a surrogate endpoint useful for one intervention may not have the same utility for all possible interventions under study.

In order for regulatory agencies to accept surrogate endpoints, they must be validated before, during, or (in some cases) after approval (CHMP, 2005; ICH Expert Working Group, 1997; Code of Federal Regulations, 2014). In essence, the validation requires that the endpoint must have a strong biological rationale and be a prognostic marker for the relevant clinical outcomes. Treatment-induced changes in the marker should predict the clinical outcome, and the effects of treatment on the marker should explain the effects of treatment on the clinical outcome (Fleming, 2005). As noted in the ICH Guideline for Small Clinical Trials, data from patient registries may provide additional evidence that the surrogate endpoint adequately represents a relevant clinical endpoint (CHMP, 2005). This can be difficult to do prior to conducting a study, and in some cases, it may be acceptable to conduct a study based on surrogate endpoints, with the understanding that the validation must be completed for full approval.

For example, with prior approval from regulatory agencies, a potential drug or therapy could be granted marketing authorization on the basis of surrogate endpoints. This accelerated approval (US) or conditional approval (EU), instituted in order to facilitate the earlier approval of drugs to treat serious diseases and fill unmet medical needs, can be based on surrogate endpoint, but still requires that clinical benefit will be established with post-approval data. This strategy can be a useful alternative to designing studies with a clear clinical endpoint that could take years to conduct properly.

Lack of accepted surrogate markers is a large challenge in designing clinical trials for orphan diseases. Very little may be known about the natural history of the disease and the clinical presentation of the disease may be complex. The heterogeneity of the disease, resulting from complicated biology and multi-faceted clinical phenotypes, may be clinically observed but not well understood. Patient groups can be a critical partner in defining relevant surrogate markers, as they are often keenly aware of the differing clinical phenotypes, clusters of clinical manifestations, and even underlying biology of the disease. More efficient communication with regulatory agencies, leading to more efficient clinical trials, can be facilitated by better understanding the relationship between surrogate and clinical endpoints.

Conclusion

It is possible to overcome the challenges of developing treatments for rare diseases. Patient groups can participate in finding solutions to these challenges, by assisting with the development of appropriate safety and efficacy endpoints that are relevant to the patient, as having the wrong endpoints can lead to studies that do not show a clear benefit. Rare diseases are often poorly characterized, and it is critically important for patients to drive their own research because they have a more direct understanding of the clinical manifestations that are important to them. Patients also often have a more clear understanding of the standard of care, changes in the standard of care, and measures of disease progression. Because the risk-benefit analysis based on surrogate markers can be difficult to quantify, having a patient perspective can help regulators appreciate the importance of certain surrogate markers.

References

CHMP (Committee for Medicinal Products for Human Use) (2005) *CHMP Guideline on Clinical Trials in Small Populations* (CHMP/EWP/83561/2005; London: CHMP, 27 July 2006)

CHMP (Committee for Medicinal Products for Human Use) (2006) *Guideline on the Procedure for Accelerated As-*

sessment Pursuant to Article 14(9) of Regulation (EC) no 726/2004 (EMEA/419127/05; London: CHMP, 17 July 2006).

Code of Federal Regulations (2014) 21 CFR Part 314 – *Applications for FDA Approval to Market a New Drug Subpart H – Accelerated Approval of New Drugs for Serious or Life-Threatening Illnesses: Section 314.510 Approval based on a surrogate endpoint or on an effect on a clinical endpoint other than survival or irreversible morbidity* (Washing, DC: US Government Printing Office).

Commission of the European Communities (2003) 'Commission Directive 2003/63/EC of 25 June 2003 amending Directive 2001/83/EC of the European Parliament and of the Council on the Community code related to medicinal products for human use' *Official Journal of the European Union* 27.6.2003.

Commission of the European Communities (2006) 'Commission Regulation (EC) No 507/2006 of 29 March 2006 on the Conditional Marketing Authorization for Medicinal Products for Human Use Falling within the Scope of Regulation (EC) No 726/2004 of the European Parliament and of the Council' *Official Journal of the European Union* 30.3.2006.

European Parliament and Council of the European Union (2004) 'Regulation (EC) No 726/2004 of the European Parliament and of the Council of 31 March 2004 Laying Down Community Procedures for the Authorisation and Supervision of Medicinal Products for Human and Veterinary Use and Establishing a European Medicines Agency' *Official Journal of the European Union* 30.4.2004.

FDA (US Food and Drug Administration) (2014) 'Guidance for Industry – Expedited Programs for Serious Conditions – Drugs and Biologics'. (Accessed 20 July 2015). www.fda.gov/downloads/drugs/guidancecomplianceregulatoryinformation/guidances/ucm358301.pdf.

Fleming TR (2005). 'Surrogate Endpoints and FDA's Accelerated Approval Process', *Health Affairs*, 24 (1):67-78.

ICH Expert Working Group (1997) *ICH Harmonised Tripartite Guideline: General Considerations for Clinical Trials* (E8; Geneva: ICH, 17 July 1997).

Chapter 20

Setting up and Running a Clinical Trial: The Regulations

Christa van Kan
PSR Orphan Experts

It is said that the field of clinical trials is the second-most regulated industry following the aviation industry. All clinical trials must be performed according to Good Clinical Practice (ICH-GCP)[1] and all applicable national laws and regulations.

GCP is a standard for the design, setup, performing, monitoring, auditing, recording, analyzing and reporting of clinical research, to assure that:

- The data and reported results are reliable and precise;
- The rights, integrity and confidentiality of subjects are protected.

Westernized countries have clinical trials legislation, which is largely based on GCP. In Europe, the EU Clinical Trial Directive ensures harmonization of clinical trial laws across the EU-countries.

Another important cornerstone of clinical trials, is the Declaration of Helsinki (first adopted in 1964), which describes ethical principles of biomedical research involving human subjects.[2]

Regulations of clinical research in humans followed several very serious incidents in the past where people were killed or severely harmed after taking medication, which had not been properly tested in humans. Examples include an incident in 1937, where Elixir Sulfanilamide (a cough syrup containing anti-freeze) killed 107 people.[3] Another infamous example is thalidomide, which was used by pregnant women to prevent morning sickness, and led to the birth of many seriously malformed babies.[4]

Strict ethical guidelines for the participation of humans in clinical research (the Nuremburg code)[5] had its origin in the Nuremburg-trials after the second World War. During these legal trials, Dr. Mengele and several others were convicted for their horrible practices of using humans as guinea pigs without obtaining their consent.

Preparing for a clinical trial

Many different stakeholders are involved in the performance of a clinical trial:

- Regulators who need to review and approve a clinical trial before it may be started;
- The pharmaceutical or biotech company that is developing the drug/device under investigation;
- Investigators; the physicians who actually perform the clinical trial;
- Patients or healthy volunteers who participate in the clinical trial; and
- Other parties, such as CROs (Contract Research Organizations), central laboratories, patient advocacy groups, home healthcare providers, etc.

Every clinical trial is based on a 'study question': What do we want to learn from this study? One or several questions may be integrated into a single clinical trial. These study questions are usually part of a larger plan, called the 'Clinical Development Plan', which describes all the clinical studies (phase I through phase III), which will need to be performed until the drug under investigation may become eligible for Market Authorization. Such a plan is often reviewed and discussed with a regulatory body (FDA in the US, or EMA in the EU), in order to ensure that the plan meets their requirements.

The study question(s) form the basis of the study protocol. The study protocol is the most important document of any clinical trial, since it describes in detail how the trial will be performed.

Key elements in a study protocol include:

- Study background: What do we already know about the disease and the drug? Why is this study being carried out? What are the main questions to be answered?
- Study design: Will the study be prospective or retrospective? Open-label or blind? Randomized or not? Placebo- or comparator-controlled? See section on study design and statistics.
- Study population: What kind of subjects (patients or healthy volunteers) will be enrolled into the trial? Which criteria (such as age, disease severity, other illnesses, use of certain medication, etc.) do they need to meet in order to participate?
- Dosing: In which dose and which frequency will the study drug be given?
- Treatment duration: How many days/weeks/months/years will the subjects be treated with the study drug?
- Comparator drug: Will some of the subjects take a placebo or active comparator drug instead of the study drug? Will the study drug be used as 'add-on therapy', on top of other existing medication?
- Visit schedule: At which time points during the study period will subjects visit the study site to have certain assessments done? Will there be a screening period and/or a follow-up period?
- Study assessments: Detailed description of all the tests,

measurements, questionnaires, etc. which will be done at the various study visits in order to collect the necessary data to answer the study question(s).

- Statistical paragraph: How will the data be analyzed? Are any interim-analyses planned?
- Safety section: How will (serious) adverse events be reported? Will there be an indepedentent Data Monitoring Committee (DMC) to oversee the safety of the patients in the trial?

Selection of investigator(s)

Another crucial element in the performance of a clinical trial is having the right investigator(s) involved. These physicians are responsible for the actual execution of the clinical trial: they perform all the study assessments (usually with assistance of other team members) and collect the study data. In contrast to common diseases, there are usually not so many physicians who are real experts in a specific rare disease and treat these patients regularly. These 'Key Opinion Leaders (KOLs)' are the main target when searching for a suitable investigator for an orphan drug trial. Often, these physicians already have a relationship with the license holder of the study drug (for instance, as a member of their advisory board) and are usually very eager to be involved in the review of the study protocol. Therefore, it is advisable to start liaising with potential investigators at an early stage and certainly before finalizing the study protocol.

Apart from their experience with the rare disease and their interest in contributing to a potential therapy, there are several other important questions to ask before making the final decision on the investigator(s) and therefore study site(s):

- Does the investigator have prior clinical trial experience?
- Does the investigator have sufficient time to perform the clinical trial? Or, does he have adequately trained

research staff (such as co-investigators and/or research nurses) to support him?

- Does the site have all the necessary facilities/equipment to properly perform all the assessments, to process and store laboratory samples, etc.?

If the answer to one or more of the above questions is no, it does not necessarily mean that the site is unfit to participate; it just means that it will take a bit more effort and training to make it work. Consider things like providing a GCP-training for the site staff, hiring additional support staff, or renting certain equipment for the duration of the trial.

As a first step in assessing the suitability and interest of clinical sites and to calculate the number of sites needed, it is advisable to perform a 'feasibility study'. This is a kind of survey, in which you send a questionnaire to all potential investigators to collect information about: number of suitable patients in their clinical practice, possible competing clinical trials, prior clinical trial experience, availability of research staff, equipment and facilities, and of course their interest to participate in the current clinical trial. Please be aware that investigators almost always over-estimate their 'recruitment potential' (how many patients they think they can enroll in a certain time frame). Investigators, who are generally very busy physicians, are not always keen to fill out a long questionnaire. A better (and more personal) approach is to schedule a phone appointment with the investigator, in which the study can be explained and the questionnaire discussed.

After collating the information from the feasibility questionnaires, the clinical sites which seem suitable for participation, are contacted to schedule a so-called Site Qualification Visit. During this visit, the study protocol is discussed in more detail, and a more thorough assessment of the site's suitability is performed. If all this is positive and the investigator is eager to participate, the procedures for 'site set-up' can be started.

Site set-up procedures

Before being allowed to start the clinical trial at a clinical site, approvals must be obtained from the applicable ethics committee and regulatory authority. In the US, ethics committees are called IRBs (Institutional Review Boards) and can be local or central. In addition, you need approval from the FDA, by submitting an IND (Investigative New Drug) application. In Europe, each country has its own Competent Authority (CA), which must review a clinical trial. For the ethics review in Europe, you need to submit to a so-called Central Ethics Committee (in each country). Submitting to these ethics committees and regulatory authorities is quite complicated and requires a vast number of forms to be completed and documents to be provided. Essential documents include: the study protocol, patient information form, detailed information about the study drug, subject insurance certificate and resumés of the investigators. Although timelines for these procedures vary from country to country, you need to allow approximately 3 to 6 months to obtain the necessary approvals. For 'Advanced Therapies'(gene therapy, cell therapy, tissue therapy) these timelines are longer.

Another item, which can take a significant amount of time, is the contract with the clinical site, which includes the fee, which the investigator and the hospital will receive for their work. Each site will have their own requirements with regard to type of contract, language of the contract, etc. The contract and budget negotiations can often be performed in parallel with the ethics and regulatory submissions, but sometimes a signed contract is needed first.

In addition to ethics and regulatory approval, some countries and/or hospitals have additional procedures to adhere to (such as radiology approvals or R&D approvals for UK sites). Please check this carefully with the study site or a local expert.

Since these site set-up procedures are so complicated and there is so much variation across countries and clinical sites, it is highly advisable to involve a CRO or consultant who has experience with these procedures, thereby avoiding unnecessary time delays.

Other study set-up procedures

There are also a number of logistical issues, which must be arranged before the study can actually start. Although these will vary from trial to trial, below are four key elements, which are applicable for almost every trial.

Patient recruitment: In addition to the patients which may be recruited directly by the selected investigators, there are many alternative methods to recruit patients who are eligible and willing to participate in a clinical trial. For rare diseases, it is highly advisable to involve the patient advocacy group(s) at an early stage to discuss their potential role in patient recruitment. Please refer to the separate section on Patient Recruitment in this book.

IMP logistics: Firstly, arrangements must be made for the proper packaging, labeling and distribution of the study drug or IMP (Investigational Medicinal Product). This is usually taken care of by the license-holder of the IMP. At each study site, arrangements for the proper storage, dispense, and drug-accountability must be made, usually with the hospital's pharmacist.

Laboratory logistics: For the analysis of body samples (blood, urine, other fluids or tissues), a choice must be made to use either the local hospital laboratories or a commercial laboratory to which all samples are sent. The advantage of such a "central laboratory" is that the samples are all analyzed in the same way, using the same equipment, and the results are therefore more comparable. If a central laboratory is involved in the study, this laboratory must be selected and decisions must be made with regard to laboratory materials to be used, as well as the proper processing, storage and transport of samples from the study sites to the central laboratory. Courier companies, which specialize in the transport of body samples are significantly more expensive than general courier companies, but should certainly be considered if the samples are crucial to the success of the study.

CRF: All the study data must be collected in a study database. To achieve this, the data collected by the study sites, must be recorded on a Case Report Form (CRF). Nowadays, CRFs are usually in electronic format: the investigator logs on to a web-based system in which he can record all the results from the study assessments. Prior to study start, the (e)-CRF must be chosen and designed.

Study execution

Once all of the above site- and study- setup-procedures have been completed, the study can finally commence. A good start of this phase (not mandatory) is a joint Investigator's Meeting, which is a very good opportunity to discuss the study in detail and to create a 'team-feeling'.

Each study site will be officially 'activated' by the performance of a Site Initiation Visit (SIV), during which all the site staff will receive further training on the study procedures and study-materials are delivered. Following this visit, the site can start recruiting patients.

An important regulatory requirement is that, during the study execution, regular 'on-site monitoring' is performed by qualified monitors or CRAs (Clinical Research Associates). In practice, this means that a designated CRA visits each study site approximately once every 1-2 months (dependent on study complexity, number of subjects enrolled, etc.). During these Monitoring Visits, the CRA will check the informed consent forms (to ensure that all subjects have given their voluntary consent), the patient's medical records, the (e)-CRFs, and all other forms and logs which are to be maintained by the site staff.

Behind the scenes, a so-called Data Manager is responsible for continuously checking the data, which is being entered into the clinical database and run checks (both automated and manual) to identify possible errors or discrepancies in the study data. In case a potential error is found, the Data Manager will issue a data query, which subsequently needs to be resolved by the respective study site.

During each clinical trial, a huge number of documents, letters, forms and logs are produced. All these documents are stored in an organized manner in the Trial Master File (TMF). The TMF may be either paper-based (in the form of multiple binders), or in electronic format (an e-TMF). Auditors or inspectors may check the contents of the TMF during or after the study, to ensure that all necessary approvals are in place, and that all applicable documentation is properly maintained.

Study closure activities

Once all subjects have completed the clinical trial, the Data Manager will need to ensure that any remaining omissions or inconsistencies in the clinical database are resolved. Usually, listings of all the data will be prepared, and these are reviewed by the key study team members, in order to check for strange values, outliers or other possible errors. Once everyone is confident that the data are 'clean', the Data Manager will 'lock'the database. This means that nobody is able to make any further changes to the data.

In case of a blind study (where it is unknown which patient is in which treatment group), the treatment code may be revealed only after the database has been locked. This is to avoid possible manipulation of the study data (bias).

The next step is the statistical analysis. This is done by an experienced Bio-statistician and in accordance with the Statistical Analysis Plan (SAP, which must be finalized before locking of the database). The Bio-statistician will program and run the applicable statistical tests, resulting in various tables and graphs which are considered the results of the study.

These results are described in the Clinical Study Report (CSR). This extensive report will form part of the Marketing Authorisation package, to be submitted to the FDA/EMA in order to obtain final marketing approval.

Conclusion

Performing a clinical trial in accordance with all applicable regulations is a complicated and time-consuming process. This is even more so for orphan drug trials, since every data point is crucial (you cannot afford to lose patients or study data) and study logistics are often complicated by the fact that patients live far from the study sites. Running a successful clinical trial also requires very specific knowledge. It is highly advisable to involve an experienced project manager to oversee all the various aspects of the clinical trial.

References

1 http://www.ich.org/fileadmin/Public_Web_Site/ICH_Products/Guidelines/Efficacy/E6/E6_R1_Guideline.pdf

2 http://www.wma.net/en/30publications/10policies/b3/index.html

3 Ballentine, C. Taste of Raspberries, Taste of Death The 1937 Elixir Sulfanilamide Incident. FDA Consumer magazine. http://www.fda.gov/AboutFDA/WhatWeDo/History/ProductRegulation/SulfanilamideDisaster/default.htm.

4 https://helix.northwestern.edu/article/thalidomide-tragedy-lessons-drug-safety-and-regulation

5 http://www.nj.gov/health/irb/documents/nuremburg_code.pdf

Chapter 21

Patient Registries

Kyle Brown
Patient Crossroads

Introduction

Collecting a critical mass of patient data represents one of the key problems in the field of rare diseases. As such, pulling information together from geographically and structurally dispersed sources, and making this information available for research and care purposes largely addresses this obstacle.

Patient registries constitute such key instruments for increasing knowledge on rare diseases, supporting fundamental clinical and epidemiological research, and post-marketing surveillance of orphan drugs and treatments used off-label. Furthermore, and of great importance for patients and their families, they can be instrumental in supporting health and social services planning. Rare Disease Patient Registries are powerful, cost-effective instruments to improve the overall quality of care, quality of life and survival of patients.

With over 7,000 known rare diseases, raising the visibility of a single disease area is a critical objective of any rare disease advocacy organization. With more than 7,000 disease communities vying for the attention of researchers and pharmaceutical companies, it can be extremely challenging for small advocacy organizations to increase their visibility.

It has also been demonstrated that patient registries are a major determinant for successful translational research in the field of rare diseases. Where well-implemented registries and active patient organizations exist, the likelihood for developing a treatment for the disease in question is increased.[1]

"Creating a registry of patients is the single most valuable action a rare disease community can take." said David Meeker, president and CEO of Genzyme, a subsidiary of Sanofi. *"The registry provides critical disease knowledge which makes that disease easier to study, increasing the probability a treatment can be developed."*

Dominique Ristori, Director-General of the Joint Research Centre and Paola Testori Coggi Director-General of the Directorate General for Health and Consumers fully agree with patients' organisations and healthcare professionals that disease registries are *"an indispensable infrastructure tool for translating basic and clinical research into improved care and therapeutic solutions"*.

Quantifying and qualifying your patient community to spur research interest

A well-organized and motivated patient community is critical. To de-risk major financial investments in orphan drug development or incentivize academic researchers to focus their careers on a rare disease, a patient registry can help generate crucial knowledge – the natural history of the disease, how many patients are affected, what symptoms they exhibit, what treatments they use or where they live.

A well-constructed, open and accessible patient registry program can unlock the door to academic research and pharmaceutical interest and investment. Patient involvement is a key element in the successful establishment and long-term maintenance of a patient registry and many patient groups are already very active and capable in this role, both in Europe and the United States.

Taking such a consolidated, patient centric approach to patient registries can mean:

- Patients can more easily find registries and provide their valuable data (including locations of blood and tissue samples as well as reports of diagnoses, disease symptoms, treatment usage, and lifestyle activities);
- Patients can be confident in the privacy of their de-identified data and the knowledge that their data will be shared to help improve lives;
- Researchers and pharmaceutical companies have a larger, more easily accessible pool of potential patients for research studies and clinical trials targeting specific rare diseases;
- Pharmaceutical companies can collect post-market surveillance data in a more scalable and cost-effective manner;
- Rare disease advocacy and research foundations can more easily organize their global patient populations for inclusion in trials and studies.

Types of Patient Registries

Depending on the audience, the term 'patient registry' carries different meanings. The chart below illustrates the different types of patient registries typically in use.

Patient Opt-in / Contact Registries

A patient opt-in registry is also referred to as a 'contact registry' because they typically contain only name, address and diagnosis information. This type of registry can be easily implemented by advocacy organizations and resembles a mailing list. These registries can be useful for raising the visibility of an individual advocacy organization, but does not provide enough detailed medical history to make it useful to pharmaceutical companies

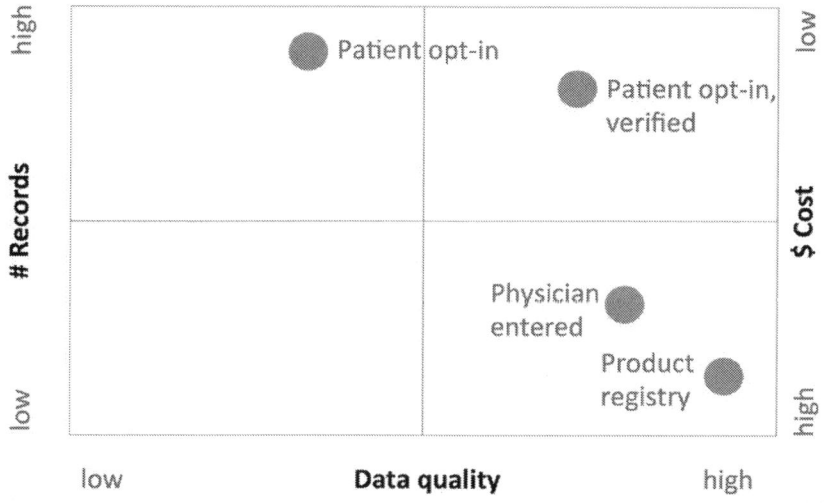

Figure 1. Different types of patient registry (PatientCrossroads, Inc.)

and academic researchers.

Contact registries have the advantage that they are easy to implement, inexpensive, and may contain large numbers of families. However, the quality of the data may be considered low. These types of registries are most often managed by patient advocacy organizations that are attempting to raise the visibility of their group and increase donations. This can result in a competitive situation with other foundations that also represent the same disease area.

Physician / Researcher Registries

Researchers must publish scientific research in respected medical journals in order to gain notoriety that can result in more funding for their research efforts.

As such, academic researchers are usually motivated to collect patient data in a patient registry to advance personal research. These registries often contain records of only those patients seen by an academic center or clinic. The data is entered into the registry by a medical professional, resulting in more detailed and accurate clinical data. The patients in these registries must sign a consent form, allowing the researcher or physician to enter data about them on their behalf.

These registries can be very detailed and contain valuable information about a disease. However, they typically have very limited access, often restricted only to researchers entering the data. These researchers benefit from the registry, but the community at large generally will not unless the data is shared with more accessible patient registry programs.

Researcher registries are expensive to implement because they are frequently managed by internal technology resources, are built from scratch and will be managed under the direction of an IRB (Institutional Review Board) or Ethics Review Board (ERB). Often the registry will be initiated through a research grant. Once the grant funding runs out (typically in two to three years), the registry will be halted and the data maybe lost or outdated.

Patient Opt-in & Verified Registries

This model, pioneered by companies such as PatientCrossroads, provides the best of patient opt-in and physician entered registries. In this model, patients opt-in and provide detailed medical history, upload confirmatory test results and agree to update their information once or twice per year. A medical professional then reviews each patient-provided history and tags each profile based on the quality of the patient-provided data. For example, a patient record without a confirmatory testing result could be tagged as 'likely diagnosis / unconfirmed', while a patient that has completed their medical history and uploaded genetic testing results may be categorized as 'confirmed diagnosis'.

By stratifying the patient provided data, a wide net can be cast – allowing anyone that believes they have the disease to participate and receive educational materials and clinical trial and study notices. Pharmaceutical companies and researchers can then use the data that is most relevant to their goals. If recruiting for a clinical trial, pharmaceutical companies would target only those patients with a confirmed diagnosis, whilst academic researchers may be searching for patients that may not have had confirmatory testing.

This model can be implemented inexpensively and contain a more representative number of patients. However, depending on the level of verification, the quality of the collected data is typically considered higher than a contact registry, but not as accurate as a physician or researcher registry.

Product Registries

Pharmaceutical and biotechnology companies most often utilize product registries. These registries may be utilized in clinical trials or post-market surveillance programs required by the FDA. These registries will most closely resemble Physician / Researcher Registries, but will be paid for by pharmaceutical companies to meet regulatory requirements. CROs (Contract Research Organizations) and funded physicians and clinics will be responsible for the execution of the trial and entry of the patient data. The data is closely guarded and is collected under rigorous protocols.

These registries may cost millions of dollars and typically benefit only the funding organization with the goal of bringing a drug to market.

Electronic Health Records

Electronic health records (EHR) are the systems utilized in a hospital to track each patient's medical history, physician notes, billing and prescriptions. These robust systems cost many millions of dollars and contain very detailed and valuable data about individual patients. However, since these systems are restricted to only authorized hospital personnel, they have limited utility as patient registries.

There are initiatives underway to make the data contained in EHRs more readily accessible to patients. Many hospital systems now have Patient Portals where patients can access testing results, refill prescriptions, schedule appointments, and even view physician notes. As these systems mature, there may be opportunities for this data to be married with the patient-provided health histories contained in patient registries.

The Importance of Data Sharing

Although patient registries and other data repositories are still traditionally managed by universities, industry or public administrations, patient data ultimately belongs to patients. More and more, rare disease patient organisations are taking a very active role in initiating, designing, funding, and even directly collecting and sharing data.

Public-private partnerships, whether between patient groups and researchers, patient groups and the drug development industry, or research institutions and industry, are also being encouraged. In the context of the current economic climate, the need for the optimal sharing of resources is an imperative. Different scenarios are being proposed to provide financial sustainability to registries and their networks. The most promising rely on the collaboration amongst all the stakeholders.[2,3] This collaborative approach has been recognized as a requirement to: avoid duplication of efforts and take advantage of economies of scale; foster improved quality and robustness of data collected; to unify patient data especially for diseases where several treatments exist; and best sustain registries as long-term endeavours. With both governments and private groups showing interest in patient registries, public-private partnerships are a promising collaborative scheme. Patient groups can be instrumental facilitators of public-private partnerships, driving the common goals of all stakeholders through a patient-centred approach and assuring optimal efficiency and transparency. Regulatory bodies can strongly encourage such collaboration in this pre-competitive space. The nature of potential public-private partnerships, the issues to consider when establishing such a partnership, and best practices enhancing the success of such efforts should be investigated in a prompt and transparent manner.

Some disease communities have demonstrated the translation of these principles in public-private partnerships into action. Yet for many others, this is not yet a reality.

TREAT-NMD is a worldwide network for neuromuscular diseases that provides an infrastructure to support the collection of data about patients with Duchene Muscular Dystrophy and delivery of promising new therapies. The harmonized implementation of national and ultimately global patient registries has been central to the success of TREAT-NMD. For the DMD registries within TREAT-NMD, individual countries have chosen to collect patient information in the form of standardized patient registries to increase the overall patient population on which clinical outcomes and new technologies can be assessed. The registries comprise more than 13,500 patients from 31 different countries and continue to grow – fostering collaboration between academia, patient organizations, and industry.[4]

There are multiple different types of possible patient registry programs each with different stakeholders and motivations. Each model should have one thing in common – patients are at the heart of the program. Most registry participants want their data shared with any researchers that can help find a treatment or can improve the lives of patients.

If each advocacy, research and drug discovery organization created their own private registries, for their own exclusive use, the rate of research and the development of life saving treatments would be delayed; no single organization would have a complete picture of the natural history of disease, or have the ability to contact patients for participation in clinical trials and studies.

For example, DuchenneConnect is the largest patient registry for Duchenne Muscular Dystrophy; the data is detailed and is shared broadly with the research community. This Opt-in / Verified registry is often held as an example of the right way to implement a patient registry program. Unfortunately, there are 50 other Duchenne Muscular Dystrophy registries around the world. Each collecting different levels of information, some entered by patients, some by physicians, some covered under IRBs, others without IRBs. The data is nearly impossible to combine to provide a truly global view of Duchenne Muscular Dystrophy.

Any patient registry program should have a data access and publication policy that protects the privacy of participants while making the data broadly available. The policy should consider the following:

- Who may access the registry data;
- For what purposes can the registry data be used;
- How researchers apply for access to the data;
- Who reviews and approves applications to utilize the data;
- How should the research cite the data in publications; and
- How the registry will contact participants and for what purposes.

Ethical, Legal and Social Issues in Patient Data Collection

Patient registries store highly personal and sensitive information. The confidentiality of the information must be guaranteed. However, the level of protection required for their personal data, when balanced with the benefits of encouraging translational research, is a particularly difficult consensus to reach. On the one hand, sharing of scarce data is an absolute priority in order to foster research and facilitate translational projects in the rare diseases field, while on the other hand, patients living with rare diseases are in a vulnerable position as they are much easier to identify (eg. through cross-cutting of databases) than patients with common conditions. The balance between protecting personal data and facilitating research into rare diseases is a particularly difficult one to strike.

Allowing access to patient registries data without breaching confidentiality requires thought and planning. In Europe, the European Commission proposed a major reform of the EU legal framework on the protection of personal data to incorporate considerations brought into play by the introduction of new technologies. The new legislation favours a high standard of protection of personal data that is widely considered detrimental to health research. As no further compromises have yet been reached by the Council on other parts of the Regulation, negotiations are expected to continue into 2015. Under the current timetable, the Regulation is unlikely to come into force until 2017.

US federal regulations, in particular the 'Sunshine Act', restrict the ability for pharmaceutical companies to have direct contact with patients and physicians, which may be seen has having undue influence over the use of their treatments.

Types of Data Collected

There is a trade-off between the rarity of a disease, and the willingness of patients to contribute to a registry program. For example, a diabetes registry may only be able to collect high level information from patients because they are plentiful and diabetes is a more manageable disease. Life-threatening or pediatric diseases on the other hand, have more motivated patient communities that will contribute vast amounts of data if they feel it will further the discovery of treatments.

Utilizing KOLs (Key Opinion Leaders) in your disease area can be a great resource for learning what types of data are the most important to collect. Including the leading researchers in the development of the patient registry will help to gain acceptance in the research community. The information should include those questions that are important to researchers, pharmaceutical companies, advocacy organizations and also the patients themselves. Collecting too much information will result in fewer participants, while collecting too little data makes the registry less valuable.

Keep in mind your community, and the level of motivation of the community, when deciding what and how much data to collect. Most registries use surveys to capture medical history. Most rare disease patients or caregivers are extremely busy caring for their disease or loved ones. Asking for too much time to participate in a registry may result in less data collected. Breaking the data collected into manageable sizes that can be completed as time allows will result in more information being provided. If possible, break your main survey into multiple, smaller surveys that are presented to the user based on their personal profile. For example, do not present a pregnancy questionnaire to men registering in your program.

The types of data most frequently collected in registries may include:

- Demographic data (name, location, date of birth, gender)
- Diagnosis (who, when, where was the patient first diagnosed)
- Symptoms
- Treatments
- Family history
- Quality of life
- Disease specific questions
- Confirmatory testing results.

A good rule of thumb is to create medical questionnaires that can be completed in 15-20 minutes. Users should have the ability to compete their history over time, so being able to log out, and come back and complete the survey is critical.

Funding and Sustainability

Longterm funding and sustainability of patient registries is a concern, particularly in rare diseases that may not have the financial resources of larger disease organizations.

Industry sponsors can help to initiate patient registries in a disease area in partnership with foundations. If a single foundation exists in any given rare disease, and a pharmaceutical company provides the bulk of that foundation's funding, the funding company may run afoul of the Sunshine Act. This concern is causing pharmaceutical companies to re-think their relationships with individual patient advocacy organizations.

Academic researchers often fund their patient registry programs through grants. As much as a third of grant funding may be earmarked for recruitment of patients into the researcher study. Because grants have a specific start and end date, when the grant is finished, the research must make a decision on the sustainability of the registry. If the data was collected in a researcher-funded and -controlled registry, there is a good likelihood the registry will end when funding runs out or the researcher retires.

There are several open, accessible registry programs that provide registries for free to advocacy and non-profit organizations. The advocacy organizations provide the marketing and outreach efforts to their community, to raise awareness of the disease. This model is gaining acceptance in the community because they often make the data more open and accessible and collect the data in a consistent fashion that can enable pan-disease analysis.

Conclusion

Rare disease organizations often struggle with raising the visibility of their disease, not only to the patient community, but also to academic researchers, government institutions and pharmaceutical companies. It is difficult for a rare disease advocacy foundation to attract research attention if they cannot answer basic questions about their disease, including:

- How many people have the disease?
- Where do they live?
- Who provides the first diagnosis?

- How do patients manage their disease?
- What is the quality of life of patients?
- What is the financial burden of the disease?

There are free patient registry programs that any advocacy foundation, regardless of size, can use to implement a patient registry. For example, PatientCrossroads offers the same high-end registries sold to government and pharmaceutical companies, free to advocacy organizations. In return, the advocacy organizations promote the registry and act as the marketing and outreach arm of the registry program. Too often, we find advocacy organizations being indecisive and wasting precious years, trying to decide if they should start a patient registry and what vendor they should use. The answer is yes, start a patient registry today!

References

1 Orphanet. Report on Rare Disease Research, Its Determinants in Europe and the Way Forward, May 2011.

2 Workshop on Natural History Studies of Rare Diseases. Feb 2014. FDA. US Food and Drug Administration. (Accessed July 2015). http://www.fda.gov/ForIndustry/Developing-ProductsforRareDiseasesConditions/OOPDNewsArchive/ucm292294.htm

3 EUCERD Workshop of Public-Private Partnerships for RD Registries.

4 Standard questionnaires developed by the authors: not published.

Chapter 22

How to Interact with Government and Lobby for Change to the Clinical Trials System

Empower: Access to Medicine – The Road to Early Access

James Hargrave and James Turgoose
Empower: Access to Medicine

Les Halpin

Les Halpin was diagnosed with Motor Neurone Disease (MND) in 2011. A gifted mathematician, with an inquisitive brain, Les quickly realised the numbers were stacked against him, and furthermore the money spent on new drugs versus the output was wildly out of kilter.

In the case of MND, Les was dismayed to discover there had been no substantial advancement in its treatment since the creation of Riluzole – a drug now decades old with the prospect of only adding a few months, at most, to a patient's life.

Rather than take on the treatment and research of MND directly, as this is catered for already by a number of associations, Les instead set his sights on taking on the system more widely.

Les, a successful businessman in his own right, marked with astonishment the exponential growth in the amount spent on trying to develop new drugs – he rapidly became of the opinion that this was due, in large part, to the regulatory and legislative environment that govern how new medicines are developed.

The Right Advice

Understanding that the system he wanted to change was governed by the regulatory and political world, Les approached JBP, a specialist communications company based in Westminster. Working together, Les established a mechanism for changing the system – and so began Empower: Access to Medicine.

Les, through his research, strongly believed that the regulatory and legal framework that governed drug development had failed to keep pace with modern science. The law had rightly developed in a way to try to maximize patient protection/safety, however in so doing it was now stifling innovation at the clinical and research level.

For the campaign to understand how to overcome these possible hurdles and address the regulatory 'log jam', it was going to need some expert advice.

Empower: Access to Medicine engaged with some of the leading minds on regulatory, legal and drug development issues, so as to chart a practical way forward for the campaign that might see real, practical benefits for patients. In doing so, Empower has worked closely with experts including Professor Sir Peter Lachmann, founding President of the Academy of Medical Sciences, Professor Richard Barker, founder of CASMI, and Sir David Cooksey, chair of the Francis Crick Institute and a long-standing adviser to UK governments on the future of biosciences.

Ready for Launch

Once having understood the areas of the regulatory and political framework that needed to change to see patients, like Les, get access to medical drugs faster, Empower: Access to Medicine was ready to launch.

At the centre of the launch was an understanding of who the campaign needed to engage with. This required a comprehensive mapping out of the patient groups, politicians, campaigners, trade bodies and pharmaceutical businesses that Empower would need to work with. Communicating with these groups required a number of communication channels, including the traditional letters of introduction, to more modern tools such as online newsletters, Twitter and Facebook. The campaign was unveiled at the House of Commons on 19th June 2012, as Les Halpin addressed a cross-section of key influencers about why he had decided to launch Empower.

The House of Commons launch set the tone for the campaign's ambitions and highlighted the campaign's first major policy debate. The debate that followed, held at the Kings Fund in September 2012, brought together the media, legal minds and academics to debate the tenets at the core of Empower's goals. The outcome of the Kings Fund debate was to raise awareness of Empower, forge the key pillars of its objectives and provide valuable content for sharing on the campaign website and through social media.

Parliamentary Engagement

As Empower: Access to Medicine built its profile in the academic and patient community, it was vital that the key issues were raised in Parliament.

Following initial meetings with the Health Minister, Earl Howe, supported by his local MP Geoffrey Clifton-Brown, Les began to build awareness of the Empower cause. The campaign achieved a significant parliamentary breakthrough in November 2012, when Baroness Masham highlighted the work of Les, and Empower's aims, in a debate in the House of Lords discussing the treatment of neurological conditions.

The House of Lords, with its range of experts, often provides a forum for debates to take place of a more detailed and nuanced complexion than the House of Commons. Baroness Masham cited many of Empower's concerns with the drug approval process, and received an undertaking from Earl Howe, the Health Minister, about the Government's plans around the issue.

Discussions in the House of Lords against a backdrop of growing patient community restlessness, combined with increasing expertise on the barriers in the system, allowed Empower to push the issue up the policy agenda. With the support of Geoffrey Clifton-Brown MP, a House of Commons debate took place in January 2013 on *access to medicine for people with terminal illnesses*.

In a matter of months, Empower had gone from its launch to a matter of public record in the House of Commons and the House of Lords.

Media Spotlight

Having now received significant parliamentary attention Empower was attracting interest from across the media.

With the help of the Sunday Times' Lois Rogers, Les' plight had been brought to the attention of the general public. On 10th February 2013, the *Sunday Times* ran a substantial interview with Les and his wife Claire, highlighting his work and the achievements of the campaign to date.[1]

The piece also provided the opportunity to draw attention to a Government e-petition that the campaign launched, which garnered thousands of signatures. The petition attracted the attention of BBC Radio 4's *Today Programme*[2] and Les was interviewed as part of a package, which saw Professor Sir Peter Lachmann and Sir Michael Rawlins (head of NICE at the time) go head-to-head over the issue. It also saw coverage in the *Daily Telegraph* and *Daily Mail*.

The Halpin Protocol

Having now raised the matter up the parliamentary and media agenda, and with a firm grounding in the issues that needed to be overcome, Empower needed to propose a constructive way forward. Working with a coalition of experts, Empower developed a protocol that the patient community could stand behind.

The protocol was formed as a charter for increased patient input in the decision to take experimental treatments. Launched as an open consultation, Empower took the protocol to experts and patient campaigners to collate their opinions and contributions.

The Health Minister responsible for such matters, Earl Howe, was by this point very familiar with Empower and Les' drive for change (having met Les in the early stages of his condition). Earl Howe led a discussion in the House of Commons (15th April 2013), where he pledged to take on board some of the key principles outlined in the protocol in the progression of the early access scheme the Department of Health and MHRA were working on (which in 2013 was already behind schedule).

Building a Coalition

Having taken the protocol to a wide range of policy makers, campaigners, patients, industry and academics, the Halpin Protocol had been heavily consulted upon; and now Empower: Access to Medicine had solid recommendations to take to Government.

Empower published its inaugural report, *Early Access – A Year On*, in July 2013.[3] The report featured high profile contributors such as MHRA Chairman, Sir Gordon Duff; Sir Peter Lachmann and Professor Richard Barker; ethicists of note, Baroness O'Neill and Professor John Harris; pharmaceutical experts, Dr Jack Scannell and Sir David Cooksey; and many more.

The authoritative report was circulated to MPs, Peers and policy makers in the relevant Government and regulatory departments at a time when substantive decisions were being made about the future structure of drug approval and licensing in the UK.

Against a backdrop of a similar drive for reform in medical innovation, being led by Lord Saatchi through his Medical Innovation Bill, Empower had helped to foster a grassroots groundswell for changes to current practice. Empower was now working with the Saatchi team and patient campaigners such as Emily Crossley (Duchenne Children's Trust) and Alex Johnson (Joining Jack), to build a coalition for change.

Influencing Early Access

Empower's *Year On* report had caused a ripple with parliamentarians and policy makers, and opened the door for high-level engagement with key decision makers.

Earl Howe, and leading MHRA officials, committed to a further meeting in January 2014 to discuss the practical reality of earlier access and how the USA's 'breakthrough' system could act as a suitable template for a streamlined system in the UK.

It was a meeting that Les Halpin would unfortunately never see the outcome of. In September 2013, Les lost his battle with Motor Neurone Disease, acting as a stark reminder of the very real consequences of a lack of progress for patients. The campaign redoubled its efforts to drive the issue forward.

The meeting in January 2014, led by Geoffrey Clifton-Brown MP, featured key influencers from across the academic, policy and industry divide, bringing together people such as the newly appointed Wellcome Trust Director, Dr Jeremy Farrar, and the chiefs of both the ABPI and the BIA, Stephen Whitehead and Steve Bates.

The meeting came at a crucial time. Dr Ian Hudson, CEO of the MHRA, and the DH advisers present, explained that the proposed early access scheme was entering its final stages – though they could not commit to a launch date.

Emily Crossley and Alex Johnson were able to explain at the meeting, to Earl Howe and Dr Hudson, that a non-specific timeline was not good enough – children, such as theirs who suffer from Muscular Dystrophy, would die without progress being made to make drugs more readily available. It was also explained that the combined campaigns (a coalition of patient groups led by Empower, Duchenne Children's Trust and Joining Jack) would be taking their concerns to Parliament in March

2014 for a patient summit where they would publically call on the Government for change.

However, rather than the Parliamentary summit becoming an event to highlight slow progress, it became a celebration of a significant positive step forward. In the months running up to the event Empower became increasingly involved in the final stages of the launch of the imminent *Early Access to Medicines Scheme*,[4] in particular what scope there may be for accelerating access to drugs at the Phase II trial stage – a key recommendation in the *One Year On* report.

Empower's high level engagement, consistent and detailed messaging, combined with the right links in the right departments came together at a critical juncture to give it a key voice in the creation of the *Early Access to Medicines Scheme*. Claire Halpin, Les' widow, was even invited to provide supporting statements alongside the Health Secretary, Jeremy Hunt, at the scheme's launch.

What Next?

The *Early Access to Medicines Scheme* presents the opportunity for drug development to take a significant step forward. The scheme, having only gone live in April 2014, still has some way to go in proving what difference it may make. One year on from its launch and there have been four drugs earmarked for approval, Empower had hoped for more by this stage. However, should these four be successful, it may perhaps drive more innovative medicines to the scheme.

Unfortunately the Medical Innovation Bill was defeated in the House of Commons in March 2015. Empower and like-minded groups will take stock and assess options for pushing for new legislation on medical innovation in the new Parliament. Though unsuccessful, the attention the Medical Innovation Bill garnered has served to widen the debate around drug access and galvanise the patient community.

Empower and its allies will work to build on this constructive spirit and continue to keep pressure on Government to ensure that the system continues to reform to fit modern medicine and patient needs.

"True innovation exists at the frontiers of scientific endeavour – this is as true for medicine as it is for physics. Clinicians and pharmacists must be allowed the space to strive for new discoveries with the support of systems that allow responsible innovation.

"The time has come for medical regulation to match modern medicine. I encourage you to sign Empower's petition, let's practically demonstrate that the system can work differently. I wish you every success and good luck".

– **Professor Stephen Hawking**

Conclusion

Les Halpin demonstrated that through a single mission, aimed at the right political and media stakeholders, he could exercise a powerful voice, even if his own was beginning to fail him. Empower: Access to Medicine worked with the right people to pull the right levers to expedite action from the Department of Health.

Though it is still early days for the Early Access to Medicines Scheme, it has opened a vital door for the patient community to potentially drive vital medicines through the system faster.

References

1 Dying tycoon fights to use untested drug. 2013. The Sunday Times. (Accessed 24 July 2015). http://www.thesundaytimes.co.uk/sto/news/uk_news/Health/article1211152.ece

2 BBC Radio 4 Today interview. 2013. AudioBoom. (Accessed 24 July 2015). https://audioboom.com/boos/1214600-i-ll-run-the-risk-on-unapproved-drugs?utm_campaign=detailpage&utm_content=retweet&utm_medium=social&utm_source=twitter

3 Early Access to Medicines: A year on – Summer 2013. 2013. Empower: Access to Medicine Policy Report. Empower. (Accessed July 2015). http://www.accesstomedicine.co.uk/news-and-events/pathways-to-progress.

4 Early Access to Medicines Scheme. Dec 2014. Medicines and Healthcare Products Regulatory Agency. (Accessed July 2015). www.gov.uk/apply-for-the-early-access-to-medicines-scheme-eams.

Chapter 23

The Saatchi Campaign Case

Dominic Nutt
The Saatchi Campaign

It's not about the money

Many who oppose Maurice Saatchi's push to increase innovation in the British health sector by dint of a change in the law have assumed that the former Tory party chairman has put the full weight of his vast global advertising agency behind the so-far hugely successful campaign.

This is not so.

Firstly, relatively little money has been spent on the campaign – a campaign that has only three part-time, freelance staff working on it. Second, Lord Saatchi's advertising agency is not in any way involved.

And therein lies the hope for all health campaigners everywhere. In my experience, you do not need much to make a lot happen.

Maurice Saatchi began his campaign to support greater medical innovation after his wife, Josephine Hart, died of ovarian cancer in 2011.

Frustrated by what he saw as too little progress in developing new treatments for some cancers over the past 40 years or so, Saatchi started to ask questions – what was getting in the way of finding cures for cancers?

Readers will know there are of course many reasons why it takes a long time to find new cures for diseases – not just cancers. To list a few, there is the cost of drug development, complexity around trials, lack of money, lack of suitable patients – not to mention the obvious, that however far medical science has developed, finding new cures is not easy.

It's complicated – but focus on a simple objective

However, Saatchi alighted on one, specific issue within a basket of complex reasons – the legal barrier to innovation. Some of the UK's most senior doctors told him that British medicine is ruled by protocols and standard procedures, developed over years by solid medical research and practical experience, and reinforced by NICE guidelines and the law.

The law is a key part of the picture. Innovating can be a high-risk enterprise, which many doctors seek to avoid. There is a culture in the NHS that drives clinicians to stick to what are known as 'standard procedures'. These are the prescribed norms of practice for any given illness. Sticking to these gives the clinician protection in law in the event of a negligence claim – irrespective of whether the standard procedures are effective or not.

In the vast majority cases, of course, standard procedures, based on experience and data derived over many years and through clinical trials, is precisely what is required.

A newly diagnosed type 1 diabetic doesn't want a doctor to 'innovate' on a random and individual basis and theorise that insulin injections are not necessary. No. For most patients, most of the time, standard procedures are the way forward.

But standard procedures may be less relevant for the terminal patient, for whom all the usual protocols have been tried and have failed.

In such a case, when there is nothing left in the toolbox, the patient and the doctor may feel that it is worth trying something that has not been laid down by any protocol, that does not have the force of a NICE guideline and for which the evidence is patchy.

An example might be the use of Zmapp – an untested potential treatment for Ebola. In August 2014, the World Health Organisation – a UN body – approved its use for those in West Africa who had picked up the fatal infection which has a mortality rate of up to 90 per cent.

There are no effective treatments and the WHO panel, which included the Wellcome Trust director Prof Jeremy Farrar, unanimously concluded that it was ethical to offer patients Zmapp, despite the fact it had not been tested on humans.

However, in the UK some doctors are unwilling to move away from standard procedures, even when their patient is dying. This is, in part, because the law and medical culture stands against those who try novel treatments and protects those who stick to accepted protocols – even when they are known to fail.

It is rather like saying to the pilot of a plane that is about to crash: "You see that parachute over there? Well, you can't use it, because it's never been tested and we don't know if it works and we don't want you to get hurt if it fails to open."

It is ridiculous, of course.

But let me pause here. Many readers will find the whys and wherefores of Lord Saatchi's Medical Innovation Campaign to be irrelevant to them. So, if you are not interested in the point of the campaign itself, you can ignore it. This chapter is about what we tried to do and how – as well as the lessons we learned as we progressed.

The campaign menu

This is a bald list of the elements incorporated into our campaign at the start. I will expand on each of these.

- Define the objective – what is victory?
- Define the stakeholders – for and against;
- Build a supporter base;
- Find the evidence – for and against;
- Build the campaign contents – in advance;
- Deliver the campaign;
- Nuance and refine the campaign in light of experience gained.

Defining the objective – what is victory?

It is so obvious that perhaps it need not be said. But you would be surprised how many campaigns fail, or are delayed because no one is clear on what they are trying to achieve. The objective defines everything you do. From your objective, you build the strategy and your tactics – constantly referring to the goal and ensuring every step you take moves you closer to victory.

It is vital that you check every move against the objective. Will it help or hinder? If you are unable to say how it will move you closer to victory, don't do it – it will be a waste of time, money and energy.

Keep it simple. Spend time thrashing it out, boiling it down and writing it down. Ensure that all key players in the team are all signed up and are clear on the goal. Do you all agree? Do you all understand? Does anyone have a furrowed brow or look uncertain? If so, get it out into the room, let them speak and openly resolve confusion and doubt.

I always ask colleagues, when starting a campaign: "What goes on the T-shirt?" If it is something straight, short and simple, like 'Save our school' or 'Yes/No to Devolution' you are off to a flying start.

If it is longwinded, and everyone umms and aahs and cannot trot out the objective at the snap of a finger, you are already failing. If you do not know what you want, then how will you persuade anyone else to follow you?

Is your objective clear? If not, you will trip up over your socks at some point; someone with doubts and confusion will inadvertently miscommunicate a key message and this will set you back or destroy you.

In our case, the headline and strategic objective was as clear as day: we wanted to pass into law the Medical innovation Bill.

This led to a series of tactical objectives, which formed part of the communication and campaign strategy.

Define the stakeholders – for and against

You need to know who is for you and against you and why. Write down all the groups and individuals who have – or might have – an interest in what you are doing. What do you think their position will be? Make contact, meet them, explain your thinking and listen. At this stage, you are only testing the water. This is often called 'stakeholder mapping'. Also, at this stage, include those who have the power to make the change for which you are campaigning – local politicians, the council chief exec, the Secretary of State for Health, for example.

Build a supporter base

As part of your stakeholder mapping, make contact with those who support you. Look for those who exemplify and personify the reason you are campaigning for change. These are called case studies; who stands up your case and who will get cut through with those you are seeking to influence?

Case studies will also be key to building your evidence – see below.

Include in this element of the project the media and social media influencers. Who are the journalists you need to talk to? And, who are the influencers on social media – those with an interest in your campaign who have big followings. You need influential bloggers, Tweeters and YouTubers.

Your supporter base will be the people who will carry the campaign for you; they will adopt it, care for it, influence it and fight for it. You will not be able to do this alone – you need to reach out to partners who want what you want and will hitch their wagons to your campaign.

However, do not assume that everyone who supports you is a bona fide 'good thing'. An example: the campaign for the Medical Innovation Bill is about doctors innovating within the mainstream health space – surgery, drugs and the like. It is not about alternative medicine.

Some opponents to the Bill claimed it was a license for quacks to operate within the standard health service, thereby endangering patients with unproven homeopathic interventions.

A handful of advocates of the Bill who supported alternative therapies within the NHS did the cause harm – they made it look like the Bill was indeed about alternative therapies. (We did not criticize such supporters, nor did we engage with them – we simply bypassed them ensuring that our topline messaging stated clearly that our Bill was about mainstream medicine only).

Find the evidence – for and against

This is crucial. Do not assume you are right. Ask yourselves the hard questions – the ones you would not want to be asked live on Newsnight – and answer them.

Know your reasons, build the evidence, challenge the evidence, leave no stone unturned. If there is a weakness in your position and you are going to be opposed, the opposition will find it. Do not wait until they do. I always have a mantra – know the opposition's arguments better than they know them themselves.

Evidence gathering overlaps with much of the other elements of the campaign-building process. It is, for example, a component of the initial meetings you will have with stakeholders – why do they support you? What is their experience of the current situation? Why do they want change?

And you will want to refresh, constantly, your evidence base and to continue to ask yourselves hard questions – as you deliver the campaign. When you go public, you will smoke out more stakeholders and they will have their views and evidence, and questions for you – which you must incorporate and build on.

As they say, no plan survives first contact with the enemy. Be ready to challenge and change.

Build the campaign contents – in advance

First, what is 'content'? Content is the stuff you use for your media and campaigns work – videos, photos, FAQs, story angles for newspapers.

You must get as much of this pre-loaded and in hand before you launch. You want to sustain your media and social media coverage, not explode in a day, spectacularly, and then fade.

It takes many months of sustained exposure just to get people aware of your existence, especially from a standing start. You need the media fuel to sustain a long campaign.

Deliver the campaign

This speaks for itself. However you launch the campaign (and many people get het up by the launch – it really might just be a nominal day in your diary where you place the first story in the local or national press), you must have a plan for what you will do over the coming weeks. See above.

There is a separate bit about how you deal with opposition – a whole book can be written on this. But here are some headline suggestions.

Do not engage with individuals on social media. Social media can be an ugly and irrational place and people feel emboldened by the relative anonymity Twitter (for example) affords them. If you wrestle with a chimney sweep, you will get covered in soot. Rise above the nasty, the petty, the silly – answer critics in the round – use blogs to answer questions you are consistently asked and to quash myths. But, do not name any critic personally.

It is tempting to take them on. Don't. Let your supporters answer them directly if they like – but the official campaign HQ must be above the fray.

Be prepared for constant setbacks. Support each other. Laugh. Think, plan and adjust. Be true to your values, stick to your objectives, speak only the truth and never spin. You will be caught out and damage your reputation.

Nuance and refine the campaign in light of experience gained.

The key thing to remember here is that you must keep refreshing your evidence and answering new questions as you go along. Be open to change – you will not be 100 per cent right about everything. Those that challenge you may raise good points. Adapt to them.

In the end, if you are right and you can get your message and arguments across calmly and clearly, you will win. Be patient.

Chapter 24

Patent Protection and Ownership of Patents

Carine van den Brink and Arber Gjunkshi[1]
Axon Lawyers

Introduction

The protection offered to orphan drugs by orphan drug market exclusivity is completely different from the protection offered by a patent. While orphan drug market exclusivity may not give exclusivity beyond the composition of the subject matter of the medicinal substance, a patent can. Therefore, the patent protection of orphan drugs is very important in securing and extending a competition-free supply of orphan drugs on the market.

An orphan drug may enjoy the best protection by a combination of patent protection and market exclusivity. In this chapter, we will discuss patent protection of medicinal products only, as regulatory exclusivity of orphan drugs is the subject of chapter 12 of this book.

The introduction will provide a basic overview of the elements of a patent, and explain how and where to file a patent application. Further on, the importance of the national patent laws will be discussed in relation to determining the ownership of Academia generated patented inventions, and we demonstrate how the United Kingdom (hereinafter referred to as 'UK') and the German national patent laws deal with the ownership of such patents.

I. Patent Protection in General

The introduction of the patent system worldwide has been revolutionary for the whole industry and has had a tremendous impact on innovation and consumer welfare. Abraham Lincoln considered the patent system to be one of the (three) most important developments in the world`s history and described patents to be "the fuel of interest to the fire of genius".

What is a Patent?

A patent is one of the most important forms of intellectual property rights. A patent is described as intangible property, because it lacks material existence. Despite this lack, its owner may still economically benefit from it, in the same way as the owner of tangible property does.

Different from tangible properties, a patent has a limited term of a certain maximum of years, starting from the date of filing of the patent application with a national or international Patent Office. During this term, the owner of the patent is supposed to be able to recover the incurred costs for the development of the subject matter of the patent and to generate income at the same time, using the monopoly right over the patent without facing any competition. The monopoly right granted to the patent owner is the incentive, which encourages inventors to develop new inventions and consequently fulfill the objective of patent law: the promotion of technological innovation in a manner conducive to social and economic welfare.

Once the limited term of a patent expires, the owner`s rights over the protected invention cease to exist and the patent`s subject matter becomes a public property pertaining to the public domain, meaning that it may be freely exploited by the society without any economic obligation to its owner.

It is also very important to mention that, while inventions may be granted a patent, provided that certain conditions are fulfilled, discoveries remain out of the scope of patent law.

How can a patent application be filed and where?

Patent Application via a National Patent Office

The national Patent Office of every country is the only responsible authority of that country for receiving patent applications and deciding whether to grant a patent.

Upon the receipt of a patent application, a national Patent Office usually conducts an examination in order to check whether the subject matter of the application fulfills the conditions for patentability. Depending on the outcome of this examination, the national Patent Office may or may not grant a patent. Should a national Patent Office grant a patent, it shall be valid and enforceable only within the borders of that country.

For geographically big countries such as the USA or China, it is very practical from a patent applicant's point of view to have to deal only with one Patent Office and enjoy patent protection for such a territory with only one single patent.

The situation becomes more complicated when patent protection is sought for a whole continent or a considerable part of a region consisting of multiple independent countries, for example Europe, where each country has different national patent laws in place. Let's keep in mind that a patent right is a national right, meaning that a patent granted in country A may never be valid and enforceable in country B. The same invention may be protected in country B only if it is granted a patent by the national Patent Office of that country.

In order to speed up the flow of innovation, and also to simplify and to render the patent applications more economically for a series of countries, various international patent treaties have been brought into existence, such as the Patent

Cooperation Treaty (hereinafter 'PCT') and the European Patent Convention (hereinafter 'EPC').

Patent application via the Patent Cooperation Treaty

The PTC is a worldwide agreement signed by almost 148 states, including the most industrialized ones. This treaty governs the so-called 'International Applications'. Through an International Application, the applicant has the option to choose for patent protection of his invention in all or some particular states, as he may designate among the signatory states to the PCT. The states from which the applicant has chosen to seek patent protection are referred to as 'Designated States'. An International Application may be filed only by nationals, or persons who are residents, of one of the signatory states of the PCT.

An International Application has two phases, an international and a national phase.

The international phase starts with filing a patent application either with the applicant`s respective national Patent Office – where it should be indicated that the application concerns an 'International Application'-, or directly with the International Bureau of WIPO in Geneva. International Applications received by the national Patent Offices shall be sent to the International Bureau, which has the role of administrating the PCT applications. The International Bureau will then ask an International Searching Authority to perform a search of the prior art. After the search, this authority will prepare an International Search Report about the patentability or not of the application in question.

Once the International Search Report is issued, it will be sent to the national Patent Offices of the Designated States. From this moment, the international phase enters the national phase. In the national phase,[2] even though the International Searching Authority has already performed a prior art search, the national Patent Office of each Designated State either accepts the International Search Report or may search again and shall exclusively decide whether the patent application in question may be patentable according to their own national patent laws.

The PCT international patent filings are very advantageous because PCT represents a worldwide system for the simplified filing and processing of patent applications. It is also advantageous because it provides a strong basis for patenting decisions by the national Patent Offices and reduces the costs.

Patent Application via the European Patent Convention

The European Patent Convention (EPC) is a regional European patent treaty, adherence to which is open to all the states of the European continent, independent whether or not they are member states of the European Union, because EPC is not a treaty of the European Union ('EU').

The EPC permits an applicant to obtain patent rights in all or in several European states with one single patent filing with the European Patent Office (hereinafter 'EPO'). EPO acts as an examination authority, meaning that it will examine whether a patent application is patentable, and if so then it will automatically, on its own discretion, grant patents on behalf of all the European states designated by the applicant in the patent application (Designated States).

When EPO grants a patent for the territory of an EPC member state, the national Patent Office of that state does not have the right to review the patentability of that patent application. The situation is different under PCT, where, once the international application enters the national phase, it would be the national Patent Office(s) of the Designated State(s) which would decide on the patentability of the patent application.

What are the patentability criteria?

The basic patentability criteria were first set by the international treaty of TRIPS ('Trade related Aspects of Intellectual Property Rights'). These basic criteria were later introduced to the national laws or regional patent treaties in the same or at stricter levels. In this section, we will discuss the basic patentability criteria under TRIPS and EPC.

In principle, according to TRIPS, patents are available for any and all inventions, in all fields of technology, provided that the invention is new, involves an inventive step and is capable of an industrial application. The EPC further explains and defines the terms 'new', 'inventive step'and 'capable of industrial application'. All these three criteria must be met by a patent application in order to be granted a patent.

Novelty

Determining the `state of the art` is the starting point to decide whether an invention is novel. According to EPC (Article 54), the state of the art comprises everything made available to the public in any way or form, prior to the date of filing of a patent application. The term 'made available to the public'refers to the exposure to the public before the filing date of the patent application, of all the technical characteristics found in the claims of the patent application. Such an exposure is novelty destroying and as such, researchers and inventors should avoid exposing or making public any of the technical characteristics of the claims of their inventions prior to the date of filing of the patent application.

Important for the pharmaceutical industry and of course for the orphan drug developers and manufacturers is to know how 'first medical use'and 'second and subsequent medical use'inventions of already existing substances or composition of substances may still qualify as novel.

A naturally occurring substance may be patentable for usage in a medical procedure only if it has not been previously known to have any medical usage.[3] This is known as a 'first medical use'invention. Such a substance may be subject to further patentable inventions if it is found to be used for the manufacture of a medicament for a new and specific therapeutic application. This new mode of use is known as 'second and subsequent medical use'. Different from the 'first medical use'inventions where the patent claims to the therapeutic use may be broad, in 'second and subsequent medical use'inventions, the patent claims must be specific to the new therapeutic use.

Inventive Step

Under the EPC, an invention is considered to involve an inventive step if the invention would not have been obvious for a person skilled in the art. 'Person skilled in the art'and 'obvious'are two key terms.

A person skilled in the art is presumed to be one or more ordinary practitioners, who are expected to know everything available in the state of the art until the date of filing of a patent application. This term refers to the examiners employed by the regional or national patent offices, who conduct a thorough search of the state of the art and, if necessary, do experiments over the subject matter of the patent application in order to prove whether, or not, an inventive step is involved.

The person skilled in the art will check, by using all the information available in the state of art prior to the filing date of the said patent application, whether he would have come to exactly the same result as the patent applicant claims in his patent application. If the answer is negative, the subject matter of the invention is not obvious, and consequently the patent application will survive the 'inventive step'test. However, if the answer is positive, the application will lack the inventive step and a patent will not be granted.

Industrial application

Besides novelty and an inventive step, the application should also fulfill the 'industrial application'requirement in order to be patentable under the EPC. In this context, the term 'industrial'refers to an activity which aims at financial benefits i.e. the invention should have a profitable use.

What rights does a patent confer to its owner?

Exclusive rights

During the patent's term, which is twenty years from the filing date of the patent application, the owner enjoys exclusive rights. When the subject matter of a patent is a product, then no third party is allowed to make, use, offer for sale, sell, or import such a product for these purposes, unless the owner gives consent for such acts. If the subject matter of a patent is a process, then the exclusive patent rights of the owner extend not only to the use of the process itself but also to end products obtained directly by that process. In other words, a third party, not having the consent of the patent owner, may not use the process and also may not use, offer for sale, sell, or import for such purposes the end product obtained directly by the patented process.

The owner of a patent may exercise such rights only within the borders of a country in which the patent has been granted and only during the term of that particular patent.

Other than making use of the exclusive patent rights himself, the owner may exploit his patent by assigning it or licensing it out to a third party.

All these exclusive rights are the basic patent ownership rights as dictated by the TRIPS Agreement. However, the national patent laws may introduce broader national patent rights, provided they comply with those of the TRIPS Agreement.

Exceptions to rights conferred

Even though a patent confers a monopoly right to its owner, exceptions to this right are provided by the TRIPS Agreement,[4] that allows the member states to introduce exceptions to the exclusive patent right in their national patent laws. Such exceptions should not unreasonably conflict with the normal exploitation of the patent and should not unreasonably prejudice the legitimate interests of the patent owner, taking account of the legitimate interests of third parties.

There are two kinds of patent right exceptions: the 'experimental use' exception and 'regulatory approval privilege' exception.

Experimental Use Exception

Neither the TRIPS Agreement nor the EPC mention what are the concrete experimental use exceptions to a patent right, leaving it to the discretion of the national law of the member states to determine the border between patent infringement and experimental use exceptions. The lack of international harmonization on this subject, has allowed divergences among the national patent laws of member states.

The experimental use exception, or also known as research exemption is of particular importance for the pharmaceutical industry, since the discovery of new drugs depends in many cases on research conducted on the subject-matter of already patented pharmaceutical substances with the aim of finding new therapeutic applications. The research exemption is the right of a third party to legitimately conduct research (during the term of a patent in a member state/country where the patent is granted and is valid) on the subject matter of the patented medicinal substance. The research on the subject matter of the patent may be conducted either to test the validity of that patent and find new therapeutic applications of the patented substance or any other aim stipulated by the national patent laws.

However, it is very important for researchers to know whether the nature of their research on the subject matter of a patented medicinal substance suits to the experimental use exception permitted by the national patent law of the country where the research will take place (provided the research is conducted in a country where the patent subject to the research enjoys protection). If the conducted research does not fit to the exceptions allowed by that national patent law, then the researchers may face patent infringement claims.

Regulatory Approval Privilege

The regulatory approval privilege allows generic drug manufacturers to conduct (free of any patent infringement threats), the necessary actions with regard to the subject matter of a patented product, within the term of that patent. This enables them to develop and submit any bioequivalence and other test data of their generics to the regulatory authorities, to obtain market authorization and bring their product to the market as soon as the patent of that particular patented medicinal product expires.

In the USA, this privilege is known with the term 'Bolar exemption'. The Hatch-Waxman Act indicates that "it shall not be an act of infringement to make, use, offer to sell, or sell within the United States or import into the United States a patented invention [...] solely for uses reasonably related to the development and submission of information under a Federal law which regulates the manufacture, use, or sale of drugs [...]".[5] As further interpreted by the US courts, this provision applies also to the pre-clinical testing of patented compounds, which is reasonably related to the submission of information to a regulatory agency (for drugs the regulatory agency is the US Food and Drugs Administration), comprising not only the late-stage safety and efficacy testing in human subjects, but also post-approval activities which are explicitly required by the agency. However, it still depends on the very specific merits of each case, whether or not the US courts shall grant exemption to activities as described above.

In Europe, the regulatory approval privilege is regulated by Directive 2001/83/EC (as amended by Directive 2004/27/EC) which is a EU legal instrument, and as such is applicable only towards the regulatory approval activities within the member states of the EU, and not to all the signatory countries of the EPC. This Directive indicates that the conduct of the necessary studies and trials with a view to the demonstration of bioequivalence and biosimilars, and the application of the consequential practical requirements, shall not be regarded as contrary to patent rights.[6]

The nature of a Directive as a EU legal instrument allows the EU member states to implement its provisions in their national law with divergence. As it is the case with Directive 2001/83/EC (as amended) some member states implanted it as strictly applicable to the regulatory activities related to generic drugs only, while other member states as comprising also regulatory activities related to innovative drugs as well. When conducting regulatory activities with regard to a patented drug in one of the EU member states, a drug manufacturer should always make sure that its regulatory approval activities comply with the national laws of that member state.

Supplementary Protection Certificates

Because of the very long time needed before a new drug reaches the market, and the very short effective patent protection time remaining once a patent on a medicinal product is granted, an optimal financial return on the investment sometimes may be achieved only by an extension of the protection period, through the grant of a supplementary protection certificate (hereinafter 'SPC'). Within the EU, an SPC may be granted for a maximum duration of five years. A six-month protection time on top of the SPC protection time may be additionally applied, if the medicinal product, subject to the SPC, is authorized for a pediatric indication.

In the EU, the grant of an SPC is regulated by Regulation 469/2009/EC, provisions of which are binding for all the Member States and no divergence is possible. Under this Regulation, an SPC may be granted only if, at the date of the application:

   i. the product is protected by a basic patent in force;
   ii. a valid authorization to place the product on the market as a medicinal product has been granted in accordance with the EU Directives on medicinal products;
   iii. the product has not already been subject of an SPC;

iv. the authorization under point (ii) above is the first authorization to place the product on the market as a
medicinal product.[7]

An SPC may be granted only to the active ingredient or
the combination of active ingredients of the basic patent of a
medicinal product which is covered by the marketing authorization. An active ingredient, which is part of the basic patent
but has not been covered by the marketing authorization may
not be subject of an SPC.

II. Protection of the Ownership of Academia generated Patents

Protection of an invention depends solely on the measures undertaken by its owner during the pre-patent grant proceedings
or after-patent grant period, in case of patent-opposition proceedings or patent invalidity claims. The question of patent
ownership is crucial and is of more significance for Academia
generated inventions, since the employer – employee relationship between the academic institution and the academic employee who has made an invention is a source of dispute over
the ownership of a patent.

According to the EPC the question of the ownership of an
employee's invention shall be subject to the law of the state
where the employee is mainly employed. If there would be any
difficulties in determining this state, then the national law of the
state where the employer has the place of business shall govern
this issue. In either case, this convention, points at the national
law, so it would be very helpful to see how the national laws of
United Kingdom ('UK') and Germany treat this issue.

It is interesting to see that while some countries treat the
inventions generated by the academic staff equal to inventions
generated by private sector employees, other countries have put
in place a different regime for academia generated inventions.

UK Law

According to Section 39 of the UK Patent Act 1977 (as amended), an invention shall always belong to the employer if the employee (i) made it in the course of his normal duties, if it was specifically assigned to him, or if the invention might reasonably be expected to result from the carrying out of his duties, or the employee (ii) made it in the course of his duties and because of the particular responsibilities arising from the nature of his duties he had a special obligation to further the interests of the employer's undertakings.

Any other employee invention not corresponding to any of the above situations, shall belong to the employee.

The UK law does not make any further distinction between inventions generated by an academia employee and those made by other private sector employees. However, attention should be paid to the UK courts' case law to see where the borderline between the ownership of these two kinds of generated inventions shall lie.

German Law

Under German law, employee inventions are not regulated by the German Patent Act. Instead, these inventions are subject to a more specific law: the German Act on Employee Inventions (Gesetz über Arbeitnehmererfindungen). According to this law, employee inventions can be either 'service inventions'(made during the term of the employment, as part of the employee's activities or based to a significant extent on the company's work), or 'free inventions', which are owned by the employee.

Apart from these general provisions, the German Act on Employee Inventions contains a specific clause[8] with regard to inventions generated by academic institutions. The amendment of this act in 2002, brought the inventions of professors in German academic institutes (which till then were considered to be 'free inventions') under the sole ownership of the academic institute. As compensation, 30% of the income generated by the invention is paid to the inventor who is a member of the academic staff.

Upon entry into force of this amendment, the industry partners who had previously collaborated with the German academic institutes were somehow reluctant to continue collaborating. Consequently, the German academic institutes compiled the so-called 'Berlin contracts', which are template agreements governing the ownership rights over the patented inventions resulting from collaboration between the German academic institutes and the industry partners.

'Berlin contracts' comprise three template contracts: the Service or Works Contract, the Contracted Research Contract and the Research Cooperation Contract.

   a. The **Service or Works Contract,** is a type of contract where the industry partner asks the German academic institute to perform a clear and well defined task, results of which are not of a publication interest to the institute. The industry partner owns the full ownership over the results with no due compensation for the institute, which receives full remuneration for its service.
   b. The **Contracted Research Contract,** is a type of contract where both the industry partner and the German academic institute have an interest in the results of the research. The institute shall interpret the obtained data and is interested in publishing them. The IP ownership of any inventions deriving from the research belongs to the industry partner. However, the industry partner is obliged to compensate the institute for such inventions.
   c. The **Research Cooperation Contract,** is a type of contract where both parties, the industry partner and the institute, have strong interest in the results of the research, and they contribute together to the costs of the research and of the personnel involved. Taking into account that both parties contribute together to the costs of the research, the question of the ownership of any generated IP shall be subject to the following scenarios:

    iv. If the invention is based on the results achieved solely by the industrial partner, without any contribution from the institute, then the IP ownership shall belong to the industrial partner.

    v. If the institute has a contribution of more than 50% to the invention, then it shall be the sole owner of the invention. However, the industry partner shall enjoy the right of an exclusive worldwide license.

    vi. If the institute has a contribution of 25% or less to the invention, the industrial partner has the ownership right over the patented invention. If the institute has a contribution of more than 25% to the invention the same rules as the Contracted Research Contract apply.

Conclusion

As seen above, the ownership issue of the patents generated by academia, exclusively belongs to the national patent laws of the state where the academic institute is located. Industry partners and patient organizations should research the national patent law of the state where the academic institution of their choice is located (which may have a system similar to the UK, Germany or other) and should explore the best possible options in securing their interests over possible patentable inventions.

References

1 Carine van den Brink and Arber Gjunkshi are lawyers at Axon Lawyers.

2 http://www.wipo.int/pct/guide/en/gdvol2/pdf/gdvol2.pdf (Accessed 11 March 2015).

3 European Patent Convention (EPC), Article 54(4).

4 Agreement on Trade-related Aspects of Intellectual Property (TRIPS), Article 30.

5 35 U.S.C. Section271(e)(1).

6 Directive 2001/83/EC on the Community code relating to medicinal products for human use, Article 10(6).

7 Regulation 469/2009/EC concerning the supplementary protection certificate for medicinal products, Article 3.

8 German Act on Employee Inventions, Article 42.

Chapter 25

Engaging Patients and Carers Online for Clinical Trials

Julie Walters and Pete Chan
Raremark and Tudor Reilly Health

Why Engage with Patients Online?

In the context of patient groups taking an active role in drug development, one of the strongest, and most positive, trends is the rise of the epatient. Definitions vary, but we understand epatient to mean someone who is empowered, internet-savvy and searching for health information online. In this sense, we are probably all epatients to some extent, and will likely become even more so in the years to come.

While individual epatients vary in the extent of their engagement online, what they have in common is a robust appetite for information and news on all things health-related. Statistics abound, but some of the most compelling include the fact that:

- Some 72% of internet users look online for health information;[1]
- 52% of consumers want to access websites or other online sources to gauge the quality of doctors and hospitals;[2]

- One-third of videos watched on YouTube are about health; that is more than the viewing figures for food or celebrities.[3]

But there are two ways of reading these numbers. On the one hand, epatients clearly have a great desire for health information. But, on the other hand, and frustratingly from a drug development standpoint, their interest is not translating into significant public awareness of how to take part in clinical research.

People are interested *in principle*: 87% of respondents to a survey by the Center for Information and Study on Clinical Research Participation (CISCRP) said they would be "somewhat willing" or "very willing" to participate in a clinical trial.[4] In a US survey, though, more than half of respondents attributed low clinical trial participation to a lack of awareness.[5]

Perhaps we should not be too surprised about this last fact. ClinicalTrials.gov,[6] a website managed by the US National Institutes of Health, is arguably one of the most reliable public databases of clinical trial information in the world. The European Medicines Agency (EMA) offers something similar for European trials in the form of the EU Clinical Trials register.[7] Yet such sites remain unknown to the majority of the general population. And those epatients who do find them have to get their heads around portals that, while comprehensive, can be difficult to navigate, with much of the language accessible only to the scientifically trained.

Could it be possible to encourage more people to take part in clinical trials by delivering better, more patient-friendly information over the internet? We believe the answer is an unequivocal yes – and for three reasons.

Firstly, the volume of information created and shared online is on a sharp upward trajectory. It is expected to reach almost eight zettabytes this year, up from around two zettabytes in 2011.[8] One zettabyte equals one trillion gigabytes and, for context, eight zettabytes is the equivalent of 18 million times the digital assets stored by the US Library of Congress today.

Secondly, more people are gaining access to the internet. A Eurobarometer study conducted in 15 EU member states found that almost all patients had accessed health information online, either directly or through friends and relatives.[9] Much the same thing is happening all over the world. Eric Schmidt, Google's executive chair, has famously predicted that everyone on Earth will be connected to the internet by the end of this decade.[10]

And, thirdly, 2013 marked a critical tipping point: patients are now informed about trials online more than through any other channel. Some 46% of respondents to the CISCRP survey said they had found out about trials over the internet, compared with 39% who got this information from the media.[4] Only 20% were told about trials by their primary physicians and the same percentage by speciality care physicians. A decade ago, only 25% of patients learnt about clinical trials from the internet.

At this rate, a conservative estimate would put over half of all clinical trial participants recruited through digital channels within one to two years. In the most developed markets, we believe this figure could easily reach 60% in the same timeframe.

Online clinical trial recruitment should be particularly effective in niche conditions. In rare diseases, a lack of relevant health information from traditional sources has turned patients into hyper-users of the internet. Online communities and patient forums provide relief from the isolation they otherwise feel, as well as the opportunity to connect with others in a similar situation.

And the same logic may apply in certain, more common, conditions. In an Australian study conducted in 2011, around four-fifths of people with a mental illness were found to be Facebook users, compared with 50% of the general population.[11]

The context for this final chapter is that there is a real opportunity to meet people's hunger for health information online and, in doing so, to recruit patients to clinical trials. We know of some great early case studies for patient groups that want to help shape the development of new drugs.

The themes we will be exploring include:

- Regulatory restrictions you need to consider when promoting clinical trials online;
- Some of the most promising online initiatives being explored by the pharmaceutical industry and specialist service providers;
- How social media and online tools have supported clinical trial recruitment in the rare metabolic disease alkaptonuria (AKU);
- Best practices for implementing Google advertising campaigns; and
- Our predictions for the future.

Online clinical trial recruitment is perhaps one of the most exciting and rapidly evolving aspects of drug development. It is also one where entrepreneurial patient groups can participate, both as driving forces and as educators of others entering the field.

Case Study: How epatient communities can be life-savers

The story of ePatient Dave is one of the most compelling accounts of how online health information can shape an individual's experience on a clinical trial. Diagnosed in 2007, with an advanced case of kidney cancer, which had metastasised and spread to his bones, lungs and muscles, this man's outlook was grim.

Fortunately, Dave deBronkart – as he is known offline – had access to expert medics at a Harvard Medical School teaching hospital. He had surgery there and took part in a clinical trial of an investigational therapy now marketed as Proleukin. Eight months after his diagnosis, he was clear of the disease.

A pivotal stage of Dave's journey was preparing for the clinical trial. He had already joined an online kidney cancer community. Knowing the drug could lead to severe side-effects, he asked his peers if any had been on the trial, and received 17 replies describing a range of experiences. The shared insights were critical to Dave's successful response. He coped with the side-effects because he knew what to expect.

Dave says the community's advice may have saved his life. His story is a striking example of how epatients, sharing information online, can drive positive experiences in clinical trials.

More recently, Dave has become a vocal advocate for participatory medicine. He wants doctors' surgeries to employ information coaches to help patients get better at finding accurate health information on the internet.[12]

Legislation

The good news is that the new media world has not changed the rules of what can be communicated to patients and carers about clinical trials: the same established rules apply. Information must be factual, balanced and without undue influence or persuasion. The end goal remains appropriate and balanced, informed consent.

In the US, regulations about information issued direct to the public about clinical trials are governed by the US Food and Drug Administration (FDA). They set the guidelines for Institutional Review Boards (IRBs) that review materials about trials issued to the general public.[13]

In Europe, new legislation was published in 2014 to guide the practice of clinical trials. This will come into effect in 2016.[14] The legislation seeks to simplify and harmonise the rules governing clinical trials in the EU. Previous legislation has not achieved a unified approach, so the revisions are welcome. The industry has responded to the previously complex rules in Europe by taking their business elsewhere. In 2006-7, the percentage of European patients in pivotal clinical trials was 44%. By 2011, the percentage had declined to 31%.[15]

The hope is that the new rules will encourage more trials in the EU and stimulate the inclusion of as many member states as possible. Different applications for permissions to perform a trial will be replaced with one application dossier for all member states through a single submission portal.

The European legislation also encourages clinical trials for the development of orphan medicinal products.

What has not changed is how the applications will be assessed within the member states. Local ethics committees will still assess the application for a clinical trial, including information direct to patients and carers. In some countries, ethics committees are better organised and resourced than in others: it is possible to have communication materials assessed and approved for use within a month; in other countries, it can take up to six months.

Ethics committees should include laypersons, in particular patients or patient organisations. Assessment should be done by a reasonable number of persons who collectively have the necessary qualifications and experience. They must be independent of the sponsor, the clinical trial site, and the investigators involved, as well as any other undue influence.

It is worth finding out early on which ethics committees will be responsible for your application, how often they meet and how long it will take on average to have materials reviewed. These factors will be important for planning.

Theory vs practice: what does Google actually allow?

Google lays out certain rules for all advertising on the Google Network, regardless of subject matter. The rules fall into the four broad policy areas listed below. All ads are reviewed against these requirements, in most cases within one business day.

- **Prohibited content** covers content advertisers aren't allowed to promote on the Google Network

- **Prohibited practices** are the things advertisers can't do if they want to advertise with Google
- **Restricted content** means material which can be advertised, albeit with limitations
- **Editorial and technical** rules cover quality standards for adverts and websites

Advertising for clinical trials falls within the **Restricted content** category. Google's current policy in this area is not to allow advertisements that promote clinical trial recruitment except in certain countries. In addition, in those countries where the practice is allowed, advertisers need to ensure their content does not "promote prescription drugs or create misleading expectations or effects of a product being tested, or imply that the product being tested is safe".

At the time of writing, there were 20 countries where Google explicitly allows clinical trial-related advertising. These included both developed markets, such as France, Germany, Italy, the UK and the US; and emerging economies, like Indonesia, Malaysia, the Philippines and Vietnam. There were only 10 countries on this list just a year ago, reflecting Google's constantly evolving rules and the need for advertisers to keep abreast of them.

As long as your website and advert copy have approval from local ethics committees, and they comply with current rules for advertising on the Google Network, the adverts should run without problems. A certification of approval from ethics committees only needs to be provided if Google disapproves an advert. The certificate does not have to be submitted if Google approves the advert in the first instance.

Even if a country isn't one of the 20 currently listed by Google, it doesn't necessarily mean Google advertising is forbidden there. From experience, we would recommend getting ethics approval, setting up a Google AdWords account (discussed in more detail below) and seeing what happens. We have run advert campaigns in other countries after gaining ethics approval and not encountered any issues with Google.

Four top tips for mitigating risk

There are always some risks when using online tools to engage patients and carers. The following points will reduce some of that risk before you get started.

- Make sure you have all clinical trial-focused copy approved by local ethics committees – this will ensure patients are not over-promised anything and are fully aware of what participating in a clinical trial involves;
- Draft your privacy policy with the help of lawyers, so that visitors to your website understand what will happen to their data and that it is protected;
- Add a tick-box requiring patients and carers to confirm that they have read the privacy policy of your website before submitting any personal information online;
- Make sure your site complies with the relevant data privacy regulations for your markets. These include: the EU Data Protection Directive (soon to be the General Data Protection Regulation), the Data Protection Act in the UK, the Safe Harbor Framework in the US, and the Health Insurance Portability and Accountability Act (HIPAA) Security Rule, a key piece of US regulation concerning personal health data.

Current Practice

Examples from the pharmaceutical industry

Despite the traditionally conservative culture of the pharmaceutical industry, some forward-thinking companies are experimenting with new ways of reaching patients directly online. This section provides a snapshot of the most promising online initiatives and their key features.

THE PATIENT GROUP HANDBOOK

Location-based clinical trial search

Visitors to www.novartisclinicaltrials.com1[6] who click on a tab labelled *Ongoing Trials* and allow the website to access their location are automatically presented with a map showing the closest open trials sponsored by Novartis. At the time of writing, the closest studies to our office in London, UK were taking place in Coventry, a city about 100 miles away.

Novartis is not unique in providing an online portal for its clinical trials; most of the world's largest pharmaceutical companies also have them (see Appendix). Novartis' innovation is to make it easy for patients to find open studies in their area. After all, there is little point telling them about studies taking place at sites they cannot feasibly reach. (The recent use of telehealth approaches in clinical research may make distance less of a challenge for particular studies).

Bristol-Myers Squibb (BMS) has taken a similar approach with its **Study Connect** website.[17] Unlike Novartis' site, it does not use a GPS locator, but it does allow US residents to enter their location and search for trials taking place within a set distance. And, addressing the fact that clinical trial information alone may not be enough to encourage people to participate, the website also provides patient stories and videos featuring others who have been through a similar journey.

Study Connect includes prominent links to two separate websites owncd by BMS: http://www.clinicalcancerstudy.com[18] and http://www.abouthepc.com.[19] These provide content about various cancers and about hepatitis C, respectively and they link back to disease-specific pages within Study Connect.

A makeover for ClinicalTrials.gov data

Most pharmaceutical companies' clinical trial portals replicate or summarise information they have already submitted to ClinicalTrials.gov, the clinical trials database managed by the US National Institutes of Health. (The most basic portals are mere landing pages featuring links to the ClinicalTrials.gov home page).

In large part, this is because strict regulations govern how companies communicate clinical trial information to the public. However, as we noted earlier, ClinicalTrials.gov can be off-putting or even intimidating to anyone without a medical background. It does little to encourage people to learn about an aspect of medical research they may barely understand to begin with.

The good news is that some pharmaceutical companies are thinking beyond the traditional way of doing things, with a view to making clinical trial information more user-friendly.

For one example, take a look at http://www.shiretrials.com[20] a website owned by Shire. The first thing you will notice is its design. It has clearly been created with non-specialists in mind, with simple navigation and images selected to emphasise the company's focus on patients.

Importantly, while descriptions of studies match those found on ClinicalTrials.gov, the way they are presented is far more appealing. Compare the ClincalTrials.gov and shiretrials.com headings in Table 1 and see how simple changes to language can make a large difference to a lay audience.

Table 1: Simple tweaks to language can go a long way.

ClinicalTrials.gov heading	shiretrials.com heading
Purpose	What is the purpose of this study?
Eligibility	Is this study right for me?
Criteria	See if you may qualify

Sources: ClinicalTrials.gov; shiretrials.com

Another positive feature of shiretrials.com is its *Connect with a Study Location* function. It provides the addresses and phone numbers for participating investigator sites and often an email address for an individual member of the site team, rather than a generic shared inbox. It leaves you with a more personal impression than you would get from a general number for a call centre.

Meanwhile Lilly, through its Lilly Clinical Open Innovation (LCOI) initiative,[21] is a proponent of learning and sharing methods to improve the drug development process, arguing that open interactions between patients, industry and innovators is fundamental to creating more patient-focused clinical trial experiences. Its past work has included making data from ClinicalTrials.gov available in a variety of useful formats through a free application programming interface (API).

Dedicated patient recruitment websites

Growing numbers of pharmaceutical companies are creating patient recruitment websites dedicated to specific clinical trials. These are by far the most direct way to communicate clinical trial information directly to patients and carers online. They are ideally suited to late-stage (Phase II or Phase III) clinical trials, where the numbers of patients required are higher.

A key feature of these websites is a pre-screener, typically a short questionnaire, allowing a patient to submit information about him- or herself, or a carer to do so on their behalf. Celgene has several of these, all following the same format and accessible at: https://celgeneclinicaltrials.com[22] To pick just one example, the questionnaire on https://celgeneclinicaltrials.com/quazar-aml[23] a website for the company's QUAZAR trial in acute myeloid leukaemia, presents visitors with the following questions:

- Are you 55 years or older?
- Were you newly diagnosed with AML or AML secondary to MDS?

- Did you have prior bone marrow or stem cell transplant?
- Were you treated with chemotherapy?
- Have you responded to the bone marrow transplant and/or drug treatments for this disease within the last 3 months?

It is possible to build clinical trial websites so that completed questionnaires are sent automatically to the closest trial centre. Alternatively, a patient or carer who completes a questionnaire might be presented with a list of the trial sites that are closest to where they live. There is little point collecting information from individuals who cannot feasibly travel to sites involved in a trial.

Using disease awareness to capture epatients

As useful as clinical trial websites are, a key consideration is that people searching for health information online generally do not do so with clinical trials in mind. Many will not even know what a clinical trial is.

On the other hand, you can expect epatients to Google their medical conditions (if they have been diagnosed) and the symptoms they experience (whether they have been diagnosed or not).

With this in mind, a complementary approach is to create what are widely referred to as disease awareness websites to capture individuals with an interest in a disease, before funnelling some of them to a trial-specific website.

To give one example, the Tudor Reilly Health (TRH) team has previously created a disease awareness website for one of the world's top 10 pharmaceutical companies working in the field of early Alzheimer's. The objective was to drive visitors, via a prominent advertisement, to a clinical trial recruitment website that the company already owned.

We optimised the disease awareness site for search engines by using the language of patients and carers rather than the vocabulary of the pharmaceutical industry. The two are very different: family members are more likely to search for memory loss or nursing homes than the term Alzheimer's itself. We also translated and optimised the content in five languages to reach epatients in key countries involved in the trial.

Consequently, we achieved some impressive metrics, including over 647,000 unique global visitors, more than 1.5 million page views, and a top 10 Google ranking for key search terms in the target recruiting markets.

Harnessing the power of video

Pharmaceutical companies such as Pfizer and AstraZeneca have experimented with creating clinical trial-specific videos for YouTube. Typically featuring employees speaking directly to camera, sponsors are essentially delivering via video the same information some people may find hard to understand in writing.

A video on AstraZeneca's YouTube channel features three members of a clinical team talking about a study in opioid-induced constipation, including its eligibility criteria and what participants in the trial can expect.[24]

Another option is to post on YouTube advertisements for particular clinical trials, as Amgen did for its Fourier Study in cardiovascular disease.[25] Brief and non-technical, the advert features a couple of actors giving an overview of the trial, while captions provided a toll-free telephone number and a link to a dedicated clinical trial website.

Roche, meanwhile, has created a video as part of its **Drawn to Science** YouTube series, explaining what clinical trials are about, and the medical jargon patients might encounter.[26] Posted in May 2014, the video has attracted more than 19,000 views and it links to a page on the Roche corporate website describing how the company conducts clinical trials.[27]

Table 2 provides links and summaries of selected clinical trial-related videos on YouTube.

Table 2: Clinical trial-related YouTube content (selected pharmaceutical and biotechnology companies).

Company	YouTube channel & URL	Notes
Amgen	Amgen Fourier Study www.youtube.com/channel/UCUiabdB63406h7YX17XAK94	Actors speak about Amgen study in cardiovascular disease; video provides URL: www.heartresearchstudy.com (now inactive)
AstraZeneca	azvideochannel www.youtube.com/watch?v=y35Vl0JhRAY	Video features AstraZeneca study leaders and clinical research director outlining details of one specific clinical trial: *Information for Patients Suffering from Opioid-Induced Constipation* (July 2011)
Pfizer	PfizerClinicalTeam www.youtube.com/user/PfizerClinicalTeam/feed	Videos feature clinicians and/or Pfizer representatives outlining details of specific clinical trials, including links to ClinicalTrials.gov listings, eg: • *New Pfizer Clinical Study for Adolescents with Fibromyalgia* (June 2010) • *Teenage Smoking Clinical Trial* (September 2011) • *Pfizer Clinical Study for Systemic Lupus Erythematosus (SLE)* (November 2011)
Roche	Roche www.youtube.com/watch?v=5zXuQN7Rue0	*Drawn to Science: Clinical Trials* video (May 2014) provides lay explanation of clinical trials

Source: Tudor Reilly Health research; October 2015

Examples from specialist service providers

In parallel with the pharmaceutical-sponsored initiatives described above, a new generation of specialist companies that are small, nimble and ideally positioned to innovate, are taking online clinical trial recruitment to new frontiers. Bridging the gap between empowered epatients and clinical trial sponsors that want to reach them, these companies are operating in a space that is seeing some of the most interesting innovations.

A patient-friendly clinical trial search engine

Established in 2010, TrialReach says it wants to make clinical trials easier for patients to find, understand and apply for.[28] The company's ultimate goal is to make new treatments available more quickly and efficiently.

In 2013, TrialReach launched a platform that allows users to search for active trials in nearby centres. Its default search function provides summaries of information sourced from ClinicalTrials.gov. TrialReach also collaborates with sponsors to convert their clinical trial protocols into simple, interactive web pages that are free of medical jargon. In addition, the platform provides simple contact forms allowing users to request the study team to get in touch.

TrialReach has gone on to sign agreements with several partners, including Healthline, CenterWatch and CureClick, to increase its ability to connect patients to clinical trials.

Connecting patient networks with clinical trials

Another innovative approach taken by specialist companies is to build and maintain active, online health communities in certain diseases, and connect them with clinical trials they might find helpful.

In our view, of all the channels available for reaching epatients, online communities are by far the most promising for the future of clinical trial recruitment. The best communities deliver high-quality content, informed by patient interest and input. They are platforms where patients can speak to each other. Naturally, some of these conversations may include clinical trial experiences.

PatientsLikeMe is one of the best-known examples.[29] Since it was founded in 2004, its network has grown to more than 2,300 disease communities with a total of over 300,000 members. They use the platform to keep track of their own health and to see aggregated data collected from others with the same diseases.

In 2013, PatientsLikeMe launched a tool that matches patients the world over with clinical trials based on their condition and location.[30] Interestingly, the fact that PatientsLikeMe members volunteer information, including their age and medical condition, when they create their profiles means the clinical tool can also indicate how many members might be eligible for specific clinical trials. At the time of writing, PatientsLikeMe said 4,773 of its members might be eligible for Pfizer's Phase III clinical trial in psoriasis with the ClinicalTrials.gov identifier NCT01163253.

Raremark: A new online service dedicated to people affected by rare diseases

Finally, one of the newest initiatives is Raremark[31], a free online service in rare disease which will make scientific and medical knowledge accessible and understandable for patients and carers. Raremark was created both to help companies that are developing new therapies for rare diseases and people who may benefit from them.

The service will be launched in English in 2015 in two therapeutic indications. More conditions and languages will be added over the next 12 months based on user feedback and experience.

Raremark will use online tools to:

- Establish the prevalence of particular rare diseases;
- Identify the locations of patients with those conditions, down to city level;
- Reach patients and carers to inform them of new treatments in development.

It is an exciting time and the Raremark team looks forward to optimising the platform and broadening its reach to multiple conditions and multiple languages.

Using Online Tools in Rare Disease – From Theory to Practice

The AKU Society, a UK-based patient advocacy group, has been a driving force in recruiting patients to clinical trials in alkaptonuria (AKU), an ultra-orphan metabolic disease with an estimated prevalence between 1 in 250,000 and 1 in 1,000,000. The society's recent work on the Phase III DevelopAKUre clinical trial demonstrates what can be achieved by entrepreneurial groups with the know-how to use online tools to drive patient recruitment.

The DevelopAKUre study aimed to enrol 200 patients at three European trial centres; in the UK, France and Slovakia. As in other rare diseases, people with AKU are few and far between; a key challenge to finding and recruiting them to clinical studies. Another major obstacle is lack of awareness of the condition, both among the general public and primary care physicians, often leading to non-diagnosis or misdiagnosis. As a result, finding enough people to take part in the trial was problematic, even for an active and engaged patient group like the AKU Society.

The society had been using its own community website, www.akusociety.org[32] to drive visitors to a separate clinical trial microsite, www.developakure.eu[31] where people could register their interest in the trial. TRH helped the patient group to optimise www.akusociety.org[33] for Google and other search engines.

We knew, for instance, that affected individuals search online for the tell-tale symptoms of AKU, including black urine and black spots in the eyes, even if they do not actually know the correct medical term for their condition. So TRH restructured the symptoms section of the AKU Society's website such that the content matched the search terms used by people interested in those symptoms. This resulted in new pages highly optimised for Google, with URLs such as www.akusociety.org/

osteoarthritis[34] www.akusociety.org/black-urine[35] and www.akusociety.org/black-spots-in-the-eyes.[36]

These changes helped drive a 14% rise in unique visitors to www.akusociety.org over a three-month period. Importantly, around a quarter of these visitors arrived directly at the newly optimised symptoms-focused pages rather than the home page.

Digitally smart Google advertising

At the same time, we devised an advertising-based online campaign to promote DevelopAKUre to patients and carers with an interest in the condition. Central to this strategy was the use of Google AdWords, the search engine's advertising service. Google AdWords campaigns involve identifying keywords that are related to a specific area of interest (see below). Internet users who Google those keywords are then presented with advertisements positioned directly above and to the right of organic search results.

Choosing AKU keywords for Google advertising campaigns

Just as certain keywords were used to optimise the symptoms section of the AKU Society's website, www.akusociety.org, the same phrases formed the basis of the Google AdWords campaign for the DevelopAKUre clinical trial. People who searched Google for black urine, black bones, discoloured ears or black spots in the eyes saw adverts that provided a click-through to the DevelopAKUre trial recruitment microsite.

The more specific you can be in your choice of keywords, the more likely you are to reach the right people. The ideal outcome is that whenever someone searches Google for your chosen terms, your advert appears as close as possible to the top of the search results.

The first set of adverts was designed to appeal to people who had been diagnosed with AKU, and their carers, who were looking online for treatments. These adverts had the headline

Clinical Trials for AKU. The keywords selected for these adverts included *AKU clinical trials, DevelopAKUre clinical trials, AKU study* and *AKU treatment.* They depended on patients knowing they had been diagnosed with AKU.

The second set of adverts targeted those who were undiagnosed or misdiagnosed, in other words, people who had symptoms of AKU, but did not know the cause. We created three adverts relating to distinct key symptoms: black urine, discoloured ears and black spots in the eyes. In this way, people searching those keywords would see an advert relating to that particular symptom and then be directed to the DevelopAKUre microsite.

Both groups of adverts were created in more than 20 languages to reach the countries considered most important for the clinical trial. We then used Google's geo-targeted advertising function to ensure that the right adverts appeared in those specific countries.

Achieving global reach

The AKU Society's geo-targeted Google advertising campaign drove a significant amount of traffic to the DevelopAKUre microsite. After six months, the adverts had been seen by just under half-a-million people worldwide, with over 6,000 people arriving at the microsite.

Considering the total (known) AKU population is just over 900 worldwide, attracting so many visitors to the DevelopAKUre microsite was no mean feat. And TRH's online tactics, combined with the AKU Society's outreach work, laid the groundwork for study teams to recruit all the required patients during the formal recruitment period. It was a landmark achievement for an ultra-orphan disease.

Already sophisticated, online tools like Google AdWords will only grow in value in the years to come. Used in the right way, these tools can empower even small, local patient groups to connect with interested people from all corners of the globe.

Cost-management, with help from Google

The cost of Google AdWords campaigns is calculated on a cost-per-click (CPC) basis, meaning advertisers pay each time someone clicks on their adverts. CPC advertisers who are active in the same field bid for specific keywords or phrases, or groups of keywords. How well an ad ranks is determined by factors such as the bid amount, the quality of the ad and the relevance of the ad to the keyword.

To maximise return on investment from advertising, it is important to identify which keywords will yield the best results. A tool called the Google AdWords Keyword Planner allows advertisers to identify:

- *The* volume of searches *for certain keywords;*
- *The level of* competition *among advertisers for those keywords relative to all other keywords; and*
- *The* suggested bid *for a keyword.*

Search volume *indicates the average number of people searching for that keyword over the past 12 months. In general, advertisers like to target high-volume keywords, but it's important to remember that they are context-specific. In rare diseases, for example, it would be natural to see a lower volume of searches, reflecting the fact there aren't many people affected by them.*

Low competition *may be preferable for some advertisers, as there are fewer competing advertisers to bid against. But another school of thought is that low competition reflects poor historical performance of a keyword for advertisers that have used it previously. High competition, on the other hand, may make it more difficult to achieve a prime position, but it is likely that there are so many advertisers bidding on the keyword because it performs well.*

The suggested bid *takes into account the CPCs that other advertisers are paying for this keyword, and thus is a good forecast of your potential CPC. It would be intuitive to target keywords with a low suggested bid, as you would pay less for each click on your advertisement and your campaign would cost less overall. However, CPC is determined by many factors; some relating to your own campaign performance or AdWords account, and others relating to the performance of a keyword. It is also a good indication of the value of that keyword (to other advertisers, at least). A keyword with a high CPC may still be worth targeting in niche markets, or if the expected return is greater than the cost.*

The reality is that there are many factors that go into crafting the optimum online advertising strategy, and advertisers need to make a series of judgement calls in each case.

CPC bidding can be expensive, so Google allows advertisers to set daily budgets for each campaign, in effect capping their advertising spend. In addition, Google offers a grant programme to non-profits, including patient groups, helping them to bid more competitively than their budgets would otherwise allow. You can find out more about Google's grants on its website.[37]

The Future

The internet is changing our world in ways that Sir Tim Berners-Lee, the inventor of the World Wide Web, could never have imagined. What began as a way for academic researchers to share information has turned into an information superhighway for us all.

As a sign for visitors to Amazon's headquarters near Seattle says:

> "There is so much stuff that has yet to be invented.
> There's so much new that's going to happen.
> People don't have any idea yet how impactful the Internet is
> going to be and that this is still Day 1 in such a big way."
> Jeff Bezos, Amazon CEO

For patients and carers, the next decade will see small steps in the availability of information on clinical trials turn into true access. For too long, information about prospective new medicines has been closely held by pharmaceutical innovators and chosen doctors, who have traditionally been the only gate-keepers to potentially life-changing treatments. If you were one of the lucky patients who happened to have one of the chosen doctors as your healthcare professional, then you might be given the chance to find out about a trial – or not. If the doctor was busy, uninformed or forgot to offer you the chance to take part, you had no way of finding out about a trial.

Thankfully, that closed loop of information is now opening up. Websites that list clinical trials such as ClinicalTrials.gov and the World Health Organization's International Clinical Trials Registry Platform[38] are a big step forward. But you need to know about these sites and the vast majority of people have no idea they exist.

Companies such as TrialReach and Raremark are helping to translate complex and often forbidding medical language into something that patients and carers have some chance of accessing and understanding.

In the future, a simple web search for the symptoms of a rare condition will provide information not just on the condition and diagnosis, but also on potential treatments that are in development. Not only that, but everyone will be able to find out what doctors, and where, are recruiting for the trial. They can then beat a path to their door and demand to find out more.

Information and power will shift from the few to the many – and that has to be good news for us all.

Julie Walters is the founder of Raremark (www.raremark.com) and Tudor Reilly Health (www.tudor-reilly.com). Pete Chan is Chief Innovation Advocate of Tudor Reilly Health.

References

1 S. Fox and M. Duggan. 2013. Health Online 2013. Pew Research Center. (Online) Available at: http://www.pewinternet.org/2013/01/15/health-online-2013/ (Accessed: 12 September 2015).

2 M. Meeker. 2014. 2014 Internet Trends. KPCB. (Online) Available at: http://www.kpcb.com/blog/2014-internet-trends (Accessed: 12 September 2015).

3 Think Insights with Google. 2009. Google. (Online) Available at: http://www.gstatic.com/ads/research/en/2009_HealthConsumerStudy.pdf (Accessed: 12 September 2015).

4 Public and Patient Perceptions and Insights Study. 2014. The Center for Information and Study on Clinical Research Participation. (Online) Available at: https://www.ciscrp.org/programs-events/research-and-studies/perceptions-and-insights/ (Accessed 12 September 2015).

5 Research!America. 2013. Poll: Majority of Americans would participate in clinical trials if recommended by doctor. Elsevier. (Online) Available at: http://www.elsevier.com/connect/poll-majority-of-americans-would-participate-in-clinical-trials-if-recommended-by-doctor (Accessed 12 September 2015).

6 ClinicalTrials.gov. US National Institutes of Health. www.clinicaltrials.gov (Accessed: 12 September 2015).

7 EU Clinical Trials register. The European Medicines Agency. https://www.clinicaltrialsregister.eu (Accessed: 12 September 2015).

8 M. Meeker., Liang Wu. 2013. 2013 Internet Trends. KPCB. (Online) Available at: http://www.kpcb.com/blog/2013-internet-trends (Accessed 12 September 2015).

9 TNS Qual+. 2012. Patient Involvement. European Commission. (Online) Available at: ec.europa.eu/public_opinion/

archives/quali/ql_5937_patient_en.pdf (Accessed 12 September 2015).

10 D. Gross. 2013. Google boss: Entire world will be online by 2020. CNN. (Online) Available at: http://edition.cnn.com/2013/04/15/tech/web/eric-schmidt-internet/ (Accessed 12 September 2015).

11 Sane Australia. 2012. Information Technology and Mental Illness. SANE Research Bulletin. (Online) Available at: https://www.sane.org/images/stories/media/2012_media_releases/SANE_Research_Bulletin_15-_Information_technology_and_mental_illness.pdf (Accessed 12 September 2015).

12 J. Payne. 2012. The rise of the e-patient. Scrip Clinical Research. (Online) Available at: http://www.scripclinicalresearch.com/patients/The-rise-of-the-e-Patient-336553 (Accessed 12 September 2015).

13 Code of Federal Regulations Title 21. US Food and Drug Administration. http://www.accessdata.fda.gov/scripts/cdrh/cfdocs/cfcfr/CFRSearch.cfm?CFRPart=56 (Accessed: 12 September 2015).

14 Medicinal Products for Human Use – Clinical Trials. 2014. http://ec.europa.eu/health/human-use/clinical-trials/index_en.htm (Accessed: 12 September 2015).

15 European Medicines Agency. 2013. Clinical trials submitted in marketing-authorisation applications to the European Medicines Agency. European Medicines Agency. (Online) Available at: http://www.ema.europa.eu/docs/en_GB/document_library/Other/2009/12/WC500016819.pdf (Accessed 12 September 2015).

16 Novartis Clinical Trials. Novartis. www.novartisclinicaltrials.com (Accessed: 12 September 2015).

17 BMS Study Connect. Bristol-Myers Squibb. http://www.bms.com/StudyConnect (Accessed: 12 September 2015).

18 Clinical Cancer Study. Bristol-Myers Squibb. http://www. clinicalcancerstudy.com (Accessed: 12 September 2015).

19 Hepatitis C Study. Bristol-Myers Squibb. http://www. abouthepc.com (Accessed: 12 September 2015).

20 Shire Clinical Trials. Shire. http://www.shiretrials.com (Accessed: 12 September 2015).

21 Lilly Clinical Open Innovation. Lilly. http://portal.lillycoi. com (Accessed: 12 September 2015).

22 Celgene Clinical Trials. Celgene. https://celgeneclinicaltrials.com (Accessed: 12 September 2015).

23 QUAZAR trial in acute myeloid leukaemia. Celgene. https://celgeneclinicaltrials.com/quazar-aml (Accessed: 12 September 2015).

24 Information for Patients Suffering from Opioid-Induced Constipation. AstraZeneca. YouTube video. https://www. youtube.com/watch?v=y3yVtcJhRAY (Accessed: 12 September 2015).

25 Amgen Fourier Study. Amgen. YouTube video. www. youtube.com/channel/UCUiabdB634o6h7YX17XAK9g (Accessed: 12 September 2015).

26 Drawn to Science: Clinical Trials. 2014. Roche. YouTube video. https://www.youtube.com/watch?v=5zXuON7Rueo (Accessed: 12 September 2015).

27 Clinical Trials. 2015. Roche. http://www.roche.com/research_and_development/who_we_are_how_we_work/clinical_trials.htm (Accessed: 12 September 2015).

28 TrialReach. http://trialreach.com (Accessed: 12 September 2015).

29 PatientsLikeMe. www.patientslikeme.com (Accessed: 12 September 2015).

30 Find Clinical Trials. PatientsLikeMe. http://www.patients-likeme.com/clinical_trials (Accessed: 12 September 2015).

31 Raremark. www.raremark.com (Accessed 12 September 2015).

32 Alkaptonuria Society Ltd. www.akusociety.org (Accessed: 12 September 2015).

33 DevelopAKUre. The AKU Society and the DevelopAKUre Consortium. www.developakure.eu (Accessed: 12 September 2015).

34 Osteoarthritis. Alkaptonuria Society Ltd. www.akusociety.org/osteoarthritis (Accessed: 12 September 2015).

35 Black Urine. Alkaptonuria Society Ltd. www.akusociety.org/black-urine (Accessed: 12 September 2015).

36 Black spots in the eyes. Alkaptonuria Society Ltd. www.akusociety.org/black-spots-in-the-eyes (Accessed: 12 September 2015).

37 Google Ad Grants Programme Details. Google. http://www.google.co.uk/intl/en/grants/details.html (Accessed: 12 September 2015).

38 The International Clinical Trials Registry Platform Search Portal. World Health Organization. http://apps.who.int/trialsearch (Accessed: 12 September 2015).

Appendix

Online clinical trial portals and related initiatives (selected pharmaceutical and biotechnology companies)

Company	Notes & URL(s)
Amgen	Website allows users to search by condition, drug name or protocol number www.amgentrials.com
Astellas	Simple landing page refers visitors to ClinicalTrials.gov and US FDA page on clinical trials www.astellas.us/therapeutic/product/clinical_trail_resources.aspx
AstraZeneca	Search function allows users to search by keyword and returns results identical to details published on ClinicalTrials.gov www.astrazenecaclinicaltrials.com Separate initiative, **Cancer Study Locator**, established by AstraZeneca and EmergingMed to increase public awareness of and access to oncology clinical trials www.emergingmed.com/networks/AstraZeneca
Bayer	**Trial Finder** function allows users to search by several criteria, including: product, country, condition and trial status www.bayerpharma.com/en/research-and-development/clinical-trials/trial-finder
Boehringer In-gelheim	Web page provides general information on clinical trials, but no trial locator www.boehringer-ingelheim.com/clinical_trials.html
Bristol-Myers Squibb	BMS Study Connect website's **Find a Study** function allows users to search by condition, location and distance they are willing to travel www.bmsstudyconnect.com
Gilead	Simple landing page refers visitors to ClinicalTrials.gov www.gilead.com/research/clinical-trials
GlaxoSmithKline	**Find Studies** function allows users to search by medical condition or compound name www.gsk-clinicalstudyregister.com
Lilly	Website provides links to useful resources including ClinicalTrials.gov, CenterWatch and WHO ICTRP www.lillytrials.com
Merck & Co	As well as a search function, site allows people to register their email addresses to be notified about trials of potential interest in future www.merck.com/clinical-trials
Novartis	**Ongoing Trials** section allows users to search for *Opportunities Near You*; *GPS search* and *Global Search* www.novartisclinicaltrials.com
Novo Nordisk	World map feature allows users to zoom in on geographical regions and countries, before presenting them with trials taking place there www.novonordisk-trials.com
Roche	Web page allows users to search by Trial Results or Protocol Registry www.roche-trials.com Separate page provides general information on clinical trials in an easy-to-understand format www.roche.com/research_and_development/who_we_are_how_we_work/clinical_trials.htm
Sanofi	Web page provides general information on clinical trials, but no trial locator or trial listings en.sanofi.com/rd/clinical_trials/clinical_trials.aspx
Shire	Trial listings provide study location maps, including contact details for participating sites www.shiretrials.com
Takeda	**Clinical Study Protocol Information** page provides trial headings automatically redirecting visitors to ClinicalTrials.gov www.takeda.com/research/ct

Source: Tudor Reilly Health research; October 2015

Conclusion

Nick Sireau and Anthony Hall
Findacure

Patient groups – especially those working on rare diseases – face many challenges. We hope this handbook will help overcome many of these. Nevertheless, it is worth concluding by looking at the wider sociological picture for patient groups. Indeed, there is a sub-set of sociology called social movement theory that develops four particularly useful concepts for our understanding of the rare disease patient group movement and how this handbook fits into it.

Political opportunities

First is that of political opportunity structures: whether the political environment is favourable or not towards the social movement. Thanks to the hard work of groups such as Eurordis (the European Organisation for Rare Diseases), NORD (the US National Organization for Rare Disorders), Global Genes™ and national alliances such as Rare Disease UK, the political opportunity structure is shifting positively towards rare diseases. For instance, the US Orphan Drug Act of 1983 and the European orphan drug legislation of 2000 set the framework for companies to invest more in orphan drug development.

Since then, and particularly in the past few years, many European countries have developed national plans for rare diseases, with France already being on its second such plan. These national plans set the scene for actions in healthcare for rare disease patients, research, centres of excellence and other areas.

Interpretive frames

Second is the concept of interpretive frames: how a social movement sees the world and defines itself, its vision and mission. This is particularly challenging for rare diseases due to the use of the term 'rare', which tends to devalue the sector and make it sound less important.

Three years ago, Findacure carried out an informal survey with students from the Judge Business School at Cambridge University in which the students asked people in the streets of Cambridge how many people they believed were affected by a rare disease. The responses were shocking: many said they expected 5,000-10,000 people to have a rare disease in the UK. When the students responded that it was more likely to be in the millions, the respondents were equally shocked.

In many cases, the rare disease movement has tried to overcome this misconception by focusing on the 'rare is common' theme. But this creates problems in that there is no agreement over just how common rare diseases are, with numbers for people affected ranging from 1 in 10, to 1 in 17, 1 in 25 and even 1 in 50.

One way of overcoming this is through the use of the concept of 'fundamental diseases' developed by Findacure. This is based on the long-held view in medicine that rare diseases are fundamental to understanding human biology and even to treating common diseases. The founder of modern medicine, William Harvey, who discovered blood circulation in the 17th century, was one of the first people to say this, followed 100 years ago by William Bateson, the father of modern genetics, and more recently by Francis Collins, head of the US National Institutes of Health.

The iconic genetic disease Alkaptonuria (also called AKU or Black Bone Disease) is a prime example of this. It is an ultra-rare disease affecting approximately one in half a million people. Symptoms include progressive joint deterioration that leaves patients severely disabled. It is an extreme form of osteoarthritis – a particularly common disease – and an excellent chemical model for it. Research by the University of Liverpool, comparing Alkaptonuria to osteoarthritis, has already led to new discoveries that are changing the way we understand both diseases.

Collective identity

The third concept is that of collective identity: whether members of a social movement feel that they are part of the same thing and what this means in terms of shared values and behaviours. Again, the rare disease movement faces a challenge here because of the 6,000-8,000 rare diseases out there, which leads to fragmentation.

Understandably, each patient group focuses exclusively on their rare disease or their group of rare diseases. But this means that it is difficult to create a sense of collective identity across the movement, despite the fact that all patient groups face similar problems.

That's again where the umbrella groups such as Eurordis and Rare Disease UK play a major role. International Rare Disease Day, which takes place on the last day of February, has been very successful in bringing together rare disease groups around the world under the same banner. It creates a sense that we are all in this together and allows the umbrella groups to increase their political pressure by underlining their role as the legitimate representatives of the rare disease movement.

Resource mobilisation

Fouth is the concept of resource mobilisation: that all social movements – including those organised by patient groups – need to mobilise resources of time, skills, people and money in order to achieve their goals.

In the case of patient groups, this is particularly difficult. Many patient groups are what we might term 'kitchen-table groups', organised by parents of children with a disease, or by the patient themselves. They have very little time available, since they spend most of it in and out of hospital and caring for their child or themselves.

They struggle to find the money available to support their patients, let alone moving ahead with research. Few of them start with the skills needed in biology and research in order to understand easily the latest developments in science relating to their disease.

Researchers – many of whom work closely with patient groups – are also finding it difficult to access resources for rare diseases. At the European level, the European Commission has a call every two years for rare disease research. In 2015, this amounted to €60m as part of the EC's Horizon 2020 call for proposals. Out of more than 400 proposals, fewer than 10 were successful, showing just how much demand for resources outstrips supply.

Yet rare disease patient groups are still managing to mobilise resources, particularly of people and patients, thanks in large part to the advent of social media. The internet has revolutionised the way patient groups operate. Thirty years ago, patient groups communicated mainly through newsletters, phone calls and the occasional meeting or conference. Now, thanks to Facebook, websites and online communities, they can mobilise themselves much faster in order to be agents of change.

This is particularly important for the success of clinical trials. The AKU Society, for instance, was the lead organisation for the recruitment of 138 patients for a major phase III clinical trial for a promising treatment called nitisinone, funded under the European Commission's previous framework protocol seven programme. Thanks to agile use of social media, as well as mobilising its sister AKU patient groups across Europe and the Middle East, it succeeded in recruiting all the patients necessary for the trial within a nine month window.

It's on this last point – of resource mobilisation – that we hope this handbook will have the biggest impact. This is not a lobbying handbook intended to modify the political opportunity structure, or a vision document that defines the interpretive frame within which we can understand our movement.

Instead, this handbook is an attempt at providing some of the knowledge needed for rare disease patient groups to mobilise their resources of people, money, skills and time more effectively. From our personal experience, we have seen how each new patient group tries to reinvent the wheel in order to move forwards. We hope this handbook will provide a shortcut to this, so that rare disease patient groups can focus effectively on what is most important for them: the quest for cures.

Nick Sireau and Anthony Hall
nick@findacure.org.uk
tony@findacure.org.uk

Author Biographies

Listed alphabetically by first name

Dr Anil Mehta

Dr Anil Mehta is a four career man – Oxford drop-out where he was reading Mathematics Physics and Engineering and switching to a degree in Medicine at University College, followed by a spell as a bioengineer at the Medical Research Council in London where he was awarded an MRC best of British Science Award for his inventions. His reward was a Fellowship to read Biochemistry at Kings College London where he was awarded two distinctions and new Fellowship support by the Wellcome Trust to work in the University of Dundee. This varied background has been applied to three rare diseases. He is an advisor on rare disease registries to many organisations including Eurordis and has been instrumental in the development of a new therapy for the disease cystic fibrosis. This discovery has highlighted the gap between academic biochemistry and the need for the synthesis of kilograms of pure safe drugs that satisfy the stringent safety profiles to ensure stability of supply to patients scattered across the globe who live in different jurisdictions. His philosophy is simple and follows the Leonardo Da Vinci dictum, first, measure what is measurable (he makes rare disease registries); next, use the data to make measurable what is currently not measureable (understand the rare disease pathways); finally combine the two measures into a best 'path-

THE PATIENT GROUP HANDBOOK

way' strategy for likely patient benefit. The fourth element is to create a ring fenced spinout to sell to industry or Angel Investment as a going concern.

Email: a.mehta@dundee.ac.uk
00441382383110

Anne R. Pariser, M.D.

Anne Pariser is the Associate Director for Knowledge Management in the Office of Translational Sciences at the US Food and Drug Administration, Center for Drug Evaluation and Research. Prior to this, she was the Associate Director for Rare Diseases in the Office of New Drugs at FDA, where she established the Rare Diseases Program, which focuses on the development of biomedical and regulatory science, rare disease-specific training and education, and policy and guidance generation for rare disease product review and regulation. Dr Pariser has also been actively involved in numerous collaborations within FDA and with drug developers, other governmental agencies, advocacy groups and other stakeholders to further the development of treatments for rare diseases. Dr Pariser has worked at FDA since 2000. Prior to founding the Rare Diseases Program, she was a Medical Officer and Team Leader in OND where she worked almost exclusively on the review and regulation of products for rare genetic disorders. Her research interests include the development of regulatory, translational and biomedical science for rare diseases, and the harnessing of FDA's extensive databases to facilitate and improve drug development.

Annemieke Aartsma-Rus, PhD

Prof. Annemieke Aartsma-Rus played an important role in the development of the antisense mediated exon skipping therapy for Duchenne muscular dystrophy. Since 2013 she has a visiting professorship at the Institute of Genetic Medicine of Newcastle

University (UK). She was work package leader in the TREAT-NMD network of excellence during FP6 funding. Currently, she is chair of he executive board of the TREAT-NMD alliance as well as the COST Action BM1207 (www.exonskipping.eu). She is a member of the TREAT-NMD project ethics counsel and of the TREAT-NMD Advisory Committee for Therapeutics (TACT).

Thus far, she has published over 100 peer-reviewed papers and 9 book chapters, as well as 14 patents and has edited one book. She has given many invited lectures at meetings, symposiums and workshops as well as patient/parent organizations meetings. She has created and maintains multiple websites on therapeutic approaches for aimed at patients and parents. In 2011 she received the Duchenne Award from the Dutch Duchenne Parent Project in recognition of this work and her dedication to the Duchenne field.

In 2013 she was elected a member of the junior section of the Dutch Royal Academy of Sciences, which consists of what are considered the top 50 scientists in the Netherlands under 45. In 2015 she was selected as most influential scientist in Duchenne muscular dystrophy in the past 10 years (2005-2015) by Expertscape based on contributions to the understanding and treatment of Duchenne muscular dystrophy.

Dr Anthony Hall

Dr Anthony (Tony) Hall graduated from King's College London with first class joint honours in physiology and pharmacology before going on to study medicine at the Royal Free Hospital. He joined the pharmaceutical industry in 1994 before starting his own company in 2001, providing drug development consultancy and other services to the biopharmaceutical industry. Since 2009, Tony has focused exclusively on the orphan drugs and rare diseases sector.

Tony is co-founder and member of the Board of Trustees and Scientific Advisory Board for Findacure. He also provides pro bono advice to a number of patient groups. From August 2014 until October 2015, he worked at Prosensa (recently acquired by Biomarin) on developing treatments for Duchenne muscular dystrophy. He recently moved to Mereo Biopharma as Therapeutic Area Head Orphan Drugs.

Tony speaks and chairs conferences on orphan drugs and publishes extensively on issues related to orphan drugs, from clinical development strategies to pricing and value issues.

Dr Bruce E. Bloom

Dr Bruce Bloom is President and Chief Science Officer of Cures Within Reach, a charity saving lives since 2005 by repurposing human approved drugs and devices to deliver more than a dozen fast, safe and affordable treatments and cures for a wide variety of diseases that had no effective therapy.

Cures Within Reach newest initiative is CureAccelerator™, the only global online repurposing research collaboration platform designed to bring together clinicians, researchers, funders, and industry to create and conduct pilot clinical trials that drive more treatments to more patients more quickly.

Dr Bloom is an Ashoka Fellow, recognized as a social entrepreneur for his system-changing solutions to one of the world's most urgent social problems.

Dr Bloom holds a JD from Chicago Kent College of Law, a DDS from University of Illinois Medical Center, and a BS in Biology from University of Illinois Urbana. His business and entrepreneurial experience spans not-for-profit and for-profit work in medical research, law, healthcare, insurance, risk management, regulatory affairs, product development, food service, art, and education.

Dr Bloom is on the Science Advisory Board (SAB) of Rediscovery Life Sciences, of the GARROD AKU Consortium, of the Dr Ralph and Marian Falk Medical Research Trust Awards Programs, the editorial board of ASSAY and Drug Development Technologies, a Trustee of the Kendall College Charitable

Trust, and a member of the Board of Councilors of Midwestern University. Dr Bloom hosts the Clinician's Roundtable on ReachMD.com, and is a facilitator for Pathways to Successful Living.

Christa van Kan PhD

Christa van Kan has more than 20 years' experience in managing clinical trials in a broad range of diseases, including many orphan and paediatric indications. In addition to her MSc in biomedical sciences, Christa has a PhD in clinical epidemiology. Christa is co-owner and Director Clinical Operations of PSR Group, a services company specialising in the clinical development of medicines for rare diseases. During her career, Christa has successfully led a department of dedicated clinical research professionals who are responsible for the set-up, management and monitoring of complex clinical trials across Europe and the US. She is currently involved in several EU-funded projects which aim to bring to market a drug for a rare disease with no current treatment. Christa has found that close collaboration with patient advocacy groups is very valuable for successfully running an orphan drug trial and adds a very interesting new dimension to her work. Christa is often asked to give presentations about the practical aspects of performing orphan drug trials.

Christian Hill

Christian Hill is Managing Director at MAP BioPharma Limited and a Director of MAP MedTech Limited and MAP Market Access Limited. Christian and his team at MAP provide market access guidance for biotech, pharmaceutical, medical device, diagnostics and vaccines businesses in the UK and beyond. MAP offer an up to date, validated, web based subscription service, which acts as a 'virtual' expert to help companies achieve pricing and reimbursement across Europe. If what companies need is not already there, they complete the additional work, usually at no extra charge. To supplement this, they offer product specific, one to one expert strategic advice on a consulting basis throughout the product lifecycle.

Christian is a seasoned market access professional with over 15 years of experience in the international life sciences industry. He has a broad range of expertise and experience including pricing, over 50 HTA submissions and their overall strategy leading to positive guidance, health economic modelling development, and relationships with access and reimbursement bodies and their influencers across Europe.

He has held a number of senior market-access-related positions in industry including National HTA and Government Affairs Manager at Pfizer, Head of Market Access and Business Development at Gilead Sciences and Head of Market Access Europe at InterMune. He is also a member of the board at EUCOPE, a trade body in Europe representing Medtech and BioPharma companies; and a member of the steering group of EMIG, a UK trade body representing primarily SMEs.

Christina Olsen

Christina Olsen works as a European grants consultant and project manager. Christina supports our European projects, including managing proposal preparation, and ensuing deliver is in line with the reporting requirements of the funder. She is currently working on 2 rare disease projects including managing the reporting, administration and dissemination activities. Christina is a charismatic and engaging trainer who has experience of funding, proposal writing and project management workshops. Before joining Ceratium, Christina worked for several years as a project co-ordinator in an analytical laboratory, specialising in air, water, soil and food testing. Her extensive project management skills and industry driven experience make her an invaluable asset to Ceratium and our clients.

Dr Craig Keenan

Dr Craig Keenan gained his PhD in Musculoskeletal Biology from the University of Liverpool in 2015. His thesis entitled "Identification of Ochronosis, its Inhibition by Nitisinone, and the use of Surgical and Chemical Interventions in Murine Models of Alkaptonuria", detailed the identification of ochronosis in alkaptonuric mice, and showed for the first time that nitisinone, a potential therapy for AKU, could prevent the onset and progression of ochronosis. He has published peer reviewed papers on the mouse model of AKU and has presented his research at conferences both nationally and internationally. He has a strong interest in cartilage and matrix biology in particular the pathogenesis of osteoarthritis which itself is associated with onset and progression of AKU. He is currently employed as a Postdoctoral Research Assistant at Liverpool John Moores University.

Dominic Nutt

A former journalist, Dominic Nutt is a communications consultant with more than 20 years' experience of media, digital strategy and stakeholder management who has built integrated, cross-organisational campaigns which change public and political opinion both nationally and internationally. Politically well-connected, he started his communications work for international aid agencies, working in Afghanistan, Syria, Lebanon, Gaza, Latin America and Iraq, often during intense periods of conflict. His motivation is to try to give a voice to those who struggle to be heard.

Elin Haf Davies RN (Child), BSc (Hons), MSc, PhD

Elin Haf Davies began her career as a Paediatric Nurse at Great Ormond Street Children's Hospital in London before going on to gain a PhD from University College London. Her PhD focused on the development of age-appropriate and disease specific biomarkers and clinical endpoints in neurometabolics.

In 2007 Elin moved to work at the European Medicine Agency Paediatric Team where, amongst other projects she evaluated over a 100 Paediatric Investigation Plans of drug trials in children. After nearly six years there Elin founded a digital health social enterprise: aparito.

In her free time Elin has a passion for extreme adventure to raise money for charities close to her heart. In 2007-2008 she rowed across the 2600 miles across the Atlantic Ocean, raising £190,000 for metabolic research at Great Ormond Street Hospital. Money that funded a PhD project that identified the value of Vitamin B6 for managing neonatal seizures, an area that Elin is now actively supporting in her professional capacity.

In 2009 Elin was part of the first all female crew to ever row across the Indian Ocean, and in 2012 she completed her hattrick of oceans by sailing 6000 miles across the north Pacific. Elin's adventures over the years have raised over £250,000 for charities. She has been acknowledged by the Welsh Assembly for Services to Wales, published an honest and gritty account of her experiences "On Tempestuous Seas", and was selected to carry the 2012 Olympic Torch.

www.elinhafdavies.co.uk
www.aparito.com

Dr Elizabeth Ludington

Elizabeth Ludington is the Vice President of Biostatistics and a co-founder of Agility Clinical, a unique consulting and contract research organization dedicated to working with virtual, small biopharma and device companies with a lean infrastructure, particularly those involved with orphan drug development. Elizabeth has 20 years of experience in the pharmaceutical and biotech industries, working for both contract research organizations and sponsor companies. She has provided statistical, technical, and strategic expertise for pre-clinical studies, investigational new drug applications, Phase 1-Phase 4 clinical studies, FDA/EMA submissions, and post-marketing requirements. Her statistical experience includes study design, protocol review, writing analysis plans and statistical reports, and representing clients at meetings with regulatory authorities. Prior to Agility Clinical, Elizabeth held positions as Vice President, Biostatistics at Synteract, Executive Director, Technical Operations and Biostatistics at Somaxon Pharmaceuticals, as well as statistical positions at Elan Pharmaceuticals, Statistics Collaborative, and the International Bariatric Surgery Registry. Elizabeth holds a PhD in Biostatistics from the University of Iowa and a MA in Mathematics/Statistics from Boston University.

Emily Crossley

Emily Crossley is founder and director of the Duchenne Children's Trust, a patient advocacy group fundraising for research into treatments and a cure for Duchenne Muscular Dystrophy, the biggest genetic killer of children.

Nick and Emily set up the Duchenne Children's Trust after their son was diagnosed with the disease. Before setting up the charity, Emily was a business correspondent and anchor for CNN International, and Channel Four News.

Flóra Raffai

Flóra Raffai is the Executive Director of Findacure, a UK charity building the rare disease community to drive research and develop treatments. She was the first hire at Findacure, developing the charity's projects, funding, and community. Flóra organises Findacure's patient group empowerment programmes, runs scientific community engagement projects, develops the charity strategy, and oversees major funding applications and online communications. She also line manages other members of staff. Flóra graduated from the London School of Economics and Political Science with a BSc (hons) in International Relations. She is a founding member of the Cambridge Rare Diseases Network and volunteers as Co-Organiser for the Cambridge Chapter of Good for Nothing.

François Houÿez

François Houÿez joined Eurordis in May 2003, and is now Director of Treatment Information and Access, Policy Advisor.

He has always been working as a patient advocate since the early 90s.

He represents Eurordis at the Patients' and Consumers' Working Party at the European Medicines Agency (EMA). He pioneered patient advocacy with the European Medicines Agency as part of the first patients' delegation that engaged dialogue with the CHMP back in April 1996 and has continuously been involved in the agency activities during the last 19 years.

He leads the Eurordis "Drug Information, Transparency and Access" task force.

He co-chairs the stakeholders' forum of the EUnetHTA2 Joint Action.

He has worked both as a volunteer and as an employee for a variety of patients' organisations at national and international levels, now in rare diseases and first HIV/AIDS.

François is also a patient.

Hanns Lochmüller, MD, FAAN

Professor Hanns Lochmüller trained as a neurologist in Munich (Germany) and Montreal (Canada). He was appointed chair of experimental myology in the neuromuscular research group at the Institute of Genetic Medicine of Newcastle University in 2007. He was the first elected Chair of the TREAT-NMD Alliance Executive Committee.

Hanns has a longstanding interest in the molecular genetics of the inherited myopathies and neuromuscular junction disorders, and is interested in the further study of animal models of these disorders as a means to understand their pathophysiology as well as to develop means to monitor disease progression and therapeutic interventions. Ongoing work in these areas in cell and animal models of muscular dystrophy is concentrating on gene transfer, pharmacological interventions and cell therapy.

Hanns is co-founder and former coordinator of the German muscular dystrophy network (MD-NET), and scientific coordinator of EuroBioBank, a European network of biobanks for rare disorders. He leads the activity on "patient registries and biobanks" for TREAT-NMD, a European Union Network of Excellence for the development of translational research in rare neuromuscular diseases.

Julie Walters

Julie Walters is the founder of Raremark, a new and free online service in rare disease, which will make scientific and medical knowledge accessible and understandable for patients and carers. She gained a first-class degree in molecular genetics from King's College London in 1999, before establishing two previous companies, including Tudor Reilly Health, a digital communications agency focused on healthcare and the development of new treatments. Previously, Julie trained as a news reporter and served as a news editor for breakfast television stations TV-am and GMTV in the 1990s. Outside Raremark, Julie is an area director with the Entrepreneurs' Organization, which helps established entrepreneurs to learn and grow. She also serves as a trustee of the rare disease patient group Findacure.

Kate Bushby, MD, FRCP

Kate Bushby is a Clinical Academic Professor with joint appointments with Newcastle University and the Newcastle Upon Tyne Hospitals. She is a leader of the team at the John Walton Muscular Dystrophy Muscular Dystrophy Research Centre and MRC Centre for Neuromuscular Diseases based at the Institute of Genetic Medicine.

Working in the field since 1989, Kate's interests are focussed on inherited muscular dystrophies from gene identification, disease characterisation and care standards to therapy development and delivery. Kate has a substantial grant portfolio from the EU, MRC and other funding organisations and over 200 publications. She has acted as PI on several industry and academic led clinical trials and natural history studies. This expertise in NMD has developed into a broader leadership role in Rare Disease Policy. Kate was a co-ordinator of the TREAT-NMD network and continues to work on its scientific secretariat, developing trial and therapy readiness in neuromuscular diseases. She led the EUCERD Joint Action on Rare Diseases and continues as policy co-ordinator on a new Rare Disease Joint Action 2015-2018. She is an NIHR Senior Investigator and 2015 recipient of the Eurordis Award for Research into Rare Diseases.

Kay Parkinson LLB (Hons)

Kay Parkinson was the mother of two children who were diagnosed with the ultra-rare disease Alström Syndrome when they were aged 18 and 15, having had four previous mis-diagnoses. Both children died following heart and heart/kidney transplantations aged 25 and 29 respectively. They received little support or understanding of their rare condition.

She qualified as a lawyer in 1996 as a mature student, specialising in charity law. In 1998 she founded the charity Alström Syndrome UK (ASUK). Kay served as their CEO for 15 years before stepping down in 2013 after ASUK was awarded EURORDIS Patient Organisation of the Year, to start up Alström Europe (AS EU) charity, where she serves as a Director. In 2015 Kay joined the steering group of Cambridge Rare Disease Network as she believes all rare diseases need to work together for better diagnosis, treatments, services and a much needed higher public profile.

From September 2015 Kay has formally set up and structured Cambridge Rare Disease Network (CRDN) as their CEO.

She is enjoying the challenge of working for a larger professional organisation and hopes to form closer links between the Cambridge "Cluster" and University with rare diseases.

Email: Kay@camraredisease.org
www.camraredisease.org

Les Halpin (James Hargrave)

Empower: Access to Medicine was founded by the businessman and statistician, Les Halpin, in 2012. Following his diagnosis of Motor Neurone Disease, he worked with the communications company JBP to develop a campaign that challenged the barriers to drug development. Les Halpin lost his battle with Motor Neurone Disease in September 2013, but the campaign continues.

Email: james.hargrave@jbp.co.uk

Dr Marc Van de Craen

Dr Marc Van de Craen has more than 20 years' experience in the Biotech sector. He earned his PhD. in Biotechnology at the famous Flemish Institute for Biotechnology (VIB, University of Gent, Belgium). Next he joined the start-up Devgen where he headed different departments for up to 3 line functions with one team based in Singapore. As a member of Devgen's Steering Committee and Business Development team Marc was instrumental in the success of Devgen which ultimately led to an IPO and an acquisition by Syngenta.

His entire career has been situated at the borderline between science and business. Conceiving, starting and running complex R&D programs in international collaborations leading to commercial products is part of his DNA. Marc consulted several companies at this level and the level to translate research to business cases.

In 2009 he founded Biotechsubsidy and in a partnership with Ritchie Head, he forms the basis of the Biotechsubsidy Group. The partnership focuses on optimizing subsidy management of biotech SMEs and other types of high tech R&D companies (eg. ICT, eHealth, biobased economy, nanotech). Currently the team consists of 5 permanent members and 3 consultants. We have already collected grant money in excess of 60 million Euros in Europe (regional and European subsidies), the US and Asia.

Marc K. Walton, MD, PhD

Marc K. Walton, MD, PhD, is a Senior Scientific Director in Quantitative Sciences at Janssen Research and Development. He is co-Chair of the QSTEPS meetings within Quantitative Sciences and also separately advises the drug/indication-specific development teams to aid design of clinical studies to best form a coherent drug development program. He has involvement with programs across the full breadth of Janssen's clinical research areas.

Dr Walton received his graduate degrees from the University of Chicago. Following a neurology residency at the University of Rochester, he joined the National Institute of Neurological Disorders and Stroke, NIH researching neurotransmitter responses in embryonic spinal cord. Dr Walton joined the Center for Biologics Evaluation and Research (CBER) at FDA in 1993 as a Medical Officer working on clinical trials of biological products for neurological disorders. His appointment as Branch Chief in the Division of Clinical Trial Design and Analysis brought additional clinical areas of experience. Dr Walton became the Division Director with clinical oversight for all non-oncology uses of biological proteins during the transfer of jurisdiction for biological protein products from CBER to CDER. A subsequent move to the Office of Policy in the Office of the Commissioner gave involvement in a broad range of agency-wide issues. He joined the Office of Translational Sciences in CDER in 2008 as the Associate Director for

Translational Medicine. In that position he fostered both internal and external science and policies to support innovative approaches to therapeutic development. His range of involvement spanned biomarkers, clinical study design and analysis methods, liaison to external consortia and other agencies, and advancing rare disease therapeutics.

Maria Mavris PhD

Maria Mavris joined EURORDIS* in 2008 in the capacity of Drug Development Programme Manager and from 2012 to 2014 as Director of Therapeutic Development.

Since September 2014, she is on secondment to the European Medicines Agency (EMA). Sharing her experience gained over her six years with EURORDIS, she now strives to improve the quality of work and communication with stakeholders in the Agency's new department dedicated to the interaction with patients and healthcare professionals.

Maria was previously EURORDIS observer on the Committee for Orphan Medicinal Products at the EMA. She was also responsible for coordinating the group of high-level EURORDIS representatives/volunteers who sit on the various scientific committees at EMA, known as the Therapeutic Action Group (TAG).

Maria was also implicated in activities of the Scientific Advice Working Party (SAWP) where she was responsible for the identification of patients' representatives to participate in Protocol Assistance and had a supportive role for EURORDIS representatives in the Patients' and Consumers' Working Party. Her current role in the EMA continues and expands on these activities from the EMA perspective.

In order to train and support patients' representatives in regulatory activities, she also co-organised the EURORDIS Summer School.

After obtaining a PhD in Molecular Microbiology from The University of Adelaide, Australia, she continued her postdoctoral studies at the Institut Pasteur, Paris and the Ecole

Veterinaire in Maison-Alfort. After this time, she worked as a medical writer in a Contract Research Organisation specialising in oncology.

Maria speaks English, French and Greek.

* EURORDIS- European Organisation for Rare Diseases

Marilyn R. Carlson, DMD, MD, RAC

Marilyn R. Carlson, DMD, MD, RAC has more than 20 years of industry experience in the development and post-marketing support of drugs, biologics, devices, and diagnostics. Her career includes academia and the pharmaceutical industry where she has held senior executive positions on the sponsor-side as well as within contract research organizations (CROs).

Dr Carlson has a bachelor's degree in anthropology/biology from Hunter College of the City University of New York in New York City; a dental degree from the Harvard School of Dental Medicine in Boston, Massachusetts; completed a dental residency in geriatrics and special patient care at Long Island Jewish-Hillside Medical Center in Long Island, New York; has a medical degree from Case Western Reserve University (Alpha Omega Alpha) in Cleveland, Ohio, completed an internal medicine residency at the Cleveland Clinic Foundation in Cleveland, Ohio; and received Regulatory Affairs Certification (RAC) from the Regulatory Affairs Professionals Society.

Dr Carlson is one of the founders of Agility Clinical, Inc., a CRO based in Carlsbad, California that provides full service support for companies that are developing treatments for rare and orphan diseases. At Agility, Dr Carlson serves as the Vice President of Medical, Regulatory & Scientific Affairs.

Dr Mark Edwards BSc (hons) MB BS FRCA FSB

Mark is a medically-qualified drug developer with 23 years' pharmaceutical R&D experience. Formerly, he was a Global Clinical R&D Director and then Director of Science and Medical Public Affairs at Pfizer in Sandwich, Kent. He has worked at all phases of clinical development across a wide variety of therapeutic areas. This includes regulatory product approval experience, having successfully led Pfizer's global clinical development team to achieve the US/EU registration of sildenafil as a first-in-class treatment for pulmonary arterial hypertension.

His experience has also included the establishment of major R&D projects at the interfaces between academia, the NHS and the biopharmaceutical industry eg. having helped lead the establishment of 1) MRC/industry pre-competitive consortia in COPD and RA and 2) the UK Government's Translational Research Partnership Programme.

Now he provides strategic and applied clinical, scientific and policy advice to mainly, small and medium-sized biopharmaceutical companies. Uppermost in his portfolio is The Ethical Medicines Industry Group (EMIG) for which he established (and now runs as R&D Director) a strong scientific & medical arm to complement the commercial interests of the association. This has been pivotal to help grow and diversify EMIG's membership to include a broad range of charitable organisations in addition to biopharma.

Mark is a Non-Executive Director & Trustee of MRC Technology and Executive Director of the Global Medical Excellence Cluster (GMEC). He also works with a number of other public or charitable sector organisations in the UK which include The Experimental Arthritis Treatment Centre for Children, The Health Research Authority, Innovate UK, NIHR CRN Children & National Research Scotland.

It follows that Mark has well-developed networks throughout the life sciences industries, academia and allied organisations.

Since moving to live in Cornwall, Mark's business interests have also diversified to other technology sectors, most notably renewable energy. He is a founding investor in Wattstor Ltd, a renewable energy storage and management systems company and was recently elected by the Board to be its Non-Executive Chairman.

Dr Nick Rhodes

Dr Nick Rhodes is a Reader in Tissue Engineering and Regenerative Medicine at the Department of Musculoskeletal Biology at the University of Liverpool. He has academic interests in medical implant biocompatibility, biomaterials, stem cells and tissue engineering, in particular those related to bone, ligament and soft tissues. He is an officer of the executive committee of the global Tissue Engineering and Regenerative Medicine International Society (TERMIS). He has reviewed European Research Council proposals for the EC and is a member of the UK Engineering and Physical Sciences Research Council (EPSRC) review college. He has coordinated a recent EC-FP7 project and is assisting in the coordination of a current EC-FP7 project and has assisted with an EC-FP6 large integrating project. He has participated in writing a large number of successful EC research proposals over the past 15 years.

Dr Nicolas Sireau

Dr Nicolas Sireau is Chairman and CEO of the AKU Society, a medical charity that works to find a cure for and support patients with AKU (also called Black Bone Disease), an ultra-rare disease that affects his two sons (www.akusociety.org). He is also Co-founder and Chairman of Findacure (www.findacure. org.uk), a new social enterprise that provides support to rare disease patient groups and seeks to develop new rare disease medicines through drug repurposing (www.findacure.org.uk). For his day job, Dr Sireau is Patient Engagement Director at AstraZeneca, one of the world's largest pharmaceutical companies. He is a founding director of the Cambridge Rare Disease Network. He has also been a director of Eurordis, the European Organisation of Rare Diseases, of DNA Digest, a social enterprise that works on collaborative data cures for genetic diseases, and of GenSeq, a bioinformatics company. He has been a committee member of Rare Disease UK, the national alliance of rare disease groups in the UK, and of the International

Rare Disease Research Consortium (IRDiRC). He is a fellow of the Ashoka fellowship of social entrepreneurs and of the Royal Society of Arts. He is the editor of 'Rare Diseases: Challenges and Opportunities for Social Entrepreneurs' (Greenleaf, 2013). Dr Sireau's previous career was in international development, where he was CEO of SolarAid and Sunny Money, two award-winning non-profit social enterprises that he set up.

Dr Sireau has a PhD in Social Psychology.

Nicole Boice

Nicole founded Global Genes Project in September 2008, with the goal of helping families affected by rare disease connect with people, tools and resources to equip them in their fight against rare disease.

Nicole has built a global organization that partners and collaborates with rare disease stakeholders that include biotech and pharmaceutical companies, patient advocacy organizations, researchers, academic institutions, etc. Her personal mission is to help ensure that those affected by rare disease have the tools and knowledge they need to tackle the complexities that comes with a rare disease diagnosis.

Nicole has held numerous consulting, sales and marketing executive roles in her 25 years in business. Nicole has worked with world-class organizations in Media, Pharmaceuticals and High Tech sectors – Schering Plough, CMP Media, United Business Media, and Burrill & Company. A Graduate of the University of California San Diego, proud wife and mother of two children.

Oliver Timmis

Oliver Timmis is the Head of Projects for the AKU Society, an entrepreneurial patient organisation supporting those diagnosed with a rare disease, alkaptonuria (AKU). Oliver leads on funding applications for new projects, allowing for the creation of a National AKU Centre for UK patients, and international phase III clinical trials called DevelopAKUre. He graduated with a BA(hons) in Natural Science (Physiology, Development and Neuroscience) from Cambridge University. Oliver volunteers at Eurordis (Rare Diseases Europe) on their DITA (Drug Information, Transparency and Access) taskforce, sits on the Patient Advisory Council at the RD Connect registries project, and is a member of the Patient-centered Special Interest Group at ISPOR. He also volunteers for Findacure, the Fundamental Diseases Partnership.

Email: oliver@akusociety.org
Twitter: @OliverTimmis

Dr Olivier Menzel

Dr Olivier Menzel graduated (BSc.) from the University of Geneva where he obtained a Master of Medical Genetics (MSc.) in 2001 and a PhD in 2006 from the University of Lausanne and EPFL at the Swiss Institute for Experimental Cancer Research (ISREC). For seven years he directed the laboratory of pediatric surgery at the University Hospital of Geneva. In parallel he created the BLACKSWAN Foundation (blackswanfoundation. ch), a Swiss foundation to support research on rare and orphan diseases. He organized an international scientific conference (RE(ACT) Congress; react-congress.org) and launched an online platform for sharing scientific knowledge and crowdfunding (RE(ACT) Community; react-community.org). For two years he was a director of a company specializing in the identification, acquisition, development, marketing and sale of research programs for rare and orphan diseases. In 2013 he obtained an Executive MBA from the HEC of Lausanne with a specialization in Healthcare Management. Since April 2014 he has been director at the second largest group of private clinics in Switzerland, Genolier Swiss Medical Network.

Pete Chan

Pete Chan is Chief Innovation Advocate of Tudor Reilly Health, a digital communications agency focused on healthcare and the development of new treatments. Pete has over a decade's experience in the pharmaceutical industry, having joined Tudor Reilly Health after a career as an industry editor and journalist. This experience included seven years with the B2B publishing and information services company Informa, including as analysis editor of Scrip Intelligence and editor of the annual Scrip 100. It was in these roles that Pete developed a strong interest in rare diseases and the orphan drug sector. Pete also likes to spend his time interrogating pharmaceutical market data to identify new trends, while keeping a keen eye on the next disruptive innovations in pharma.

Professor Lakshminarayan Ranganath

Professor Lakshminarayan Ranganath (LRR) is a busy full time consultant in the NHS at Royal Liverpool University Hospital. He was appointed a Professor in Musculo-skeletal Biology in 2012 at the University of Liverpool. There was no NHS service available for rare disease Alkaptonuria in the UK when he developed an interest. At the time, systematic assessment of patients with this crippling disease was lacking. Exact numbers of AKU patients were unknown in UK and overseas. There was no effective treatment for AKU. To address these issues, he established an NHS Highly Specialised Services funded National Alkaptonuria Centre (NAC), which is being carried out as a long-term observational interventional study employing off-label use of nitisinone. LRR is the inaugural Director of the NAC. Patients in the NAC are able to access nitisinone free of charge and access to a multidisciplinary team of experts. LRR has carried out a national survey that identified 81 UK, 450 European and 1000 patients worldwide. He has pioneered an assessment of AKU patients. LRR is also co-ordinating an EC-funded international research programme that involves 3 studies in AKU. This will bring advances in AKU to all patients with AKU worldwide. In recognition of his contribution to AKU, he was awarded the inaugural 2012 RARE Champion of Hope for Medical Care and Treatment.

Dr Ritchie Head

Dr Ritchie Head is Director of Ceratium Limited (www.ceratium.eu) a successful research financing and project management business. He has worked on European research and innovation projects since 1996 as a coordinator, researcher, project manager and funding expert. A well networked consultant he is experienced in working with companies, academic organisations and health care providers assisting them with research and innovation strategies, and connecting them with UK and European sources of funding. Ritchie was director of a Regional Contact point for FP6 and FP7 whilst working for RTC North, providing in-depth funding advice and support to businesses; academics; and the Public and Third Sectors. He became a self-confessed EC funding geek and has a detailed knowledge of Horizon 2020 funding and project management rules and regulations. Ritchie has provided advice on FP7 to UK government, and through successful proposal writing and support, has helped clients secure over 100 million euros of funding in the last 10 years. Since writing the successful FP7 ODAK project he has worked on multiple Rare Disease projects as part of the Biotechsubsidy Group. Ritchie also leads Ceratium training workshops to share best practice with stakeholders including patient groups.

Stephen Lynn, PhD

Stephen has been the manager of the TREAT-NMD Neuromuscular Network (now called the TREAT-NMD Alliance) since early 2007 and was involved in the development of the TREAT-NMD infrastructure and the sustainability of TREAT-

NMD and its tools and resources. In addition, since early 2012, Stephen has managed the EUCERD Joint Action project which supports the mandate of the European Commission and Expert Group on Rare Diseases in formulating and implementing the Community's activities in the rare disease field, and foster exchange of experience, policies and practices. This policy work will be continued in a new Joint Action called RD-Action (2015-2018). Stephen previously worked on science policy in the Science and Innovation Network in San Francisco as part of the UK Government's Foreign and Commonwealth Office. Stephen has a PhD in Physiology and Genetics from Newcastle University and has published on rare mitochondrial diseases and work from the TREAT-NMD initiative.

Virginie Hivert

Virginie Hivert joined EURORDIS in 2014 as Therapeutic Development Director.

Virginie is responsible for following the development of orphan drugs as an observer on the Committee for Orphan Medicinal Products at the European Medicines Agency.

She coordinates the group of high-level EURORDIS representatives/volunteers who sit on the various scientific committees/working party at EMA, known as the Therapeutic Action Group (TAG).

She is responsible of two activities areas in EURORDIS, one being related to the training of patients' representatives in therapeutic development activities (EURORDIS Summer School, EUPATI) and the other being related to their engagement in these activities (in Protocol Assistance in Scientific Advice Working Party (SAWP) at the EMA for example)

She is a member of the Therapies Scientific Committee of IRDiRC (International Rare Disease Research Consortium).

Prior to joining EURORDIS, Virginie worked for Orphanet as coordinator of data collection of the resources related to rare diseases (such as expert centers, medical laboratories, patient organisations, research projects, clinical trials, etc.) in the 37 countries of the Orphanet Consortium.

Virginie holds a PharmD and a PhD in Biological Sciences and has previously worked in basic research, particularly on pathophysiological pathways in oncology.

Virginie speaks French and English.

Email: virginie.hivert@eurordis.org

Volker Straub, MD, PhD

Volker Straub is The Harold Macmillan Professor of Medicine and Professor of Neuromuscular Genetics at the Institute of Genetic Medicine at Newcastle University, United Kingdom. He is a director of the university's John Walton Muscular Dystrophy Research Centre and holds honorary clinical appointments with the Newcastle upon Tyne Hospitals NHS Foundation Trust and the North Tees and Hartlepool NHS Foundation Trust. He is part of the steering committee of the MRC Centre for neuromuscular diseases and an executive board member of the World Muscle Society. He was founding joint coordinator of TREAT-NMD, which has as its ultimate goal accelerating the development of curative treatments for patients with neuromuscular diseases.

Professor Straub was trained as a paediatric neurologist at the University of Düsseldorf and the University of Essen in Germany. He wrote his PhD thesis on Duchenne muscular dystrophy and worked as a postdoctoral research fellow at the Howard Hughes Medical Centre at the University of Iowa, USA.

Within the John Walton Muscular Dystrophy Research Centre Professor Straub has a long-standing interest in the pathogenesis of muscular dystrophies, with research using zebrafish and mouse models. His current research also involves the application of next generation sequencing and other –omics technologies for the characterization of primary muscle diseases.

He is a steering group member of several EU funded projects and is coordinating the FP7 funded EU project SCOPE-NMD. Professor Straub also chairs the MYO-MRI COST-Action (BM1304) studying the applications of MR imaging and spectroscopy techniques in neuromuscular disease.

Yann le Cam, CEO Eurordis

Yann Le Cam is a patient advocate who has dedicated 25 years of professional and personal commitment to health and medical research non-governmental organisations in France, Europe and the United States in the fields of cancer, HIV/AIDS and rare diseases.

He has three daughters, the eldest of whom has cystic fibrosis. Yann is one of the founders of EURORDIS in 1996-1997 and its Chief Executive Officer since 2001. He has participated in the revision and adoption of European regulations having an impact on rare disease patients' life, including the EU Regulation on Orphan Drugs, December 1999.

He was one of the first patient representatives appointed to the Committee for Orphan Medicinal Products (COMP) at the European Drug Agency (EMA) where he served for 9 years and was its Vice Chairman for 6 years. He served on the Management Board and Executive Committee of the French HTA agency for 5 years, on the DIA Advisory Committee Europe for 3 years. He was the Vice Chairman of the EU Committee of Experts on Rare Diseases (EUCERD) from 2011 to July 2013, and he is nominated on the current Commission Experts Group on Rare Diseases.

In November 2013, Yann Le Cam was elected Chair of the Therapies Scientific Committee of the IRDIRC – International Rare Diseases Research Consortium.

Telephone: +(33) 1 56 53 52 11
Email: yann.lecam@eurordis.org

Made in the USA
Charleston, SC
31 January 2016